Pharmacology for Physiotherapy Students

Pharmacology for Physiotherapy Students

Fourth Edition

Padmaja Udaykumar MD
Professor and Head
Department of Pharmacology
Father Muller Medical College Hospital
Mangaluru, Karnataka, India

Foreword
M Shantharam Shetty

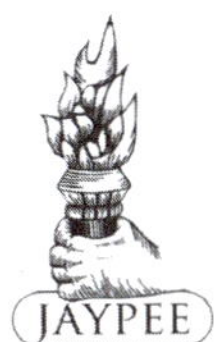

JAYPEE BROTHERS MEDICAL PUBLISHERS
The Health Sciences Publisher
New Delhi | London

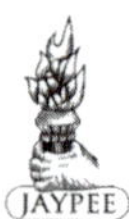

Jaypee Brothers Medical Publishers (P) Ltd

Headquarters
Jaypee Brothers Medical Publishers (P) Ltd
EMCA House, 23/23-B
Ansari Road, Daryaganj
New Delhi 110 002, India
Landline: +91-11-23272143, +91-11-23272703
+91-11-23282021, +91-11-23245672
Email: jaypee@jaypeebrothers.com

Corporate Office
Jaypee Brothers Medical Publishers (P) Ltd
4838/24, Ansari Road, Daryaganj
New Delhi 110 002, India
Phone: +91-11-43574357
Fax: +91-11-43574314
Email: jaypee@jaypeebrothers.com

Overseas Office
J.P. Medical Ltd
83 Victoria Street, London
SW1H 0HW (UK)
Phone: +44 20 3170 8910
Fax: +44 (0)20 3008 6180
Email: info@jpmedpub.com

Website: www.jaypeebrothers.com
Website: www.jaypeedigital.com

Inquiries for bulk sales may be solicited at: jaypee@jaypeebrothers.com

Pharmacology for Physiotherapy Students

First Edition: 2004

Second Edition: 2011

Third Edition: 2017

Fourth Edition: **2023**

ISBN: 978-93-5696-182-1

Printed at: Sterling Graphics Pvt. Ltd. India

Dedicated to

My dear students

Foreword

Happy to note that the popular book has reached fourth edition. It is a reflection that the book is serving its purpose.

Textbook is the most important companion, tool and light of a learning student to lead him, to shape him, enlighten him to perfect himself in the chosen subject of his studies. So, it should be reader-friendly, descriptive and analytical, to reach those goals, to fit into the mind of the learner. It should also be tailored to the needs of the student to pass his examination, which is also one of the primary goals of a student.

Pharmacology to many, including me, is one of the tough subjects, to learn amongst the medical curriculum. Most of the textbooks in pharmacology have been written, tailored to the needs of a medical student. Dr Padmaja Udaykumar in her own inimitable style has penned this textbook fully looking into the needs of a physiotherapy student. Physiotherapy is one of the most dynamic fields in medicine today to put back the patient to his physical perfection and the student ought to know the pharmacodynamics of the musculoskeletal and neurovascular systems. This book has met all these goals and I find it useful to an orthopedic, physical medicine and for postgraduate students as well.

I have known Dr Padmaja for many years. Her tenacity of purpose, vision and enthusiasm has culminated as yet another masterpiece. She is a source of inspiration to the younger generation for academic excellence.

I am sure this textbook will be of immense help to its user and I strongly recommend it, especially to physiotherapy students.

With best wishes

M Shantharam Shetty
Pro-Chancellor and Professor
Department of Orthopedics
KS Hegde Medical Academy, Nitte University
Mangaluru, Karnataka, India

Preface to the Fourth Edition

Physiotherapy has come a long way. Patients now recognize and appreciate physiotherapy as one of the useful modes of rehabilitation and pain relief.

Patients would be receiving drugs and many of them would influence the treatment course of physiotherapy too. Hence basic knowledge of drugs and their adverse effects are essential for all physiotherapists.

The text in the book has been thoroughly revised. Many figures, flowcharts and tables are added wherever necessary. Keeping the physiotherapy students in mind, importance is given for the information necessary for physiotherapists—students as well as professionals. Many mnemonics are added to help memorizing.

The pharmacology syllabus for physiotherapy students varies in each university. Therefore the students are requested to read the topics as per their prescribed syllabus.

Hope the book makes reading and studying pharmacology an enjoyable experience for physiotherapy students.

Please share your valuable feedback to *padmajaudaykumar@gmail.com*

Padmaja Udaykumar

Preface to the First Edition

Pharmacology is a science that is rapidly growing. Basic knowledge of pharmacology is required for all those who deal with patients. Since there is no standard textbook meant exclusively for physiotherapy students, they are faced with the hardship of having to refer medical pharmacology books. Such volume and depth of pharmacology is unnecessary for physiotherapists and also difficult to comprehend. Hence this book is written to make pharmacology simple for physiotherapy students. The presentation has been simple so that the students easily understand the subject. Guidelines of the University syllabus has been followed. More importance has been given for topics like analgesics, skeletal muscle relaxants and other musculoskeletal disorders which are emphasized for physiotherapy students. Syllabus of some universities have recommended topics like 'drugs and exercise', 'vasoconstrictors and vasodilators' for physiotherapy students. They have also been discussed briefly.

I hope this book reduces the burden of students in learning pharmacology.

Padmaja Udaykumar

Acknowledgments

I am extremely grateful to Dr M Shantharam Shetty, Pro-Chancellor and Professor, Department of Orthopedics, KS Hegde Medical Academy, Nitte University, Mangaluru, Karnataka, India for writing Foreword to this book.

I am highly indebted to Dr Abir Pattanayak, Senior Resident (SR), Chhatna Superspeciality Hospital, Bankura, West Bengal for his suggestions and constructive criticism.

I am sincerely thankful to the management of Father Muller Medical College, Director, Rev Fr Richard Coelho; Administrators, Rev Fr Ajith Menezes and Rev Fr Jeevan Crasta and Dean, Dr Antony Sylvan D'Souza for their encouragement and support. I am also thankful to my colleagues for their whole hearted support.

I owe a special note of thanks to my husband, Dr Udaykumar K, Medical Superintendent, Father Muller Medical College Hospital, Mangaluru Karnataka, for his constant encouragement and valuable suggestions, which made this work possible.

I am very grateful to the whole team of M/s Jaypee Brothers Medical Publishers (P) Ltd, New Delhi, India, who helped and guided me, Shri Jitendar P Vij (Group Chairman), Mr Ankit Vij (Managing Director), Mr MS Mani (Group President), Dr Madhu Choudhary (Director–Educational Publishing), Ms Pooja Bhandari [Director–Production (Books and Journals)], Ms Sunita Katla (Executive Assistant to Group Chairman and Publishing Manager), Dr Sangeeta Yadav (Development Editor), Mr Rajesh Sharma (Production Coordinator), Ms Seema Dogra (Cover Visualizer), Mr Binay Kumar (Proof reader), Mr Deepak Saxena (Typesetter), Mr Nitin Bhardwaj (Graphic Designer) and their team members, for all their support to work in this project and make it a success. Without their cooperation, I could not have completed this project.

Contents

1

CHAPTER

General Pharmacology

CHAPTER HIGHLIGHTS

- Introduction
- Routes of Drug Administration
- Special Drug Delivery Systems
- Pharmacokinetics
- Absorption
- Distribution
- Biotransformation (Metabolism)
- Pharmacodynamics
- Factors that Modify the Effects of Drugs
- Adverse Drug Reactions
- Drug Allergy
- Drug Interactions

INTRODUCTION

Pharmacology is the science that deals with the study of drugs and their interaction with the living systems.

Early man recognized the benefits and toxic effects of many plants and animal products. India's earliest pharmacological writings are from the 'Vedas.' An ancient Indian physician Charaka and then Sushruta and Vagbhata described many herbal preparations included in 'Ayurveda' (meaning the science of life). James Gregory recommended harsh and dangerous remedies like blood-letting, emetics and purgatives to be used until the symptoms of the disease subsided (such remedies often resulted in fatality). This was called 'Allopathy' meaning the other suffering. This word, still being used for the modern system of medicine, is a misnomer. Hannemann introduced the system of Homoeopathy meaning 'similar suffering' in the early 19th century. The principles of this include 'like cures like' and 'dilution enhances' the action of drugs. Thus, several systems of therapeutics were introduced, of which only few survived. The basic reason for failure of many systems is that man's concepts about diseases were incorrect and baseless in those days. By the end of the 17th century the importance of experimentation and observation became clear and many physicians applied these to the traditional drugs. Francois Magendie and Claude-Bernard popularized the use of animal experiments to understand the effects of drugs. The development of physiology also helped in the better understanding of pharmacology. The last century has seen a rapid growth of the subject with new concepts and techniques being introduced.

Definitions

The word pharmacology is derived from the Greek word—*Pharmacon* meaning an active principle or drug and *logos* meaning a discourse or study.

Drug (Drogue—a dry herb in French) is a substance used in the diagnosis, prevention or treatment of a disease. WHO definition—'A drug is any substance or product that is used or intended to be used to modify or explore physiological systems or pathological states for the benefit of the recipient.'

Pharmacodynamics is the study of the effects of the drugs on the body and their mechanisms of action, i.e., what the drug does to the body.

Pharmacokinetics is the study of the absorption, distribution, metabolism and excretion of drugs, i.e., what the body does to the drug (in Greek *Kinesis* = movement).

Therapeutics deals with the use of drugs in the prevention and treatment of diseases.

Toxicology deals with the adverse effects of drugs and also the study of poisons, i.e., detection, prevention and treatment of poisonings (*Toxicon = poison in Greek*).

Pharmacovigilance is the science and activities relating to the detection, assessment, understanding and prevention of adverse effects or any other drug-related problems. It deals with the epidemiologic study of adverse drug effects.

Chemotherapy is the use of chemicals for the treatment of infections. The term now also includes the use of chemical compounds to treat malignancies.

Pharmacy is the science of identification, compounding and dispensing of drugs. It also includes collection, isolation, purification, synthesis and standardization of medicinal substances.

Over-the-counter (OTC) drugs are the drugs that can be sold to a patient without a prescription. Examples paracetamol, ranitidine.

Prescription drugs: Many drugs can be sold only on producing a doctor's prescription. Such prescription drugs are classified as 'Schedule H' drugs as per the 'Drugs and Cosmetics Act' of India. Examples include diazepam, atenolol and antibiotics.

Pharmacopoeia (in Greek *Pharmacon* = drug; *poeia* = to make) is the official publication containing a list of drugs and medicinal preparations approved for use, their formula and other information needed to prepare a drug; their physical properties, tests for their identity, purity and potency. Each country may follow its own pharmacopoeia to guide its physicians and pharmacists. We thus have the Indian Pharmacopoeia (IP), the British Pharmacopoeia (BP) and the United States Pharmacopoeia (USP). The list is revised at regular periods to delete old useless drugs and to include newly introduced ones.

Sources of Drugs

The sources of drugs could be **natural** or **synthetic**.

Natural Sources

- **Plants**, e.g., atropine, morphine, quinine, and digoxin.
- **Animals**, e.g., insulin, heparin, gonadotrophins and antitoxic sera.
- **Minerals**, e.g., magnesium sulfate, aluminium hydroxide, iron, sulfur and radioactive isotopes.
- **Microorganisms:** Antibacterial agents like penicillin, cephalosporins, tetracyclines are obtained from some bacteria and fungi.
- **Human:** Some drugs are obtained from human beings, e.g., immunoglobulins from blood; growth hormone from anterior pituitary and chorionic gonadotrophins from the urine of pregnant women.

Synthetic

Drugs can be manufactured in large quantities and therefore cost can be less.

Most drugs are now synthesized, e.g., quinolones, omeprazole, sulfonamides, pancuronium, neostigmine.

Biotechnology

- By **cell cultures,** e.g., urokinase from cultured human kidney cells.
- By **recombinant DNA technology,** e.g., human insulin, tissue plasminogen activator
- By **Hybridoma Technique,** e. g., monoclonal antibodies.
- **Nanotechnology:** Nanomedicines are minute particles of 1–100 nm size which can be used as carriers for drugs. They can be administered parenterally for systemic effects or into the lesions as with anticancer drugs.
- **Stem cell therapy:** Stem cells have been used for regeneration of cells like in osteoarthritis. Embryonic cell or adult

pluripotent cells are used and is an upcoming field.

- **Gene therapy:** It is replacement of the defective gene by insertion of a normal, functional gene. Gene transfer may be done to replace a missing or defective gene or provide extra-copies of a normal gene.

ROUTES OF DRUG ADMINISTRATION

Drugs may be administered by various routes (Flowchart 1.1). The choice of the route in a given patient depends on the properties of the drug and the patient's requirements. A knowledge of the advantages and disadvantages of the different routes of administration is essential.

The routes can be broadly divided into:

Systemic routes: Drug given through these routes reach the systemic circulation. They include enteral and parenteral routes.

ENTERAL ROUTE

Enteral routes (intestinal) include oral, sublingual and rectal routes.

1. Oral Route

Oral route is the most commonly used, oldest and safest route of drug administration. The large surface area of the gastrointestinal tract, the mixing of its contents and the differences in pH at different parts of the gut help effective absorption of the drugs given orally. However, the acid and enzymes secreted in the gut and the biochemical activity of the bacterial flora of the gut can destroy some drugs before they are absorbed.

Advantages

1. Safest route
2. Most convenient
3. Most economical
4. Drugs can be self-administered
5. Non-invasive route

Flowchart 1.1: Routes of drug administration.

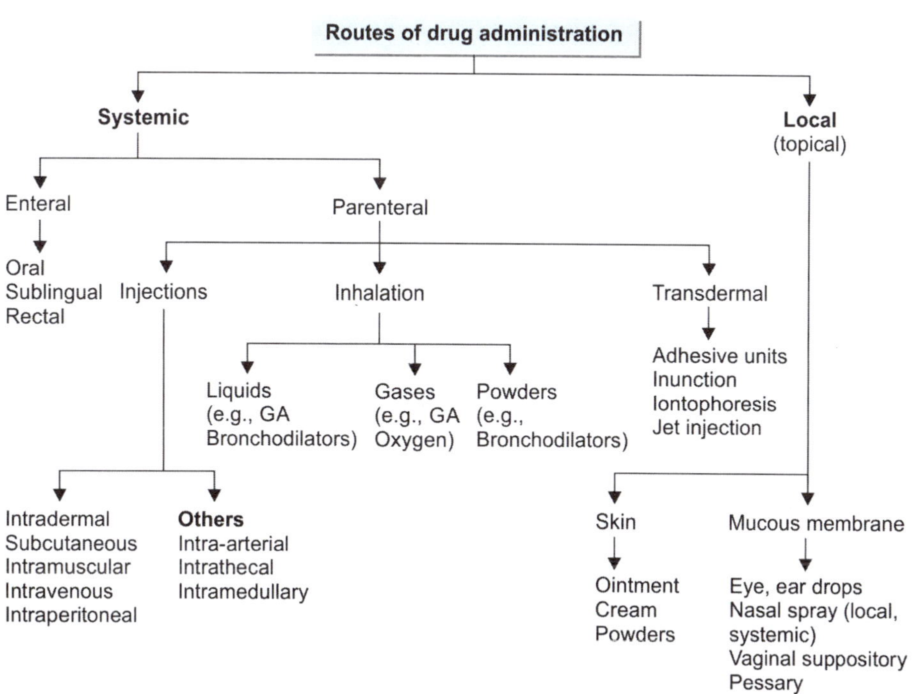

Disadvantages

1. **Slow action:** Onset of action is slower as absorption needs time.
2. **Drug properties:** Irritant and unpalatable drugs cannot be administered.
3. **Poor absorption:** Some drugs may not be absorbed due to certain physical and chemical characteristics, e.g., streptomycin is not absorbed when given orally.
4. **GI irritation:** Irritation to the gastrointestinal tract may lead to vomiting.
5. **Irregular absorption:** There may be irregularities in absorption.
6. **Metabolism:** Some drugs may be destroyed by gastric juices, e.g., insulin.
7. **Unsuitable situation:** Cannot be given to unconscious and uncooperative patients.
8. **First pass effect:** Some drugs may undergo extensive first pass metabolism in the liver.
9. **Non-compliance:** Patients may forget to take the tablet which is a practical problem.

To overcome some of the disadvantages, irritants are given in capsules, while bitter drugs are given as sugar coated tablets. Sometimes drugs are coated with substances, such as synthetic resins, gums, sugar, coloring and flavoring agents thus making them more acceptable.

Enteric Coated Tablets

Some tablets are coated with substances like cellulose-acetate, phthalate, gluten, etc., which are not digested by the gastric acid but get disintegrated in the alkaline juices of the intestine (Fig. 1.1). Enteric coating will:

- Prevent gastric irritation.
- Avoid destruction of the drug by the stomach.
- Provide higher concentration of the drug in the small intestine.
- Slow the absorption, and thereby prolong the duration of action.

However, if the coating is inappropriate, the tablet may be expelled without being absorbed at all.

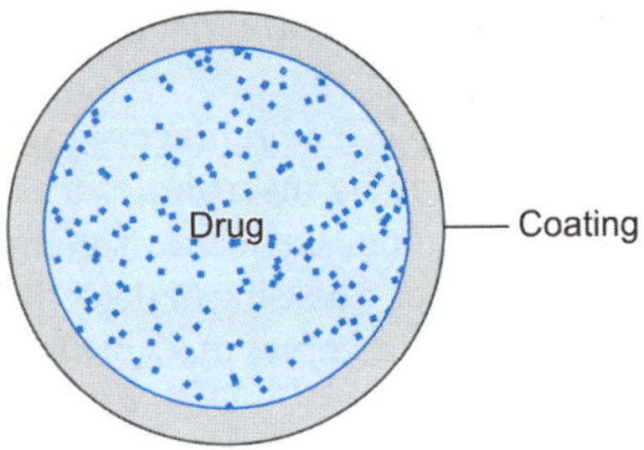

Fig. 1.1: Enteric coating.

Controlled-release or sustained-release preparations are designed to prolong the rate of absorption and thereby the duration of action of drugs. This is useful for short-acting drugs. In newer controlled release formulations, the tablet is coated with a semipermeable membrane through which water enters and displaces or pushes the drug out.

Advantages

- Frequency of administration may be reduced
- Therapeutic concentration may be maintained for a long time specially when nocturnal symptoms are to be treated.

Disadvantages

- There may be release of the entire amount of the drug in a short time leading to toxicity
- It is more expensive.

Precautions are to be taken during oral administration of drugs:

- Capsules and tablets are to be swallowed with a glass of water, with the patient in upright posture—either sitting or standing. This helps the passage of the tablet into the stomach and its rapid dissolution. It also minimizes chances of the drug getting into larynx or behind the epiglottis.
- Recumbent patient should not be given drugs orally as some drugs may remain in the esophagus due to the absence of gravitational force which helps the passage of the drug into the stomach.

Such drugs can damage the esophageal mucosa, e.g., iron salts, tetracyclines.
- The tablets should not be directly touched to avoid contamination.
- For elderly patients who are unable to swallow tablets, the tablets may be crushed and mixed with fruit juice or water for swallowing. However, enteric coated forms and sustained-release tablets should not be crushed.
- History of allergy should be taken before parenteral administration of drugs especially intravenously.

2. Sublingual

Here, the tablet or pellet containing the drug is placed under the tongue. It dissolves and the drug is absorbed across the sublingual mucosa, e.g., nitroglycerin, nifedipine, buprenorphine.

Advantages

- Absorption is rapid—within minutes the drug reaches the circulation.
- First pass metabolism is avoided.
- After the desired effect is obtained, the drug can be spat out to avoid the unwanted effects.

Disadvantages

- Buccal ulceration can occur.
- Lipid insoluble drugs cannot be given.

Nasal: Drugs can be administered through nasal route either for systemic absorption or for local effects. For example:
- For systemic absorption—oxytocin spray is used.
- For local effect—decongestant nasal drops, e.g., oxymetazoline; budesonide nasal spray for allergic rhinitis.

3. Rectal

Rectum has a rich blood supply and drugs can cross the rectal mucosa to be absorbed for systemic effects. Drugs absorbed from the upper part of the rectum are carried by the superior hemorrhoidal vein to the portal circulation (can undergo first pass metabolism), while that absorbed from the lower part of the rectum is carried by the middle and inferior hemorrhoidal veins to the systemic circulation. Drugs, such as—indomethacin, chlorpromazine, diazepam and paraldehyde can be given rectally.

Some irritant drugs are given rectally as *suppositories:*

Advantages

- Gastric irritation is avoided
- Can be administered by unskilled persons
- Useful in geriatric patients and others with vomiting and those unable to swallow
- Also useful in unconscious patients.

Disadvantages

- Irritation of the rectum can occur
- Absorption may be irregular and unpredictable.

Drugs may also be given by rectal route as enema.

Enema is the administration of a drug in a liquid form into the rectum. Enema may be evacuant or retention enema.

Evacuant enema: In order to empty the bowel, about 600 mL of soap water is administered per rectum. While water distends and thus stimulates the rectum, soap lubricates. Enema is given prior to surgeries, obstetric procedures and radiological examination of the gut.

Retention enema: The drug is administered with about 100 mL of fluids and is retained in the rectum for local action, e.g., prednisolone enema in ulcerative colitis.

PARENTERAL ROUTES

Routes of administration other than the enteral (intestinal) route are known as parenteral routes. Here the drugs are directly delivered into tissue fluids or blood.

Advantages

1. Action is more rapid and predictable than oral administration
2. These routes can be employed in an unconscious or uncooperative patient
3. Gastric irritants can be given parenterally and therefore irritation to the gastrointestinal tract can be avoided
4. It can be used in patients with vomiting or those unable to swallow
5. Digestion by the gastric and intestinal juices and the first pass metabolism are avoided.

Therefore, in emergencies parenteral routes are very useful routes of drug administration because the action is rapid and predictable and are useful in unconscious patients.

Disadvantages

1. Asepsis must be maintained
2. Injections may be painful
3. More expensive, less safe and inconvenient
4. Injury to nerves and other tissues may occur.

Parenteral routes include:

- Injections
- Inhalation
- Transdermal route

INJECTIONS

Injections are given with the help of a syringe and needle.

Intradermal

The drug is injected into the layers of the skin by:

- Raising a bleb, e.g., BCG vaccine, tests for allergy.
- By multiple punctures of the epidermis through a drop of the drug, e.g., smallpox vaccine.

Only a small quantity can be administered by this route and it may be painful.

Subcutaneous (SC) Injection

Here the drug is deposited in the SC tissue, e.g., insulin, heparin. As this tissue is less vascular, absorption is slow and largely uniform and this makes the drug long-acting. It is reliable and patients can be trained for self-administration. Absorption can be enhanced by the addition of the enzyme hyaluronidase.

Disadvantages

- As SC tissue is richly supplied by nerves, irritant drugs cannot be injected
- In shock, absorption is not dependable because of vasoconstriction
- Repeated injections at the same site can cause lipoatrophy resulting in erratic absorption.

Hypodermoclysis is the SC administration of large volumes of saline employed in pediatric practice.

Drugs can also be administered subcutaneously as:

- **Dermojet:** In this method, a high velocity jet of drug solution is projected from a fine orifice using a gun. The solution gets deposited in the SC tissue from where it is absorbed. As needle is not required, this method is painless. It is suitable for vaccines.
- **Pellet implantation:** Small pellets packed with drugs are implanted subcutaneously. The drug is slowly released for weeks or months to provide constant blood levels, e.g., testosterone, desoxy-corticosterone acetate (DOCA).
- **Silastic implants:** The drug is packed in silastic tubes and implanted subcutaneously. The drug gets absorbed over months to provide constant blood levels, e.g., hormones and contraceptives. The empty nonbiodegradable implant has to be removed.

Intramuscular (IM)

Aqueous solution of the drug is injected into one of the large skeletal muscles—deltoid, triceps, gluteus or rectus femoris. Absorption into the plasma occurs by simple diffusion. Larger molecules enter through the lymphatic channels. As the muscles are vascular, absorption is rapid and quite uniform.

Drugs are absorbed faster from the deltoid region than gluteal region especially in women. The volume of injection should not exceed 10 mL. For infants, rectus femoris is used instead of gluteus which is not well-developed till the child starts walking. If the drug is injected as an oily solution or suspension, the absorption is slow and steady. The deltoid muscle is used for injection of smaller volume (1-2 mL) while if larger volumes are to be given, gluteal muscles should be used. Once the needle is pushed into the muscle, the plunger should be pulled back to make sure that the needle is not in a blood vessel. Soluble substances, mild irritants, depot preparations, suspensions and colloids can be injected by this route.

Advantages

1. Intramuscular route is reliable
2. Absorption is rapid
3. Has all the advantages of the parenteral route—*See* page 6.

Disadvantages

1. Intramuscular injection may be painful.
2. It may even result in an abscess-local infection and tissue necrosis are possible
3. Risk of nerve injury—irritant solutions can damage the nerve if injected near a nerve.
4. The needle may puncture a blood vessel.
5. In case of some drugs, absorption by IM route is slower than oral, e.g., diazepam, phenytoin.
6. For some drugs, IM route should be avoided, e.g., heparin, calcium gluconate, tetracycline.

Intravenous (IV)

Here, the drug is injected into one of the superficial veins so that it directly reaches the circulation and is immediately available for action.

Drugs can be given IV as:

- **A bolus:** Where an initial large dose is given, e.g., heparin. The drug is dissolved in a suitable amount of vehicle and injected slowly.
- **Slow injection:** Over 15-20 minutes, e.g., aminophylline.
- **Slow infusion:** When constant plasma concentrations are required, e.g., oxytocin in labor or when large volumes have to be given, e.g., dextrose, saline. Generally about one liter of solution is infused over 3 to 4 hours—but the rate of infusion depends on the condition of the patient.

Advantages

1. Most useful route in emergencies because the drug is immediately available for action
2. Provides predictable blood concentrations with 100% bioavailability
3. Large volumes of solutions can be given.
4. Irritants can be given by this route as they get quickly diluted in blood.
5. Rapid dose adjustments are possible—if unwanted effects occur, infusion can be stopped; if higher levels are required, infusion rate can be increased—specially for short-acting drugs.

Disadvantages

1. Once injected, the drug cannot be withdrawn
2. Irritation of the veins may cause thrombophlebitis
3. Extravasation of some drugs may cause severe irritation and sloughing
4. Only aqueous solutions can be given IV but not suspensions, oily solutions and depot preparations
5. Self-medication is difficult
6. The solution should be sterile and strict aseptic measures should be taken.

Intraperitoneal: Peritoneum offers a large surface area for absorption. Fluids are injected intraperitoneally in infants. This route is also used for peritoneal dialysis.

Intrathecal: Drugs can be injected into the subarachnoid space for action on the CNS, e.g., spinal anesthetics. Some antibiotics and corticosteroids are also injected by this route to produce high local concentrations. Strict aseptic precautions are a must.

Drugs are also given **extradurally.** Morphine can be given epidurally to produce analgesia. Direct intraventricular administration of drugs may be employed in brain tumors.

Intra-articular: Drugs are injected directly into a joint for the treatment of arthritis and other diseases of the joints. **Strict aseptic precautions are required**, e.g., hydrocortisone is injected into the affected joint, in rheumatoid arthritis.

Intra-arterial: Here the drug is injected directly into the arteries. It is used only in the treatment of:

- Peripheral vascular diseases
- Local malignancies
- Diagnostic studies, such as angiograms.

Intramedullary: This route involves injection into a bone marrow—now this route is rarely used.

Syringes and Needles

Syringes

Drugs are administered as injections using a needle and a syringe. A syringe consists of a barrel and a plunger (piston). A type of syringe known as Luer-Lock syringe has the advantage that the needle can be locked in position. Intravenous injections are given with the help of an infusion set. All syringes are now disposable.

Sizes: Syringes are available in various sizes 1, 2, 5, 10, 20 and 50 mL.

Special Syringes

Insulin syringe has markings in units—(40 in 1 mL (red) or 80 in 1 mL (green) and are suitable for administration of insulin.

Tuberculin syringe is a syringe of 1 mL capacity with 0.01 mL markings. It is useful for administration of very small volumes.

Needles

Needles are made of stainless steel, which is rust-proof. The tip which is at the end of the shaft is bevelled. The bevelling may be short, very short or regular. Needle is available in different gauge thickness and length. The gauge numbers are from 13 (thickest) to 27 (finest). Depending on the route of administration and the thickness of the solution to be injected, the needle is selected.

Route	*Preferred size*	
Subcutaneous	5/8 inch	25 gauge
IM, IV	1–3 inch	22–24 gauge
Intradermal	1/2 inch	26 gauge

INHALATION

Volatile liquids and gases are given by inhalation, e.g., general anesthetics. In addition, drugs can be administered as solid particles, i.e., as solutions of drug particles and the fine droplets are inhaled as aerosol, e.g., salbutamol. These inhaled drugs and vapors may act on the pulmonary epithelium and mucous membranes of the respiratory tract and are also absorbed through these membranes.

Advantages

- Almost instantaneous absorption of the drug is achieved because of the large surface area of the lungs
- In pulmonary diseases, it serves almost as a local route as the drug is delivered at the desired site making it more effective and less harmful.
- Hepatic first pass metabolism is avoided
- Because the drug is directly delivered to the target tissue, smaller dose is needed.
- Blood levels of volatile anesthetics can be conveniently controlled as their absorption and excretion through the lungs are governed by the laws of gases.

Disadvantages

- Irritant gases may enhance pulmonary secretions and should be avoided by this route
- Drug particles may induce cough (e.g., cromolyn sodium)
- This is an important route of entry of certain drugs of abuse.

TRANSDERMAL ROUTE

Highly lipid soluble drugs can be applied over the skin for slow and prolonged absorption, e.g., nitroglycerin ointment in angina pectoris. Adhesive units, inunction, iontophoresis and jet injection are some forms of transdermal drug delivery.

Adhesive units (transdermal therapeutic systems) are adhesive patches of different sizes and shapes made to suit the area of application. The drug is held in a reservoir between an outer layer and a porous membrane. This membrane is smeared with an adhesive to hold on to the area of application. The drug slowly diffuses through the membrane and percutaneous absorption takes place. The rate of absorption is constant and predictable. Highly potent (because small quantity is sufficient) and short acting (effect terminates quickly after the unit is removed) drugs are suitable for use in such systems (Fig. 1.2).

Sites of application are chest, abdomen, upper arm, back or mastoid region, e.g., hyoscine, nitroglycerin fentanyl, estrogen, testosterone transdermal patches.

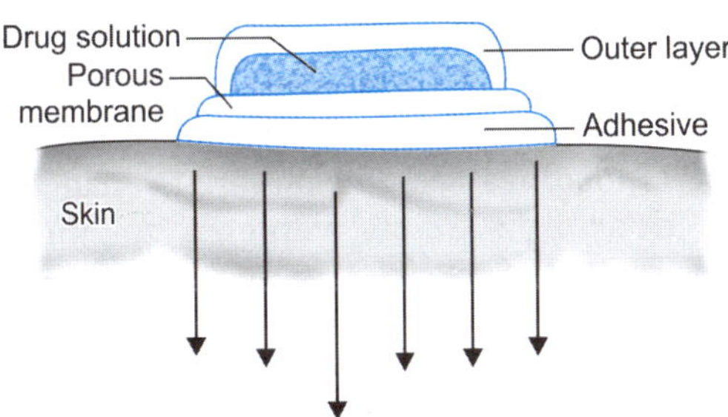

Fig. 1.2: Transdermal adhesive unit.

Advantages

- Duration of action is prolonged
- Provides constant plasma drug levels
- Patient compliance is good.

Disadvantages

- Large doses of the drug cannot be loaded into the system
- Can cause irritation to the skin
- Expensive.

Inunction: In this route of administration, the drug is rubbed into the skin and it gets absorbed to produce systemic effects.

Iontophoresis: In this procedure, galvanic current is used for bringing about penetration of lipid insoluble drugs into the deeper tissues where its action is required, e.g., salicylates. Fluoride iontophoresis is used in the treatment of dental hypersensitivity.

Jet injection: As absorption of drug occurs across the layers of the skin, dermojet may also be considered as a form of transdermal drug administration (*see* dermojet on page 6).

LOCAL/TOPICAL APPLICATION

Drugs may be applied on the skin for local action as ointment, cream, gel, powder, paste, etc. Drugs may also be applied on the mucous membrane as in the eyes, ears and nose as ointment, drops and sprays.

Nasal route: Drugs are administered through nasal route either for systemic absorption or for local effects, e.g., for systemic absorption—oxytocin spray.

For local effect—decongestant nasal drops, e.g., oxymetazoline; budesonide nasal spray for allergic rhinitis.

Drugs may be administered as **suppository** for rectum, **bougie** for urethra and **pessary** and **douche** for vagina. Pessaries are oval-shaped tablets to be placed in the vagina to provide high local concentrations of the drug at the site, e.g., antifungal pessaries in vaginal candidiasis.

SPECIAL DRUG DELIVERY SYSTEMS

In order to improve drug delivery, to prolong duration of action and thereby improve patient compliance, special drug delivery systems are being tried. Drug targeting, i.e., to deliver drugs at the site where it is required to act is also being aimed at, especially for anticancer drugs. Some such systems are ocusert, progestasert, transdermal adhesive units, prodrugs, osmotic pumps, computerized pumps and methods using monoclonal antibodies and liposomes as carriers.

1. **Ocusert** systems are thin elliptical units that contain the drug in a reservoir which slowly releases the drug through a membrane by diffusion at a steady rate, e.g., pilocarpine ocusert used in glaucoma is placed under the lid and can deliver pilocarpine for 7 days.
2. **Progestasert** is inserted into the uterus where it delivers progesterone constantly for over one year.
3. **Transdermal adhesive units:** (*See* page 9).
4. **Prodrug** is an inactive form of the drug which gets metabolized to the active derivative in the body. Using a prodrug may overcome some of the disadvantages of the conventional forms of drug administration as follows:
   i. ***Increase availability at the site,*** e.g., dopamine does not cross the blood-brain barrier (BBB); levodopa, a prodrug crosses the BBB and is then converted to dopamine in the CNS
   ii. ***Prolong duration of action:*** Prodrug may be used to achieve longer duration of action, e.g., bacampicillin (a prodrug of ampicillin) is longer acting than ampicillin
   iii. ***Improve tolerability,*** e.g., cyclophosphamide, an anticancer drug gets converted to its active metabolite aldophosphamide in the liver. This allows oral administration of cyclophosphamide without causing much gastrointestinal toxicity
   iv. ***Drug targeting:*** Zidovudine is taken up by the virus infected cells and gets activated in these cells. This results in selective toxicity to infected cells
   v. ***Improve stability:*** A prodrug may be more stable at gastric pH, e.g., aspirin is converted to salicylic acid which is the more stable active drug and aspirin also is better tolerated than salicylic acid.
   vi. ***Reduce side effects:*** For example, bacampicillin a prodrug of ampicillin is better absorbed and therefore causes less diarrhea than ampicillin.

   Disadvantages:
   - Not suitable in emergencies due to slower action
   - In liver diseases prodrug may not be activated.
5. **Osmotic pumps** are small tablet shaped units consisting of the drug and an osmotic substance placed in two chambers. The osmotic layer swells and pushes the drug slowly out of a small hole. Iron and prazosin are available in this form.
6. **Computerized miniature pumps:** These are programmed to release drugs at a definite rate either continuously as in case of insulin or intermittently in pulses as in case of gonadotropin-releasing hormone (GnRH).

   Various methods of drug targeting are tried especially for anticancer drugs to reduce toxicity.
7. **Monoclonal antibodies** against the tumor specific antigens are used to deliver anticancer drugs to specific tumor cells.
8. **Liposomes** are phospholipids suspended in aqueous vehicles to form minute vesicles. Drugs encapsulated in liposomes are taken up mainly by the reticuloendothelial cells of the liver and are also concentrated in malignant tumors.

Thus, site-specific delivery of drugs may be possible with the help of liposomes.

PHARMACOKINETICS

Pharmacokinetics is the study of the absorption, distribution, metabolism and excretion of drugs, i.e., the movement of the drugs into, within and out of the body. For a drug to produce its specific response, it should be present in adequate concentrations at the site of action. This depends on various factors apart from the dose. Once the drug is administered, it is absorbed, i.e., enters the blood, is distributed to different parts of the body, reaches the site of action, is metabolized and excreted (Fig. 1.3). All these processes involve passage of the drug molecules across various barriers—like the intestinal epithelium, cell membrane, renal filtering membrane, capillary barrier and so on. To cross these barriers the drug has to cross the cell membrane or pass in-between the epithelial or endothelial cells.

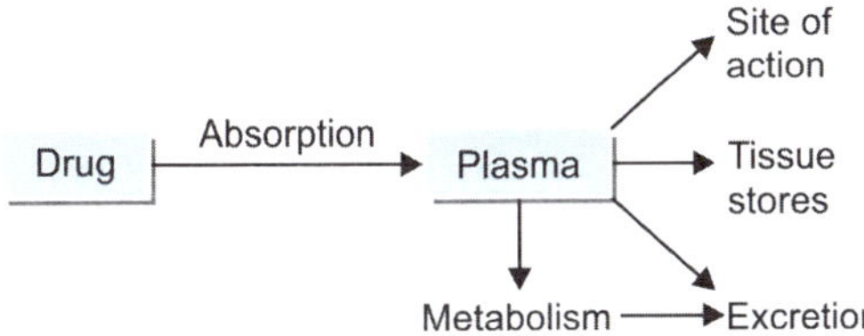

Fig. 1.3: Schematic representation of movement of drug in the body.

The cell membrane/biological membrane is made up of two layers of phospholipids with intermingled protein molecules (Fig. 1.4). All lipid soluble substances get dissolved in the cell membrane and readily permeate into the cells. The junctions between epithelial or endothelial cells have pores through which small water-soluble molecules can pass. Movement of some specific substances is regulated by special carrier proteins. The passage of drugs across biological membranes involves processes like passive (filtration, diffusion) and active transport.

Mechanisms of Transport of Drug Across Biological Membranes

Passive transfer	Carrier-mediated transport	Endocytosis
• Simple diffusion • Filtration	• Active transport • Facilitated diffusion	

Passive Transfer

The drug moves across the membrane without any need for energy either by *simple diffusion* in the direction of its concentration gradient, i.e., from higher concentration to a lower concentration or by *filtration* through

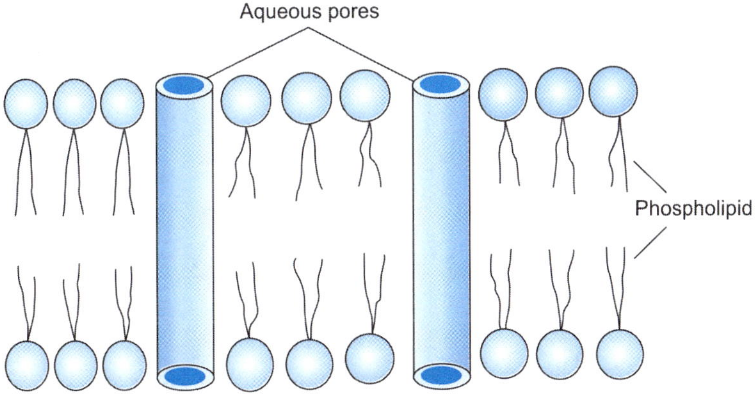

Fig. 1.4: Cell/biological membrane (schematic).

aqueous pores in the membrane. Most drugs are absorbed by simple diffusion.

Carrier-mediated Transport

Active transport is the transfer of drugs against a concentration gradient and needs energy. It is carried by a specific carrier protein. Only drugs related to natural metabolites are transported by this process, e.g., levodopa, iron, amino acids.

Facilitated diffusion is a unique form of carrier transport which differs from active transport in that it is not energy dependent and the movement occurs in the direction of the concentration gradient. The carrier facilitates diffusion and is highly specific for the substance, e.g., uptake of glucose by cells, vitamin B_{12} from intestines.

Endocytosis

Endocytosis is the process where small droplets are engulfed by the cell. Some proteins are taken up by this process (like pinocytosis in ameba).

ABSORPTION

Absorption is defined as the passage of the drug from the site of administration into the circulation. For a drug to reach its site of action, it must pass through various membranes depending on the route of administration. Absorption occurs by one of the processes described above, i.e., passive diffusion or carrier-mediated transport. Except for intravenous route, absorption is important for all other routes of administration.

Absorption from the gut: Drugs taken orally may be absorbed from any part of the gut. Acidic drugs are absorbed from the stomach while basic drugs from the intestines.

Rate and extent of absorption by all other routes is influenced by several factors (Fig. 1.5). They are:

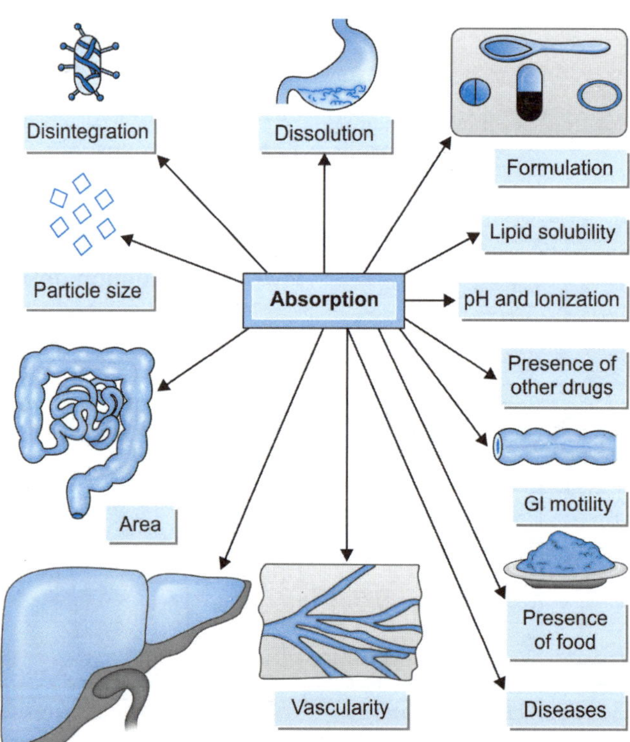

Fig. 1.5: Factors affecting absorption of drugs.

A. Pharmaceutical Factors

1. **Disintegration and dissolution time:** The drug taken orally should break up into individual particles (disintegrate) to be absorbed. It then has to dissolve in the gastrointestinal fluids. In case of drugs given subcutaneously or intramuscularly, the drug molecules have to dissolve in the tissue fluids. Liquids are absorbed faster than solids. Delay in disintegration and dissolution as with poorly water-soluble drugs like aspirin, result in delayed absorption.
2. **Formulation:** Pharmaceutical preparations are made to produce desired absorption. Inert substances used with drugs as diluents like starch and lactose may sometimes interfere with absorption.
3. **Particle size:** Small particle size is important for better absorption of drugs. Drugs like corticosteroids, griseofulvin, digoxin, aspirin and tolbutamide are better absorbed when given as small particles. On the other hand, when a drug has to act on the gut and its absorption is not desired, then particle size should be kept large, e.g., anthelmintics like bephenium hydroxynaphthoate.

B. Drug Factors

4. **Lipid solubility:** Lipid soluble drugs are absorbed faster and better by dissolving in the phospholipids of the cell membrane.
5. **pH and ionization:** Ionized drugs are poorly absorbed while unionized drugs are lipid soluble and are well absorbed. Most drugs are weak electrolytes and ionize according to pH. Thus acidic drugs remain unionized in acidic medium of the stomach and are rapidly absorbed, e.g., aspirin, barbiturates. Basic drugs are unionized when they reach the alkaline medium of intestine from where they are rapidly absorbed, e.g., pethidine, ephedrine.

   Strong acids and bases are highly ionized and therefore poorly absorbed, e.g., streptomycin.

C. Biological Factors

6. **Area and vascularity of the absorbing surface:** The larger the area of absorbing surface and more the vascularity—better is the absorption. Thus most drugs are absorbed from small intestine.
7. **Gastrointestinal motility:**

   Gastric emptying time: if gastric emptying is faster, the passage of the drug to the intestines is quicker and hence absorption is faster.

   Intestinal motility: When highly increased as in diarrheas, drug absorption is reduced.
8. **Presence of food:** In the stomach delays gastric emptying, dilutes the drug and delays absorption. Drugs may form complexes with food constituents and such complexes are poorly absorbed, e.g., tetracyclines chelate calcium present in food. Moreover, certain drugs like ampicillin, roxithromycin and rifampicin are well-absorbed only on empty stomach.
9. **Diseases** of the gut like malabsorption and achlorhydria result in reduced absorption of drugs.
10. **First pass metabolism:** Some drugs may be degraded in the gastrointestinal (GI) tract, e.g., nitroglycerine, insulin. Such drugs should be given by alternate routes.

First pass metabolism is the metabolism of a drug during its passage from the site of absorption to the systemic circulation. It is also called **presystemic metabolism** or **first pass effect** and is an important feature of oral route of administration.

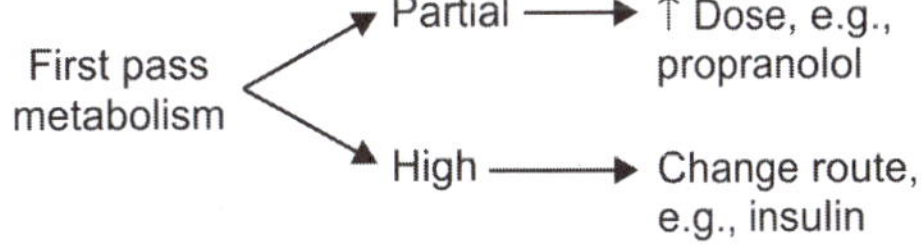

- Drugs given orally may be metabolized in the gut wall and in the liver before reaching the systemic circulation.
- The extent of first pass metabolism differs from drug to drug and among individuals, from partial to total inactivation.
- When it is partial, it can be compensated by giving higher dose of the particular drug, e.g., nitroglycerine, propranolol, salbutamol.
- For drugs that undergo extensive first pass metabolism, the route of administration has to be changed, e.g., isoprenaline, hydrocortisone, insulin.

First pass metabolism

- Is metabolism of a drug during its first passage through gut wall and liver
- Reduces bioavailability
- Extent of metabolism depends on the drug and individuals
- Significance:
  - Dose has to be increased for some drugs like propranolol
  - Route has to be changed for some others like hydrocortisone
- Examples: morphine, chlorpromazine, nitroglycerine, verapamil, testosterone, insulin, lignocaine

Absorption from parenteral routes: On intravenous administration, the drug directly reaches the circulation. On intramuscular injection, the drug molecules should dissolve in the tissue fluids and then be absorbed. Since muscles have a rich blood supply, absorption is fast. Drug molecules diffuse through the capillary membrane and reach the circulation. Lipid-soluble drugs are absorbed faster. Absorption from subcutaneous administration is slower but rate of absorption is somewhat steady.

Inhaled drugs particularly the lipid soluble ones are rapidly absorbed from the pulmonary epithelium.

On topical application, highly lipid soluble drugs are absorbed from the intact skin, e.g., nitroglycerine; but absorption is relatively slow because of the multiple layers of closely-packed cells in the epidermis. Most drugs are readily absorbed from the mucous membranes.

Bioavailability

Bioavailability is the fraction of the drug that reaches the systemic circulation following administration by any route. Thus for a drug given intravenously, the bioavailability is 100 percent. On IM/SC injection, drugs are almost completely absorbed while by oral route, bioavailability may be low due to incomplete absorption and first pass metabolism. All the factors which influence the absorption of a drug also alter bioavailability.

For example, bioavailability of chlortetracycline is 30%, carbamazepine 70%, chloroquine 80%, minocycline and diazepam 100%. Transdermal preparations are absorbed systemically and may have 80–100% bioavailability.

Factors Affecting Bioavailability

All the ten factors including particle size, disintegration and dissolution time, lipid solubility, ionization, first pass metabolism, area and vascularity of the absorbing surface, presence of food and GI motility, which influence the absorption of a drug also alter the bioavailability. Large bioavailability variations of a drug, particularly when it is unpredictable can result in toxicity or therapeutic failure as in case of halofantrine.

Bioequivalence

Comparison of bioavailability of different formulations of the same drug is the study of bioequivalence (Fig. 1.6). Often oral formulations containing the same amount of a drug from different manufacturers may result in different plasma concentrations, i.e., there is no bioequivalence. Such differences occur with poorly soluble, slowly absorbed drugs mainly due to differences in the rate of disintegration and dissolution. Variation in bioavailability (nonequivalence) can result in toxicity or therapeutic failure in drugs

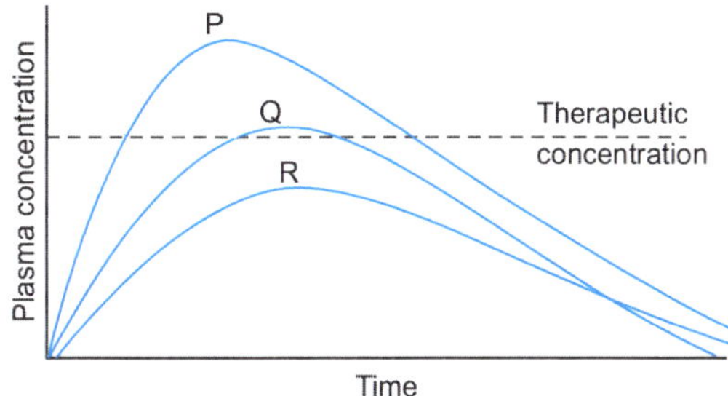

Fig. 1.6: Study of bioequivalence. Three different oral formulations—P, Q and R of the same drug yield different bioavailability values.

that have low safety margin like digoxin and drugs that need precise dose adjustment like anticoagulants and corticosteroids. For such drugs, in a given patient, the preparations from a single manufacturer should be used.

DISTRIBUTION

After a drug reaches the systemic circulation, it gets distributed to other tissues. It should cross several barriers before reaching the site of action. Like absorption, distribution also involves the same processes, i.e., filtration, diffusion and specialized transport. Various factors determine the rate and extent of distribution, *viz* lipid solubility, ionization, blood flow and binding to plasma proteins and cellular proteins. Unionized lipid soluble drugs are widely distributed throughout the body.

Plasma Protein Binding

On reaching the circulation most drugs bind to plasma proteins; acidic drugs bind mainly albumin and basic drugs to alpha-acid glycoprotein. The free or unbound fraction of the drug is the only form available for action, metabolism and excretion while the protein bound form serves as a reservoir. The extent of protein binding varies with each drug, e.g., warfarin is 99% and morphine is 35% protein bound while binding of ethosuximide and lithium is 0 percent, i.e., they are totally free.

Clinical Significance of Plasma Protein Binding

- Only free fraction is available for action, metabolism and excretion.
- Protein binding serves as a store (reservoir) of the drug and the drug is released when free drug levels fall.
- Protein binding prolongs duration of action of the drug.
- Many drugs may compete for the same binding sites. Thus one drug may displace another from the binding sites resulting in toxicity. For example, indomethacin displaces warfarin from protein binding sites leading to increased warfarin levels.
- Chronic renal failure and chronic liver disease result in hypoalbuminemia with reduced protein binding of drugs.

Some Highly Protein Bound Drugs

Warfarin	Tolbutamide	Phenytoin
Frusemide	Clofibrate	Sulfonamides
Diazepam	Salicylates	Phenylbutazone
Indomethacin		

Tissue binding: Some drugs get bound to certain tissue constituents because of special affinity for them. Tissue binding delays elimination and thus prolongs duration of action of the drug. For example, lipid soluble drugs are bound to adipose tissue. Tissue binding also serves as a reservoir of the drug.

Tissue	*Binding drug*
Adipose tissue	Thiopentone sodium, benzodiazepines
Muscles	Emetine
Bone	Tetracyclines, lead
Retina	Chloroquine
Thyroid	Iodine

Redistribution: When highly lipid soluble drugs are given intravenously or by inhalation, they get rapidly distributed into highly perfused tissues like brain, heart and kidney. But soon they get redistributed into less vascular tissues like the muscle and fat resulting in termination of the action of these drugs. The best example is the intravenous anesthetic thiopental sodium which induces anesthesia in 10–20 seconds but the effect stops in 5–15 minutes due to redistribution.

Blood-brain barrier (BBB): The endothelial cells of the brain capillaries lack intercellular pores and instead have tight junctions. Moreover, glial cells envelope the capillaries and together these form the BBB. Only lipid soluble, unionized drugs can cross this BBB. During inflammation of the meninges, the barrier becomes more permeable to drugs, e.g., penicillin readily penetrates during meningitis. The barrier is weak at some areas like chemoreceptor triggor zone (CTZ), posterior pituitary and parts of hypothalamus and allows some compounds to diffuse.

Placental barrier: Lipid soluble, unionized drugs readily cross the placenta while lipid insoluble drugs cross to a much lesser extent. Thus drugs taken by the mother can cause several unwanted effects in the fetus.

Volume of Distribution (V)

Volume of distribution is defined as the volume necessary to accommodate the entire amount of the drug, if the concentration throughout the body were equal to that in plasma. It relates the amount of the drug in the body to the concentration of the drug in plasma. It is calculated as

$$V = \frac{\text{Amount of drug in the body}}{\text{Plasma concentration}}$$

For example, if the dose of a drug given is 500 mg and attains a uniform concentration of 10 mg in the body, its V = 50 liters.

The knowledge of V of drugs is clinically important in the treatment of poisoning. Drugs with large V like pethidine are not easily removed by hemodialysis.

BIOTRANSFORMATION (METABOLISM)

Biotransformation is the process of biochemical alteration of the drug in the body. Body treats most drugs as foreign substances and tries to inactivate and eliminate them by various biochemical reactions. These processes convert the drugs into more polar, water-soluble compounds so that they are easily excreted through the kidneys. Some drugs may be excreted largely unchanged in the urine, e.g., frusemide, atenolol.

Site: The most important organ of biotransformation is the liver. Many drugs are also metabolized to some extent by the kidney, gut mucosa, lungs, blood and skin.

Result of biotransformation: Though biotransformation generally inactivates the drug, some drugs may be converted to active or more active metabolites (Table 1.1).

When the metabolite is active, the duration of action gets prolonged. **Prodrug** is an inactive drug which gets converted into an active form in the body (Table 1.1).

Enzymes in biotransformation: The biotransformation reactions are catalyzed by specific enzymes located either in the liver microsomes (microsomal enzymes) or in the cytoplasm and mitochondria of the liver cells and also in the plasma and other tissues (non-microsomal enzymes).

The chemical reactions of biotransformation can take place in two phases (Fig. 1.7).

1. Phase I (Non-synthetic reactions)
2. Phase II (Synthetic reactions).

Table 1.1: Result of biotransformation with examples.

Active drug to inactive metabolite	*Active drug to active metabolite*	*Inactive drug to active metabolite (prodrug)*
Morphine Chloramphenicol	Primidone → Phenobarbitone Digitoxin → Digoxin Diazepam → Oxazepam	Levodopa → Dopamine Prednisone → Prednisolone Enalapril → Enalaprilat

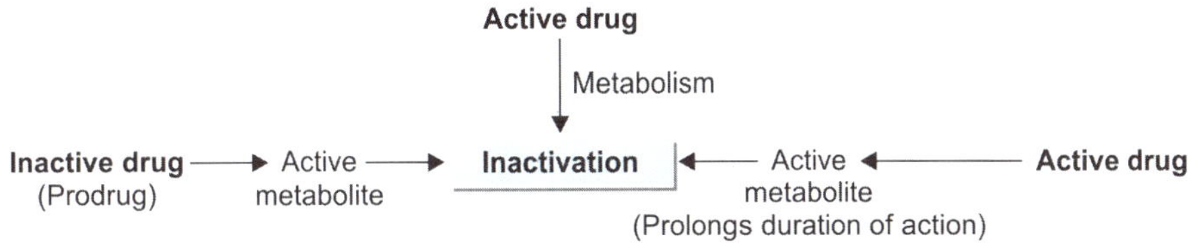

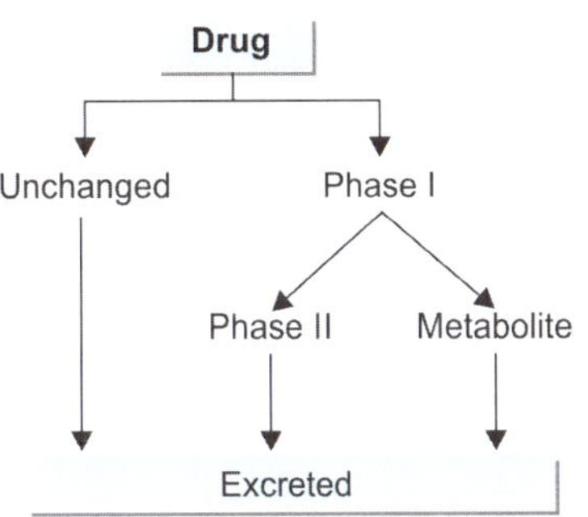

Fig. 1.7: Phases in metabolism of drugs. A drug may be excreted as phase I metabolite or as phase II metabolite. Some drugs may be excreted as such.

Phase I reactions convert the drug to a more polar metabolite by oxidation, reduction or hydrolysis. Oxidation reactions are the most important metabolizing reactions, mostly catalyzed by mono-oxygenases present in the liver. If the metabolite is not sufficiently polar to be excreted, they undergo phase II reactions.

Phase II reactions are conjugation reactions where water-soluble substances present in the body like glucuronic acid, sulfuric acid, glutathione or an amino acid, combine with the drug or its phase I metabolite to form a highly polar compound. The compound so formed is inactive and gets readily excreted by the kidneys. Large molecules are excreted through the bile. Thus, phase II reactions invariably inactivate the drug.

Glucuronide conjugation is the most common type of metabolic reaction (Flowchart 1.2).

Enzyme Induction

Microsomal enzymes are present in the microsomes of the liver cells. The synthesis of these enzymes can be increased by certain

Flowchart 1.2: Important drug biotransformation reactions with examples.

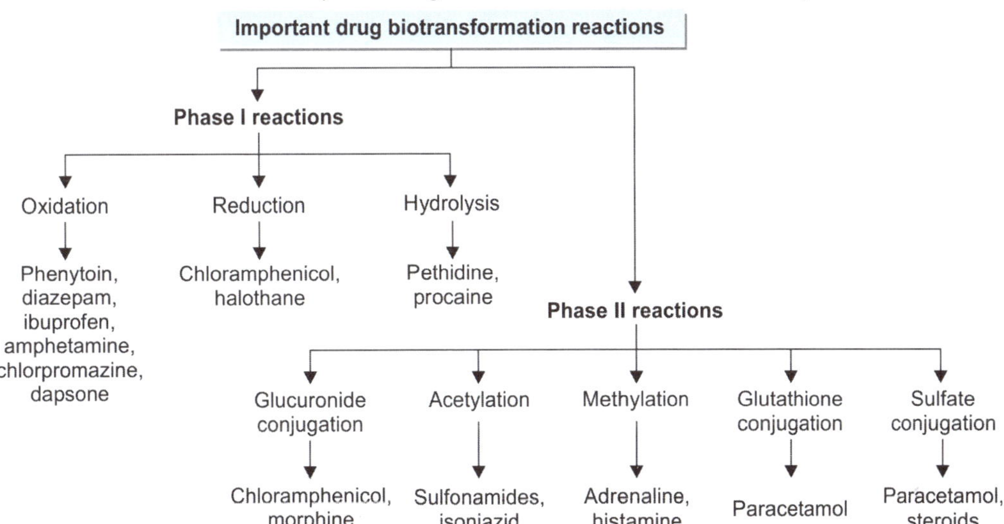

drugs and environmental pollutants. This is called *enzyme induction* and this process speeds up the metabolism of the inducing drug itself and other drugs metabolized by the microsomal enzymes, e.g., phenobarbitone, rifampicin, alcohol, cigarette smoke, dichloro-diphenyl-trichloroethane (DDT), griseofulvin, carbamazepine and phenytoin are some enzyme inducers.

Clinical importance of enzyme induction:

1. **Drug interactions:** Enzyme induction can result in drug interactions when drugs are given together because one drug may increase the metabolism of the other drug resulting in therapeutic failure.
2. **Toxicity:** Due to enzyme induction, higher amount of toxic metabolite may be produced rapidly. For example, a patient undergoing treatment with rifampicin is likely to develop hepatotoxicity with paracetamol because a higher amount of the toxic intermediate metabolite of paracetamol is formed due to enzyme induction.
3. **Tolerance to drugs** may develop as in case of carbamazepine because it increases its own metabolism.
4. **Clinical application of enzyme induction:** Neonates are deficient in both microsomal and nonmicrosomal enzymes. Hence their capacity to conjugate bilirubin is low which results in jaundice. Administration of phenobarbitone—an enzyme inducer, helps in rapid clearance of jaundice in them by enhancing bilirubin conjugation.

Enzyme Inhibition

Some drugs like cimetidine and ketoconazole inhibit cytochrome P450 enzyme activity. Hence, metabolism of other drugs get reduced and can result in toxicity. Therefore, enzyme inhibition by drugs is also the basis of several drug interactions. Chloramphenicol, cimetidine, erythromycin, ketoconazole, ciprofloxacin and verapamil are some enzyme inhibitors.

Drugs can also inhibit non-microsomal enzymes. Example

- Allopurinol inhibits xanthine oxidase
- NSAIDs inhibit cyclo-oxygenase.

Excretion

Drugs are excreted from the body after being converted to water-soluble metabolites while some are directly eliminated without metabolism. The major organs of excretion are the kidneys, the intestines, the biliary system and the lungs. Drugs are also excreted in small amounts in the saliva, sweat and milk.

Renal Excretion

Kidney is the most important route of drug excretion. The three processes involved in the elimination of drugs through kidneys are glomerular filtration, active tubular secretion and passive tubular reabsorption.

Glomerular filtration: The rate of filtration through the glomerulus depends on glomerular filtration rate (GFR), concentration of free drug in the plasma and its molecular weight. Ionized drugs of low molecular weight (< 10,000) are easily filtered through the glomerular membrane.

Active tubular secretion: Cells of the proximal tubules actively secrete acids and bases by two transport systems. Thus, acids like penicillin, salicylic acid, probenecid, frusemide; bases like amphetamine and histamine are so excreted. Drugs may compete for the same transport system resulting in prolongation of action of each other, e.g., penicillin and probenecid.

Passive tubular reabsorption: Passive diffusion of drug molecules can occur in either direction in the renal tubules depending on the drug concentration, lipid solubility and pH. As highly lipid soluble drugs are largely reabsorbed, their excretion is slow. Acidic drugs get ionized in alkaline urine and are easily excreted while bases are excreted faster in acidic urine. This property is useful in the treatment of poisoning. In poisoning with acidic drugs like salicylates and barbiturates, forced alkaline diuresis (diuretic + sodium bicarbonate + IV fluids) is employed to hasten drug excretion. Similarly, elimination of basic drugs like quinine and amphetamine is enhanced by forced acid diuresis.

Fecal and Biliary Excretion

Unabsorbed portion of the orally administered drugs are eliminated through the feces. Liver transfers acids, bases and unionized molecules into bile by specific acid transport processes. Some drugs may get reabsorbed in the lower portion of the gut and are carried back to the liver. Such recycling is called *enterohepatic circulation* and it prolongs the duration of action of the drug; examples are chloramphenicol, tetracycline, oral contraceptives and erythromycin.

Pulmonary Excretion

The lungs are the main route of elimination for gases and volatile liquids, viz. general anesthetics and alcohol. This also has legal implications in medicolegal practice.

Other Routes of Excretion

Small amounts of some drugs are eliminated through the **sweat** and **saliva**. Excretion in saliva may result in a unique taste of some drugs, e.g., metronidazole and phenytoin. Drugs like iodide, rifampicin and heavy metals are excreted through sweat.

The excretion of drugs in the **milk** is in small amounts and is of no significance to the mother. But, for the suckling infant, it may be sometimes important especially because of the infant's immature metabolic and excretory mechanisms. Though most drugs can be taken by the mother without significant toxicity to the child, there are a few exceptions (Table 1.2).

Table 1.2: Example of drugs that could be toxic to the suckling infant when taken by the mother.

Sulphasalazine	Doxepin
Theophylline	Amiodarone
Anticancer drugs	Primidone
Salicylates	Ethosuximide
Chloramphenicol	Phenobarbitone
Nalidixic acid	Phenothiazines
Nitrofurantoin	β-blockers

Drugs are metabolized/eliminated from the body by:

- **First-order kinetics:** In first order kinetics, a constant *fraction* of the drug is metabolized/eliminated per unit time. Most drugs follow first order kinetics and the rate of metabolism/excretion is dependant on their concentration (exponential) in the body. It also holds good for absorption of drugs.
- **Zero order kinetics (saturation kinetics):** Here a constant *amount* of the drug present in the body is metabolized/eliminated per unit time. The metabolic enzymes get saturated and hence with increase in dose, the plasma drug level increases disproportionately resulting in toxicity.

Some drugs like phenytoin and warfarin are eliminated by both processes, i.e., by first order initially and by zero order at higher concentrations.

Plasma Half-life

Plasma half-life (t½) is the time taken for the plasma concentration of a drug to be reduced to half its value (Fig. 1.8). Four to five half-lives are required for the complete elimination of a drug. Each drug has its own t½ and is an important pharmacokinetic parameter that guides the dosing regimen. It helps in calculating loading and maintenance doses of a drug. It also indicates the duration of action of a drug.

Importance of Plasma Half-life

Plasma half-life is needed:

- to know the duration of action of a drug
- for frequency of drug administration
- to guide the dosing regimen
- to know time needed for action, steady state concentration
- for calculating loading and maintenance doses of a drug

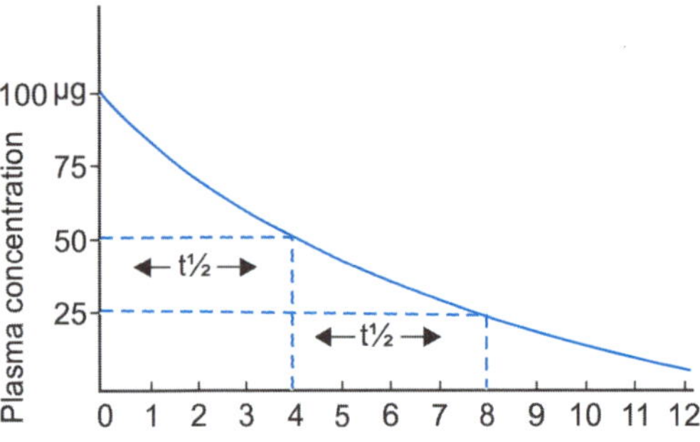

Fig. 1.8: Plasma concentration-time curve following intravenous dose. Plasma t½ = 4 hours.

Biological half-life is the time required for total amount of the drug in the body to be reduced to half.

Biological effect half-life is the time required for the biological effect of the drug to reduce to half. In some drugs like propranolol, the pharmacological effect of the drug may last much longer, i.e., even after its plasma levels fall. In such drugs, biological effect half life gives an idea of the duration of action of the drug.

Steady State Concentration

If a drug is administered repeatedly at short intervals before complete elimination, the drug accumulates in the body and reaches a 'state' at which the rate of elimination equals the rate of administration. This is known as the *'Steady-state'* or plateau level (Fig. 1.9). After attaining this level, the plasma concentration fluctuates around an average steady level. It takes 4–5 half-lives for the plasma concentration to reach the plateau level.

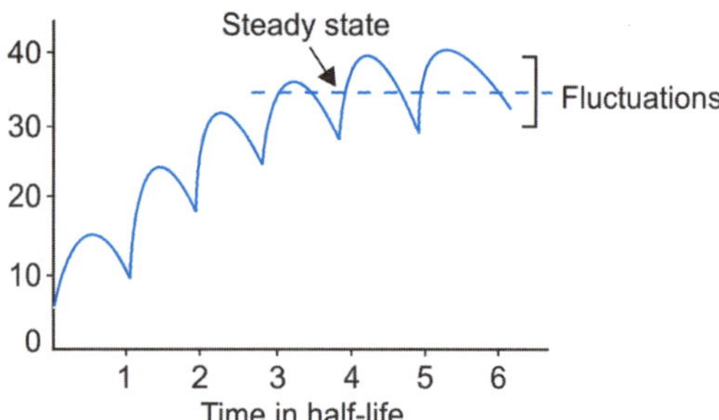

Fig. 1.9: Drug accumulation and attainment of steady state concentration on oral administration.

Drug Dosage

Depending on the patient's requirements and the characteristics of the drug, drug dosage can be of the following kinds:

Fixed dose: In case of reasonably safe drugs, a fixed dose of the drug is suitable for most patients, e.g., analgesics like paracetamol—500 mg to 1000 mg 6 hourly is the usual adult dose.

Individualized dose: For some drugs especially the ones with low safety margin, the dose has to be 'tailored' to the needs of each patient, e.g., anticonvulsants, antiarrhythmic drugs.

Loading dose: In situations when rapid action is needed, a loading/bolus dose of the drug is given at the beginning of the treatment. A loading dose is a single large dose or a series of quickly repeated doses given to rapidly attain target concentration, e.g., heparin given as 5000 IU bolus dose. Once the target level is reached, a *maintenance dose* is sufficient to maintain the drug level and to balance the elimination.

The disadvantage with the loading dose is that the patient is rapidly exposed to high concentrations of the drug which may result in toxicity.

Therapeutic Drug Monitoring

The response to a drug depends on the plasma concentration attained in the patient. In some situations it may be necessary to monitor treatment by measuring plasma drug concentrations.

Indications for TDM

- While using drugs with low safety margin—to avoid therapeutic failure, e.g., digoxin, theophylline, lithium.
- To reduce the risk of toxicity, e.g., aminoglycosides.
- To treat poisoning.

TDM is not Required in

- Drugs whose response can be easily measured, e.g., blood pressure for anti-hypertensives
- For 'hit and run' drugs whose effects persist for a long time even after the drug is eliminated
- Drugs to which tolerance develops.

Methods of Prolonging Drug Action (Table 1.3)

In several situations it may be desirable to use long-acting drugs. But when such drugs are not available, the duration of action of the available drugs may be prolonged.

The duration of action of drugs can be prolonged by interfering with the pharmacokinetic processes, i.e., by

- Slowing absorption.
- Using a more plasma protein bound derivative.
- Inhibiting metabolism.
- Delaying excretion.

PHARMACODYNAMICS

Pharmacodynamics is the study of actions of the drugs on the body and their mechanisms of action, i.e., to know what drugs do and how they do it.

Drugs produce their effects by interacting with the physiological systems of the organisms. By such interaction, drugs merely modify the rate of functions of the various systems. But they cannot bring about qualitative changes, i.e., they cannot change the basic functions of any physiological system. Thus drugs act by:

- Stimulation
- Depression

Table 1.3: Methods of prolonging duration of action of drugs.

Processes	*Methods*	*Examples*
Absorption		
Oral	Sustained release preparation, coating with resins, etc.	Iron, deriphylline
Parenteral	• Reducing solubility —Oily suspension • Altering particle size • Pellet implantation —Sialistic capsules • Reduction in vascularity of the absorbing surface • Combining with protein • Chemical alteration —Esterification	Procaine + Penicillin Depot progestins Insulin zinc suspension as large crystals that are slowly absorbed Deoxycorticosterone acetate (DOCA) Testosterone Adrenaline + lignocaine (vasoconstrictor) Protamine + zinc + insulin Estrogen Testosterone
Dermal	Transdermal adhesive patches, Ointments Ocuserts (transmucosal)—used in eye	Scopolamine Nitroglycerine Pilocarpine
Distribution	Choosing more protein bound member of the group	Sulfonamides-like sulfamethoxypyridazine
Metabolism	Inhibiting the metabolizing enzyme cholinesterase By inhibiting enzyme peptidase in renal tubular cells	Physostigmine prolongs the action of acetylcholine Cilastatin—prolongs action of imipenem
Excretion	Competition for same transport system —for renal tubular secretion	Probenecid prolongs the action of penicillin and ampicillin

- Irritation
- Replacement
- Anti-infective or cytotoxic action
- Modification of the immune status.

Stimulation: Stimulation is the increase in activity of the specialized cells, e.g., adrenaline stimulates the heart.

Depression: Depression is the decrease in activity of the specialized cells, e.g., quinidine depresses the heart; barbiturates depress the central nervous system. Some drugs may stimulate one system and depress another, e.g., morphine depresses the CNS but stimulates the vagus.

Irritation: This can occur on all types of tissues in the body and may result in inflammation, corrosion and necrosis of cells.

Replacement: Drugs may be used for replacement when there is deficiency of natural substances like hormones, metabolites or nutrients, e.g., insulin in diabetes mellitus, iron in anemia, vitamin C in scurvy.

Anti-infective and cytotoxic action: Drugs may act by specifically destroying infective organisms, e.g., penicillins, or by cytotoxic effect on cancer cells, e.g., anticancer drugs.

Modification of immune status: Vaccines and sera act by improving our immunity while immunosuppressants act by depressing immunity, e.g., glucocorticoids.

Mechanisms of Drug Action

Most drugs produce their effects by binding to specific target proteins like receptors, enzymes and ion channels. Drugs may act *on* the cell membrane, *inside* or *outside* the cell to produce their effect. Drugs may act by one or more complex mechanisms of action. Some of them are yet to be understood. But the fundamental mechanisms of drug action may be:

1. Through Receptors

Drugs may act by interacting with specific receptors in the body.

2. Through Enzymes and Pumps

Drugs may act by inhibition of various enzymes, thus altering the enzyme-mediated reactions, e.g., allopurinol inhibits the enzyme xanthine oxidase; acetazolamide inhibits carbonic anhydrase.

Membrane pumps like H^+ K^+ ATPase, Na^+ K^+ ATPase may be inhibited by drugs, e.g., omeprazole, digoxin.

3. Through Ion Channels

Drugs may interfere with the movement of ions across specific channels, e.g., calcium channel blockers, potassium channel openers.

4. Physical Action

The action of a drug could result from its physical properties like:

Adsorption	- Activated charcoal in poisoning
Mass of the drug	- Bulk laxatives like psyllium, bran
Osmotic property	- Osmotic diuretics—mannitol
	- Osmotic purgatives—magnesium sulfate
Radioactivity	- ^{131}I
Radio-opacity	- Barium sulfate contrast media.

5. Chemical Interaction

Drugs may act by chemical reaction.

Antacids	- neutralise gastric acids
Oxidizing agents	- like potassium permanganate—germicidal
Chelating agents	- bind heavy metals making them nontoxic.

6. Altering Metabolic Processes

Drugs like antimicrobials alter the metabolic pathway in the microorganisms resulting in destruction of the microorganism, e.g., sulfonamides interfere with bacterial folic acid synthesis.

Receptor

A receptor is a site on the cell with which an agonist binds to bring about a change, e.g., histamine receptor, α and β adrenergic receptors.

Affinity is the ability of a drug to bind to a receptor.

Intrinsic activity or efficacy is the ability of a drug to produce a response after binding to the receptor.

Agonist: An agonist is a substance that binds to the receptor and produces a response. It has affinity and intrinsic activity.

Antagonist: An antagonist is a substance that binds to the receptor and prevents the action of agonist on the receptor. It has affinity but no intrinsic activity.

Partial agonist binds to the receptor but has low intrinsic activity.

Ligand is a molecule which binds selectively to a specific receptor.

Site: The receptors may be present in the cell membrane, in the cytoplasm or on the nucleus.

Nature of receptors: Receptors are proteins.

Synthesis and life-span: Receptor proteins are synthesized by the cells. They have a definite life span after which the receptors are degraded by the cell and new receptors are synthesized.

Last three decades have seen an explosion in our knowledge of the receptors. Various receptors have been identified, isolated and extensively studied.

Functions of Receptors

The two functions of receptors are:

1. Recognition and binding of the ligand
2. Propagation of the message.

For the above function, the receptor has two sites (domains):

i. **A ligand binding site:** The site to bind the drug molecule.
ii. **An effector site:** Which undergoes a change to propagate or convey the message.

Drug-receptor interaction has been considered to be similar to 'lock and key' relationship where the drug specifically fits into the particular receptor (lock) like a key. Interaction of the agonist with the receptor brings about changes in the receptor which in turn conveys the signal to the effector system. The final response is brought about by the effector system through second messengers. The agonist itself is the first messenger. The entire process involves a chain of events triggered by drug receptor interaction.

Receptor Families

Four families (types) of cell surface receptors are identified. The receptor families are:

- Ion channels
- G-protein coupled receptors
- Enzymatic receptors
- Nuclear receptors (receptors that regulate gene transcription).

Receptor Regulation

The number of receptors (density) and their sensitivity can be altered in many situations:

- **Upregulation:** Denervation or prolonged absence of the agonist or constant action of the antagonist all result in an increase in the number and sensitivity of the receptors. This phenomenon is called '**upregulation**.'

  Prolonged use of a β-adrenergic antagonist like propranolol results in upregulation of β-adrenergic receptors.
- **Downregulation:** On the other hand, continued stimulation of the receptors causes desensitization and a decrease in the number of receptors—known as '**downregulation**' of the receptors.

Clinical importance of receptor regulation: After prolonged administration, a receptor antagonist should always be tapered. For example, if propranolol—a β adrenoceptor blocker is suddenly withdrawn after long-term use, it precipitates angina due to upregulation of β receptors.

Constant use of β adrenergic agonists in bronchial asthma results in reduced therapeutic response due to down regulation of β_2 receptors.

Dose Response Relationship

The response to different doses of a drug can be plotted on a graph to obtain the dose response curve.

The clinical response to the increasing dose of the drug is defined by the shape of the dose response curve (DRC). Initially the extent of response increases with increase in dose till the maximum response is reached. After the maximum effect has been obtained, further increase in doses does not increase the response. If the dose is plotted on a logarithmic scale, the curve becomes sigmoid or 'S' shaped (Fig. 1.10).

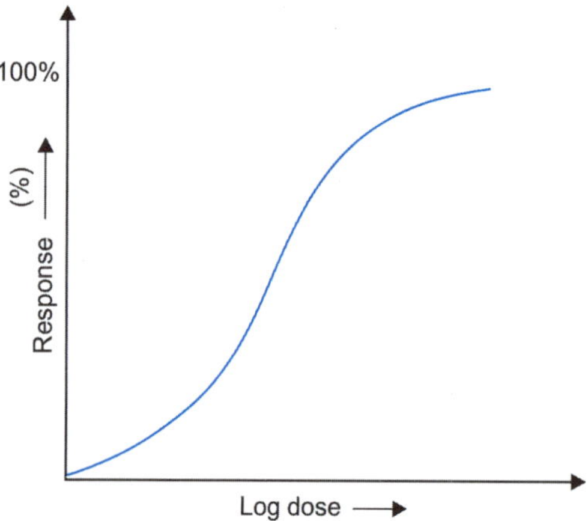

Fig. 1.10: Log dose response curve.

Drug Potency

The amount of drug required to produce a response indicates the **potency**. For example, 1 mg of bumetanide produces the same diuresis as 50 mg of frusemide. Thus, bumetanide is more potent than frusemide. In Figure 1.11, drugs A and B are more potent than drugs C and D, drug A being the most potent and drug D—the least potent. Hence higher doses of drugs C and D are to be administered as compared to drugs A and B. Generally potency is of little clinical significance.

Efficacy: Drug efficacy or **maximal efficacy** indicates the maximum response produced by a drug, e.g., frusemide produces powerful diuresis, not produced by any dose of amiloride. In Figure 1.11, drugs B and C are more efficacious than drugs A and D. Drug A is more potent but less efficacious than drugs B and C. Such differences in efficacy are of great clinical importance.

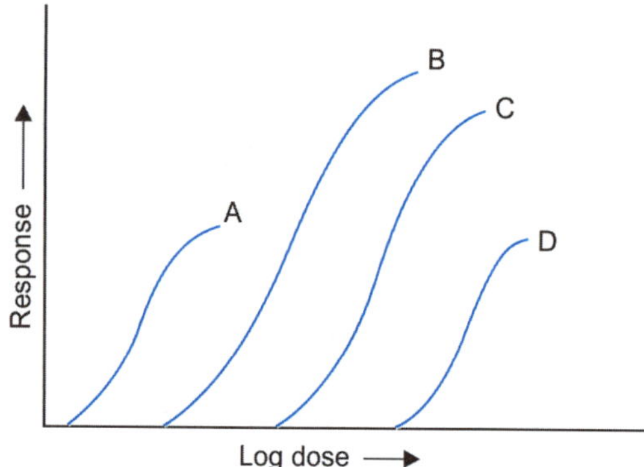

Fig. 1.11: Dose response curves of four drugs showing different potencies and maximal efficacies. Drug A is more potent but less efficacious than B and C. Drug D is less potent and less efficacious than drugs B and C.

Therapeutic index: Therapeutic index indicates the safety of the drug. The dose response curves for different actions of a drug could be different. Thus salbutamol may have one DRC for bronchodilation and another for tachycardia. The distance between beneficial effect DRC and unwanted effect DRC indicates the safety margin of the drug (Fig. 1.12).

Median lethal dose (LD_{50}) is the dose which is lethal to 50 percent of animals of the test population.

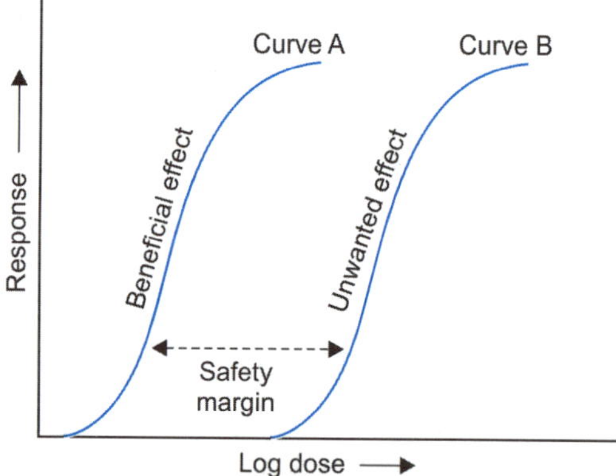

Fig. 1.12: The distance between curves A and B indicates safety margin of the drug.

Median effective dose (ED_{50}) is the dose that produces a desired effect in 50 percent of the test population.

Therapeutic index (TI) is the ratio of the median lethal dose to the median effective dose.

$$\textbf{Therapeutic index} = \frac{LD_{50}}{ED_{50}}$$

It gives an idea about the safety of the drug.

- The higher the therapeutic index, the safer is the drug
- TI varies from species to species
- For a drug to be considered reasonably safe, it's TI must be > 1
- Penicillin has a high TI while lithium and digoxin have low TI.

Drug Synergism and Antagonism

When two or more drugs are given concurrently the effect may be additive, synergistic or antagonistic.

Additive Effect

The effect of two or more drugs get added up and the total effect is equal to the sum of their individual actions.

Examples are ephedrine with theophylline in bronchial asthma; nitrous oxide and ether as general anesthetics.

Synergism

When the action of one drug is enhanced by another drug, the combination is **synergistic**. In Greek, *ergon* = work; *syn* = with. Here, the total effect of the combination is greater than the sum of their independent effects. It is often called 'potentiation' or 'supra-additive' effect.

Examples of synergistic combination are:

- Acetylcholine + physostigmine
- Levodopa + carbidopa.

Antagonism

One drug opposing or inhibiting the action of another is antagonism. Based on the mechanisms, antagonism can be:

Chemical antagonism: Two substances interact chemically to result in inactivation of the effect, e.g., chelating agents inactivate heavy metals like lead and mercury to form inactive complexes; antacids like aluminium hydroxide neutralize gastric acid.

Physiological antagonism: Two drugs act at different sites to produce opposing effects. For example, histamine acts on H_2 receptors to produce bronchospasm and hypotension while adrenaline reverses these effects by acting on adrenergic receptors.

Insulin and glucagon have opposite effects on the blood sugar level.

Receptor antagonism: The antagonist inhibits the binding of the agonist to the receptor. Such antagonism may be reversible or irreversible.

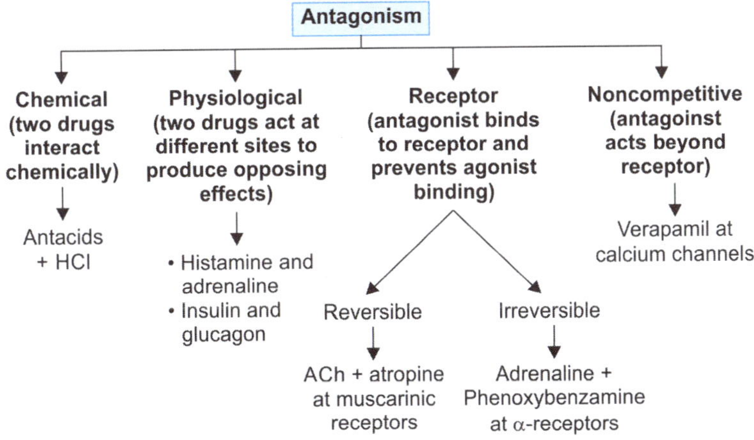

Reversible or competitive antagonism: The agonist and antagonist compete for the same receptor. By increasing the concentration of the agonist, the antagonism can be overcome. It is thus *reversible antagonism*. Acetylcholine and atropine compete for the muscarinic receptors. The antagonism can be overcome by increasing the concentration of acetylcholine at the receptor. d-tubocurarine and acetylcholine compete for the nicotinic receptors at the neuromuscular junction.

Irreversible antagonism: The antagonist binds firmly by covalent bonds to the receptor. Thus it blocks the action of the agonist and the blockade *cannot* be overcome by increasing the dose of the agonist and hence it is irreversible antagonism, e.g., adrenaline and phenoxybenzamine at alpha adrenergic receptors (Fig. 1.13).

Noncompetitive antagonism: The antagonist blocks at the level of receptor-effector linkage. For example, verapamil blocks the cardiac calcium channels and inhibits the entry of Ca^{++} during depolarization. It thereby antagonizes the effect of cardiac stimulants like isoprenaline and adrenaline.

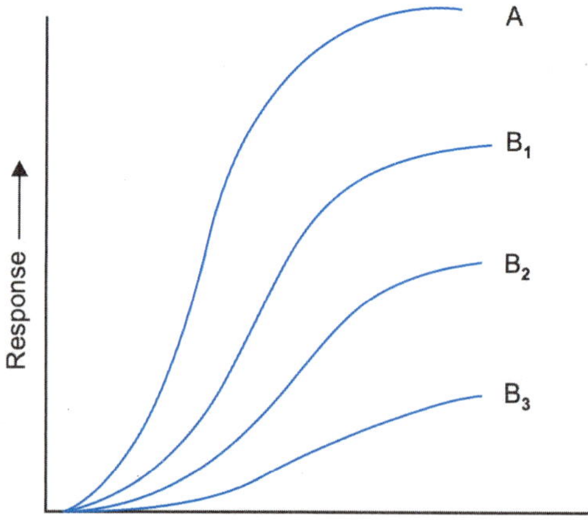

Fig. 1.13: Dose response curves of an agonist: (A) in the absence of antagonist. B_1, B_2 and B_3 in the presence of increasing doses of an irreversible antagonist.

FACTORS THAT MODIFY THE EFFECTS OF DRUGS

The same dose of a drug can produce different degrees of response in different patients and even in the same patient under different situations.

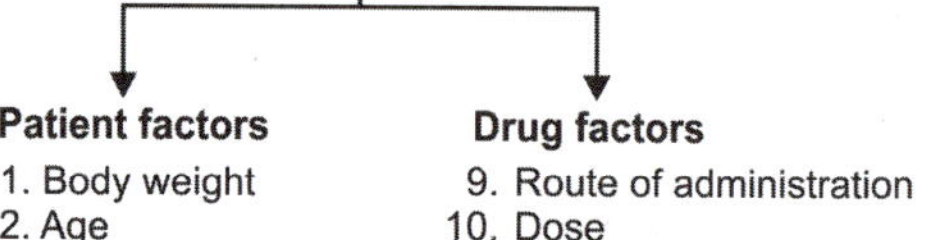

Patient factors
1. Body weight
2. Age
3. Sex
4. Species and race
5. Diet and environment
6. Genetic factors
7. Diseases
8. Psychological factor

Drug factors
9. Route of administration
10. Dose
11. Cumulation/repeated dosing
12. Presence of other drugs

Patient Factors

1. **Body weight:** The recommended dose is calculated for medium built persons. For the obese and underweight persons, the dose has to be calculated individually. Though body surface area is a better parameter for more accurate calculation of the dose, it is inconvenient and hence not generally used.

Formula:

$$\text{Dose} = \frac{\text{Body weight (kg)}}{70} \times \text{average adult dose}$$

2. **Age:** The pharmacokinetics of many drugs change with age resulting in altered response in extremes of age. In the newborn, the liver and kidneys are not fully mature to handle the drugs, e.g., chloramphenicol can produce grey baby syndrome. The blood-brain barrier is not well-formed and drugs can easily reach the brain. The gastric acidity is low, intestinal motility is slow, skin is delicate and permeable to drugs applied topically. Hence calculation of the appropriate dose, depending on body weight is important to avoid toxicity. Also pharmacodynamic differences could exist, e.g., barbiturates which produce sedation in adults may produce excitation in children.

Formula for calculation of dose for children

Young's formula

$$\text{Child's dose} = \frac{\text{Age (years)}}{\text{Age} + 12} \times \text{Adult dose}$$

In the elderly, the capacity of the liver and kidney to handle the drug is reduced and are more susceptible to adverse effects. Hence lower doses are recommended, e.g., elderly are at a higher risk of ototoxicity and nephrotoxicity by streptomycin.

3. **Sex:** The hormonal effects and smaller body size may influence drug response in women. Special care is necessary while prescribing for pregnant and lactating women and during menstruation.

4. **Species and race:** Response to drugs may vary with species and race. For example, rabbits are resistant to atropine. Then it becomes difficult to extrapolate the results of animal experiments. Blacks need higher doses of atropine to produce mydriasis.

5. **Diet and environment:** Food interferes with the absorption of many drugs. For example, tetracyclines form complexes with calcium present in the food and are poorly absorbed.

Polycyclic hydrocarbons present in cigarette smoke may induce microsomal enzymes resulting in enhanced metabolism of some drugs.

6. **Genetic factors:** Variations in an individual's response to drugs could be genetically mediated. **Pharmacogenetics** is concerned with the genetically mediated variations in drug responses. The differences in response is most commonly due to variations in the amount of drug metabolizing enzymes since the production of these enzymes are genetically controlled.

Examples

- ***Acetylation of drugs:*** The rate of drug acetylation differs among individuals who may be fast or slow acetylators, e.g., isoniazid (INH), sulfonamides and hydralazine are acetylated. Slow acetylators treated with hydralazine are more likely to develop lupus erythematosus.
- ***Atypical pseudocholinesterase:*** Succinylcholine is metabolized by pseudocholinesterase. Some people inherit atypical pseudocholinesterase and they develop a prolonged apnea due to succinylcholine.
- ***Glucose-6-phosphate dehydrogenase (G6PD) deficiency:*** Primaquine, sulfones and quinolones can cause hemolysis in such people.
- ***Malignant hyperthermia:*** Halothane and succinylcholine can trigger malignant hyperthermia in some genetically predisposed individuals.

7. **Diseases:** Presence of certain diseases can influence drug responses, e.g.

- **Malabsorption:** Drugs are poorly absorbed.
- **Liver diseases:** Rate of drug metabolism is reduced due to dysfunction of hepatocytes. Also protein binding is reduced due to low serum albumin.
- **Cardiac diseases:** In congestive cardiac failure (CCF), there is edema of the gut mucosa and decreased perfusion of liver and kidneys. These may result in cumulation and toxicity of drugs like propranolol and lignocaine.
- **Renal dysfunction:** Drugs mainly excreted through kidneys are likely to accumulate and cause toxicity, e.g., streptomycin, amphotericin B—dose of such drugs need to be reduced.

8. **Psychological factor:** The doctor patient relationship influences the response to a drug often to a large extent by acting on the patient's psychology. The patients confidence in the doctor may itself be sufficient to relieve a suffering, particularly the psychosomatic disorders. This can be substantiated by the fact that large number of patients respond to placebo. **Placebo** is the inert dosage

form with no specific biological activity but only resembles the actual preparation in appearance. *Placebo* = 'I shall be pleasing' (in Latin).

Placebo medicines are used in:

- Clinical trials as a control
- To benefit or please a patient psychologically when he does not actually require an active drug as in mild psychosomatic disorders and in chronic incurable diseases.

In fact all forms of treatment including physiotherapy and surgery have some placebo effect. Substances used as placebo include lactose, some vitamins, minerals and distilled water injections.

Drug Factors

9. **Route of administration:** Occasionally route of administration may modify the pharmacodynamic response, e.g., magnesium sulfate given orally is a purgative, but given intravenously causes CNS depression and has anticonvulsant effects. Applied topically (poultice), it reduces local edema. Hypertonic magnesium sulfate retention enema reduces intracranial tension.

10. **Dose:** It is fascinating that the response to a drug may be modified by the dose administered. Generally as the dose is increased, the magnitude of the response also increases proportionately till the 'maximum' is reached. Further increases in doses may with some drugs produce effects opposite to their lower-dose effect, e.g., (i) in myasthenia gravis, neostigmine enhances muscle power in therapeutic doses, but in high doses it causes muscle paralysis, (ii) physiological doses of vitamin D promotes calcification while hypervitaminosis D leads to decalcification.

11. **Repeated dosing** can result in:

- Cumulation
- Tolerance
- Tachyphylaxis.

Cumulation: Drugs like digoxin which are slowly eliminated may cumulate resulting in toxicity.

Tolerance: Tolerance is the requirement of higher doses of a drug to produce a given response. Tolerance may be natural or acquired.

Natural tolerance: The species/race shows less sensitivity to the drug, e.g., rabbits show tolerance to atropine; Black race are tolerant to mydriatics.

Acquired tolerance: Develops on repeated administration of a drug. The patient who was initially responsive becomes tolerant, e.g., barbiturates, opioids, nitrites produce tolerance.

Tolerance may develop to some actions of the drug and not to others, e.g., morphine—tolerance develops to analgesic and euphoric effects of morphine but not to its constipating and miotic effects.

Barbiturates—tolerance develops to sedative but not antiepileptic effects of barbiturates.

Mechanisms: The mechanisms of development of tolerance could be:

Pharmacokinetic: Changes in absorption, distribution, metabolism and excretion of drugs may result in reduced concentration of the drug at the site of action and is also known as dispositional tolerance, e.g., barbiturates induce microsomal enzymes and enhance their own metabolism.

Pharmacodynamic: Changes in the target tissue, may make it less responsive to the drug. It is also called functional tolerance. It could be due to down regulation of receptors as in opioids or due to compensatory mechanisms of the body, e.g., blunting of response to some antihypertensives due to salt and water retention.

Cross tolerance is the development of tolerance to pharmacologically related drugs, i.e., to drugs belonging to a particular group. Thus chronic alcoholics also show tolerance to barbiturates and general anesthetics.

Tachyphylaxis: It is the rapid development of tolerance. When some drugs are administered repeatedly at short intervals, tolerance develops rapidly and is known as tachyphylaxis or acute tolerance, e.g., ephedrine, amphetamine, tyramine and 5-hydroxytryptamine. This is thought to be due to depletion of noradrenaline stores as the above drugs act by displacing noradrenaline from the sympathetic nerve endings. Other mechanisms involved may be slow dissociation of the drug from the receptor thereby blocking the receptor. Thus ephedrine given repeatedly in bronchial asthma may not give the desired response.

12. **Presence of other drugs:** When two or more drugs are used together, one of them can alter the response of the other resulting in drug interactions (*See* Drug Interactions page 32).

ADVERSE DRUG REACTIONS

All drugs can produce unwanted effects. WHO has defined an adverse drug reaction as **'any response to a drug that is noxious and unintended and that occurs at doses used in man for prophylaxis, diagnosis or therapy.'** Some patients are more likely to develop adverse effects to drugs.

Adverse drug reactions (ADRs) are classified as follows (Flowchart 1.3):

Type A (augmented) reactions are related to the known pharmacological effects of the drug and are predictable, dose-related and quantitative adverse effects. For example, hypotension following alpha blockers, insulin induced hypoglycemia, bleeding following anticoagulants. Most ADRs are of this category and are mostly reversible by dose reduction or stopping the drug. Type A reactions include side effects, secondary effects and toxic effects.

- **Side effects:** Side effects are unwanted effects of a drug that are extension of pharmacological effects and are seen with the therapeutic dose of the drug. They are predictable, common and can occur in all people, e.g., hypoglycemia due to insulin; hypokalemia following frusemide.
- **Secondary effects:** Secondary effects are the indirect results of a primary drug action. Example: superinfection on

Flowchart 1.3: Adverse drug reactions.

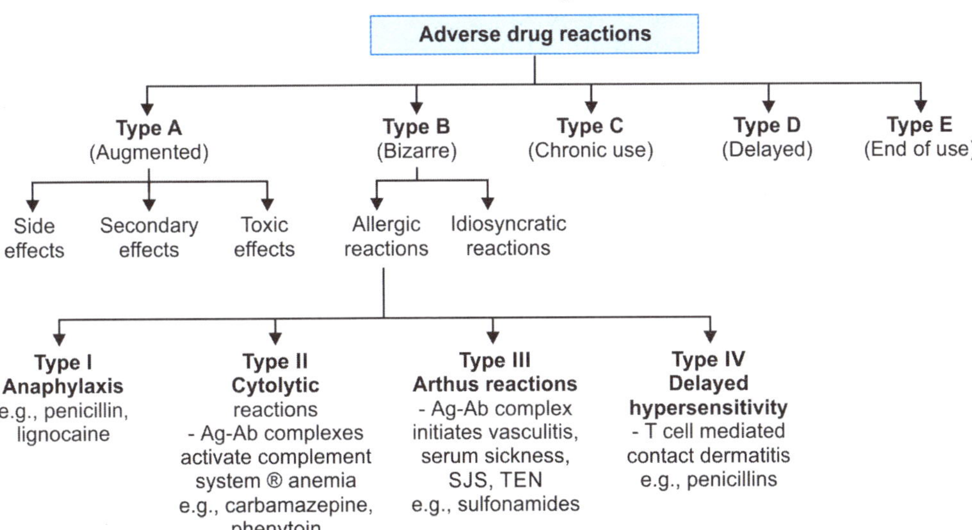

(Ag-Ab: antigen-antibody; SJS: Stevens-Johnson syndrome; TEN: toxic epidermal necrolysis)

treatment of a primary infection by broad spectrum antibiotics.

- **Toxic effects:** Toxic effects are seen with higher doses of the drug and can be serious, e.g., morphine causes respiratory depression in overdosage which can be fatal.

Type B (bizarre) reactions are unrelated to the primary pharmacological effects of the drug and are therefore not predictable. They are less common, not tolerated and are an abnormal reaction to the drug. They could be allergic reactions (immunologically mediated) or idiosyncratic (genetically mediated) reactions.

Allergic reactions to drugs are immunologically-mediated reactions which are not related to the therapeutic effects of the drug. The drug or its metabolite acts as an antigen to induce antibody formation. Further exposure to the drug may result in allergic reactions. The manifestations of allergy are seen mainly on the target organs *viz.* skin, respiratory tract, gastrointestinal tract, blood and blood vessels.

Idiosyncratic reactions are genetically determined abnormal reactions to a drug, e.g., primaquine and sulfonamides induce hemolysis in patients with G6PD deficiency; some patients show excitement with barbiturates. In addition, some responses like chloramphenicol-induced agranulocytosis, where no definite genetic background is known, are also included under idiosyncrasy. In some cases the person may be highly sensitive even two low doses of a drug (e.g. a single dose of quinine can produce cinchonism in some) or highly insensitive even to high doses of the drug.

Type C (Continuous or Chronic use) reactions occur on prolonged use of drugs and both dose and duration of drug use influence these ADRs, e.g., chloroquine retinopathy, Cushing's syndrome, analgesic nephropathy.

Type D (Delayed effects) occur long after stopping treatment, sometimes after years, e.g., leukemia following treatment of Hodgkin's lymphoma; teratogenic effects.

Type E (End of use): These effects are due to sudden discontinuation of a drug after prolonged use, e.g., acute adrenal insufficiency after sudden cessation of glucocorticoids: angina after sudden withdrawal of atenolol. Withdrawal syndrome to opioids and other drugs of abuse also are categorized as Type E ADRs.

Pharmacovigilance is the science and activities relating to the detection, assessment, understanding and prevention of adverse effects or any other drug-related problems. It deals with the epidemiologic study of adverse drug effects.

The aim of pharmacovigilance is to ensure safe and rational use of medicines.

DRUG ALLERGY

Drugs can induce allergic reactions which could range from mild itching to anaphylaxis. They can induce both types of allergic reactions viz. humoral and cell-mediated immunity. Mechanisms involved in Type I, II and III are humoral while Type IV reactions are by cell-mediated immunity.

Types of Allergic Reactions and their Mechanisms

Drugs can induce both types of allergic reactions *viz* humoral and cell-mediated immunity. Mechanism involved in type I, II and III are humoral while type IV is by cell-mediated immunity.

Type I (anaphylactic) reaction: Certain drugs induce the synthesis of IgE antibodies which are fixed to the mast cells. On subsequent exposure, the antigen-antibody complexes cause degranulation of mast cells releasing the mediators of inflammation like histamine, leukotrienes, prostaglandins and platelet-activating factor. These are responsible for the characteristic signs and symptoms of anaphylaxis like bronchospasm, laryngeal edema and hypotension which could be fatal. Allergy develops within minutes and is called immediate hypersensitivity reaction, e.g., penicillins. Skin tests may predict this type of reactions.

Type II (cytolytic) reactions: The drug binds to a protein and together they act as antigen and induce the formation of antibodies. The antigen antibody complexes activate the complement system resulting in cytolysis causing thrombocytopenia, agranulocytosis and aplastic anemia.

Type III (arthus) reactions: The antigen binds to circulating antibodies and the complexes are deposited on the vessel wall where it initiates the inflammatory response resulting in vasculitis. Rashes, fever, arthralgia, lymphadenopathy, serum sickness and Stevens Johnson syndrome are some of the manifestations of arthus type reaction.

Type IV (delayed hypersensitivity) reactions are mediated by T-lymphocytes and macrophages. The antigen reacts with receptors on T-lymphocytes which produce lymphokines leading to a local allergic reaction, e.g., contact dermatitis.

Other Forms of Adverse Drug Reactions

1. **Drug intolerance:** Drug intolerance is the inability of a person to tolerate a drug even in therapeutic doses and is unpredictable. It could be quantitative or qualitative. Patients show exaggerated response to even small doses of the drug—quantitative, e.g., vestibular dysfunction after a single dose of streptomycin may be seen in some patients. Intolerance could also be qualitative, e.g., idiosyncrasy and allergic reactions.

2. **Iatrogenic (Physician induced) diseases:** These are drug induced diseases. Even after the drug is withdrawn toxic effects can persist, e.g., isoniazid induced hepatitis; chloroquine induced retinopathy.

3. **Photosensitivity:** Drugs could sensitize the skin to sunlight and the UV rays of the Sun.

4. **Drug dependence:** Drugs that influence the behavior and mood are often misused to obtain their pleasurable effects. Repeated use of such drugs result in dependence. Several words like drug abuse, addiction and dependence are used confusingly. Drug dependence is a state of compulsive use of drugs in spite of the knowledge of risks associated with its use. It is also referred to as drug addiction. Dependence could be 'psychologic' or 'physical' dependence. Psychologic dependence is compulsive drug-seeking behavior to obtain its pleasurable effects, e.g., cigarette smoking.

Physical dependence is said to be present when withdrawal of the drug produces adverse symptoms. The body undergoes physiological changes to adapt itself to the continued presence of the drug in the body. Stopping the drug results in 'withdrawal syndrome.' The symptoms of withdrawal syndrome are disturbing and the person then craves for the drug, e.g., alcohol, opioids and barbiturates.

Mild degree of physical dependence is seen in people who drink too much of coffee.

5. **Teratogenicity:** Teratogenicity is the ability of a drug to cause fetal abnormalities when administered to the pregnant lady. *Teratos* in Greek means monster. The sedative—thalidomide taken during early pregnancy for relief from morning sickness resulted in thousands of babies being born with phocomelia (seal limbs). This thalidomide disaster (1958–61) opened the eyes of various nations and made it mandatory to impose strict teratogenicity tests before a new drug is approved for use.

Depending on the stage of pregnancy during which the teratogen is administered, it can produce various abnormalities.

- Conception to 16 days — Usually resistant to teratogenic effects. If affected, abortion occurs.
- Period of organogenesis (17–55 days of gestation) — Most vulnerable period; major physical abnormalities occur.

- Fetal period —56 days onwards — Period of growth and development—hence developmental and functional abnormalities result.

Therefore, in general drugs should be avoided during pregnancy especially in the first trimester. The type of malformation also depends on the drug, e.g., thalidomide causes phocomelia; tetracyclines cause deformed teeth; sodium valproate causes spina bifida.

6. **Carcinogenicity and mutagenicity:** Some drugs can cause cancers and genetic abnormalities. For example anticancer drugs can themselves be carcinogenic; other examples are radioactive isotopes and some hormones.

7. **Toxicity to organ systems:** Drugs can also damage various organ systems.

Organ system affected	Examples
• Hepatotoxicity	Isoniazid, pyrazinamide, paracetamol, chlorpromazine, 6-Mercaptopurine, halothane, ethanol, phenylbutazone
• Nephrotoxicity	Analgesics, aminoglycosides, cyclosporine, cisplatin, cephelexin, penicillamine, gold salts
• Ototoxicity	Aminoglycosides, frusemide
• Ocular toxicity	Chloroquine, ethambutol
• Gastrointestinal systems	Opioids, broad spectrum antibiotics
• Cardiovascular system	Digoxin, doxorubicin
• Respiratory system	Aspirin, bleomycin, busulfan, amiodarone, methotrexate
• Musculoskeletal system	Corticosteroids, heparin
• Behavioral toxicity	Corticosteroids, reserpine
• Neurological system	INH, haloperidol, ethambutol, quinine, doxorubicin vincristine
• Dermatological toxicity	Doxycycline, sulfonamides
• Electrolyte disturbances	Diuretics, mineralocorticoids
• Hematological toxicity	Chloramphenicol, sulfonamides
• Endocrine disorders	Methyldopa, oral contraceptives

DRUG INTERACTIONS

Definition: Drug interaction is the alteration in the duration or magnitude of the pharmacological effects of one drug by another drug.

When two or more drugs are given concurrently, the response may be greater or lesser than the sum of their individual effects. Such responses may be beneficial or harmful. For example, a combination of drugs is used in hypertension—hydralazine + propranolol for their beneficial interaction. But unwanted drug interactions may result in severe toxicity. Such interactions can be avoided by adequate knowledge of their mechanisms and by judicious use of drugs.

Site: Drug interactions can occur:

- *In vitro* in the syringe before administration—mixing of drugs in syringes can cause chemical or physical interactions—such drug combinations are incompatible in solution, e.g., penicillin and gentamicin should never be mixed in the same syringe.
- *In vivo,* i.e., in the body after administration.

Pharmacological basis of drug interactions: The two major mechanisms of drug interactions include pharmacokinetic and pharmacodynamic mechanisms.

1. **Pharmacokinetic mechanisms:** Alteration in the extent or duration of response may be produced by influencing absorption, distribution, metabolism or excretion of one drug by another.

Absorption of drugs from the gut may be affected by:

i. **Binding:** Tetracyclines chelate iron and antacids resulting in reduced absorption
ii. Altering gastric pH
iii. Altering GI motility.

Distribution: Competition for plasma protein binding results in displacement interactions, e.g., warfarin is displaced by phenylbutazone from protein binding sites.

Metabolism: Enzyme induction and inhibition of metabolism can both result in drug interactions, e.g., phenytoin, phenobarbitone, carbamazepine and rifampicin are enzyme inducers while chloramphenicol and cimetidine are some enzyme inhibitors.

Excretion: When drugs compete for the same renal tubular transport system, they prolong each other's duration of action, e.g., penicillin and probenecid.

2. **Pharmacodynamic mechanisms:** Drugs acting on the same receptors or physiological systems result in additive, synergistic or antagonistic effects. Many clinically important drug interactions have this basis. Examples:

- Atropine opposes the effects of physostigmine;
- Naloxone antagonises morphine;
- Antihypertensive effects of β-blockers are reduced by ephedrine or other vasoconstrictors in cold remedies.

2

CHAPTER

Autonomic Nervous System

CHAPTER HIGHLIGHTS

- Introduction to Autonomic Pharmacology
- Cholinergic System
- Cholinergic Drugs
- Anticholinergic Drugs
- Adrenergic System
- Adrenergic Drugs (Sympathomimetics)
- Adrenergic Antagonists

INTRODUCTION TO AUTONOMIC PHARMACOLOGY

The nervous system is divided (Flowchart 2.1) into central and peripheral nervous systems. The peripheral nervous system consists of autonomic and somatic nervous systems.

The autonomic nervous system (ANS) (Fig. 2.1) is **not under voluntary control** and therefore was so named by Langley *(Autos* = self, *nomos* = governing—in Greek). The ANS innervates the heart, the smooth muscles, the glands and the viscera and controls the functions of these organs.

The centers for autonomic reflexes are present in the hypothalamus, medulla and spinal cord. Hypothalamus coordinates the autonomic activity.

The ANS consists of 2 major divisions—the **sympathetic** and the **parasympathetic**. Most of the viscera have both sympathetic and parasympathetic innervation. The two divisions have opposing effects and normally their effects are in a state of equilibrium. The prime function of the sympathetic system is to help the person to adjust to stress and prepare the body for fight or flight reactions, while the parasympathetic mainly participates in tissue building reactions. Man can still survive without sympathetic system but not without parasympathetic.

Autonomic innervation (Fig. 2.2): The autonomic afferents are carried in visceral nerves through nonmyelinated fibers. For example, the parasympathetic afferents are carried by the 9th and 10th cranial nerves. The autonomic efferent innervation consists of a myelinated preganglionic fiber which synapses with the axon of a nonmyelinated postganglionic fiber. The postganglionic fiber in turn forms a junction with the receptors of

Flowchart 2.1: Nervous system.

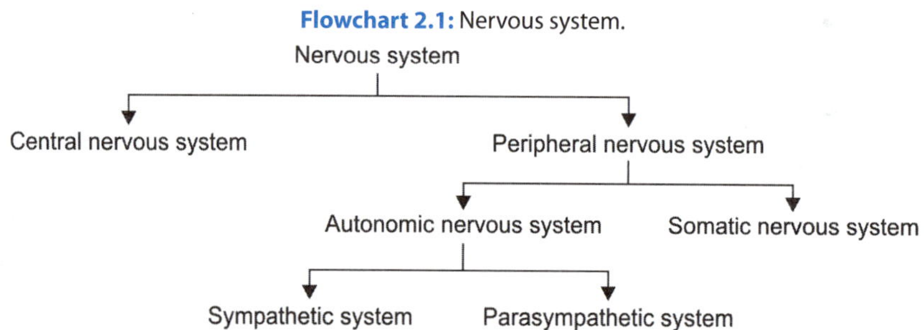

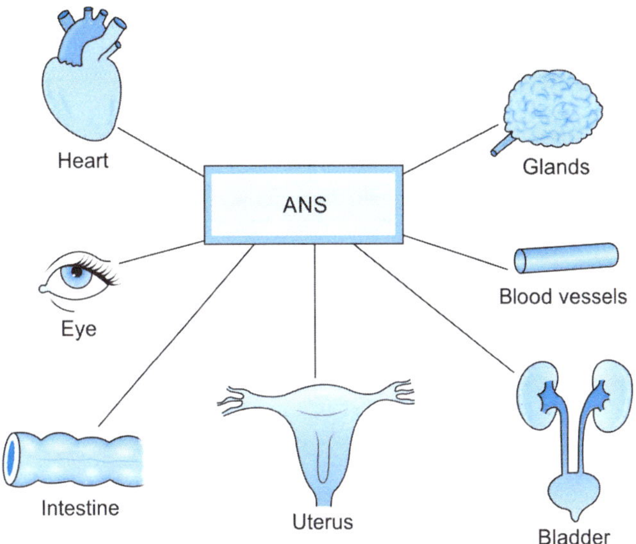

Fig. 2.1: Structures under the control of autonomic nervous system.

the organs supplied by it. The junction between the pre and postganglionic fibers is called a *ganglion* and that between the postganglionic fibers and the receptors is the *neuroeffector junction*. The traveling of an impulse along the nerve fiber is known as *conduction* while its passage across a synapse is known as *transmission*.

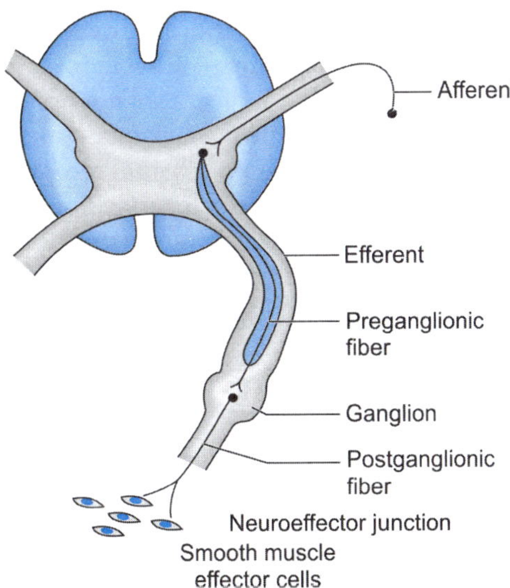

Fig. 2.2: Autonomic innervation.

The autonomic efferent is divided into sympathetic and parasympathetic divisions. The parasympathetic efferents are carried through the craniosacral outflow. The sympathetic efferents extend from the first thoracic to second or third lumbar segments (T_1-L_3) of the spinal cord. Adrenal medulla is also considered as sympathetic ganglia and differs from the other sympathetic ganglion in that the principal catecholamine that is released is adrenaline.

Neurotransmitters: For the transmission of an impulse across a synapse, a neuro-humoral transmitter substance is released into the synaptic cleft. In the ANS, the neurotransmitters released are acetylcholine, noradrenaline, dopamine and in adrenal medulla, it is adrenaline.

CHOLINERGIC SYSTEM

Acetylcholine (ACh) an ester of choline, is an important neurotransmitter of the ANS. The nerves that synthesize, store and release ACh are called *'cholinergic.'* Acetylcholine is released in response to cholinergic stimulation.

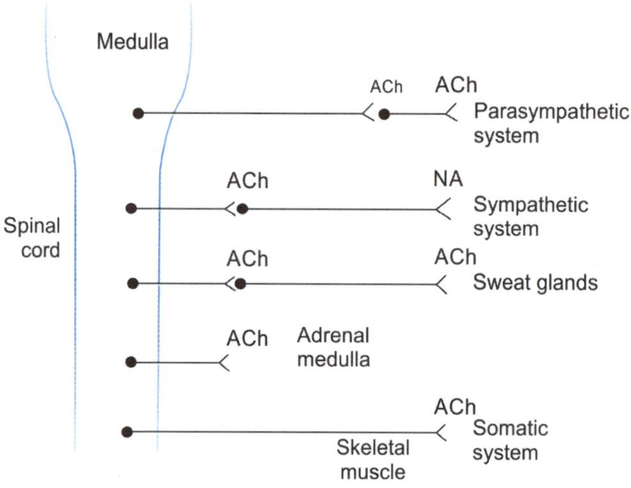

Fig. 2.3: Sites of release of neurotransmitters—acetylcholine and noradrenaline (NA) in the peripheral nervous system.

The **sites** of release of acetylcholine are (Fig. 2.3):

- **Ganglia:** All the preganglionic fibers of ANS, i.e., at both the sympathetic and parasympathetic ganglia.
- The postganglionic parasympathetic nerve endings.
- **Sweat glands:** The sympathetic post-ganglionic nerve endings supplying the sweat glands.
- **Skeletal muscles:** Somatic nerve endings supplying skeletal muscles.
- Adrenal medulla.
- **Central nervous system (CNS):** Brain and spinal cord.

Synthesis of ACh: Acetylcholine is synthesized from acetyl-CoA and choline, catalyzed by the enzyme choline acetyltransferase. This ACh is stored in small oval vesicles in the cholinergic nerve terminals.

Transmission of an impulse: When an action potential reaches the presynaptic membrane, ACh is released into the synaptic cleft (Fig. 2.4). This ACh binds to and activates the cholinergic receptor on the postsynaptic membrane leading to the depolarization of this membrane. Thus the impulse is transmitted across the synapse.

ACh released into the synaptic cleft is rapidly destroyed by the acetylcholinesterase (AChE) enzyme. Then the postsynaptic membrane is repolarized.

Cholinesterases: Acetylcholine is hydrolyzed to choline and acetic acid by the enzymes cholinesterases. Two types of AChE are present:

1. True cholinesterase—at neurons, ganglia and neuromuscular junction.
2. Pseudocholinesterase—in plasma, liver and other organs.

Cholinergic receptors: There are two classes of cholinergic receptors—**muscarinic** and **nicotinic**. Muscarinic receptors are present in the heart, smooth muscles, glands, eyes and CNS. Five subtypes of muscarinic receptors, M_1-M_5 are recognized (Flowchart 2.2).

Nicotinic receptors are present in the neuromuscular junction, autonomic ganglia and adrenal medulla. Two subtypes of nicotinic receptors are identified. N_m receptors are present at the skeletal muscle end plate and N_n receptors at the autonomic ganglia and adrenal medulla.

CHOLINERGIC DRUGS

Cholinergic drugs are chemicals that act at the same site as acetylcholine and thereby mimic its actions (Flowchart 2.3). They are

Flowchart 2.2: Subtypes and location of cholinergic receptors.

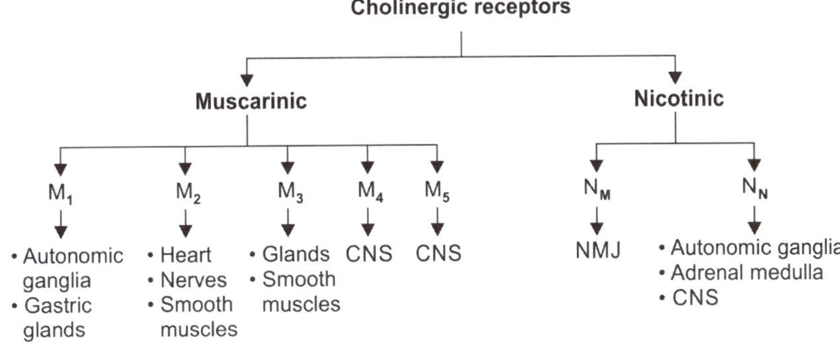

(CNS: central nervous system; NMJ: neuromuscular junction)

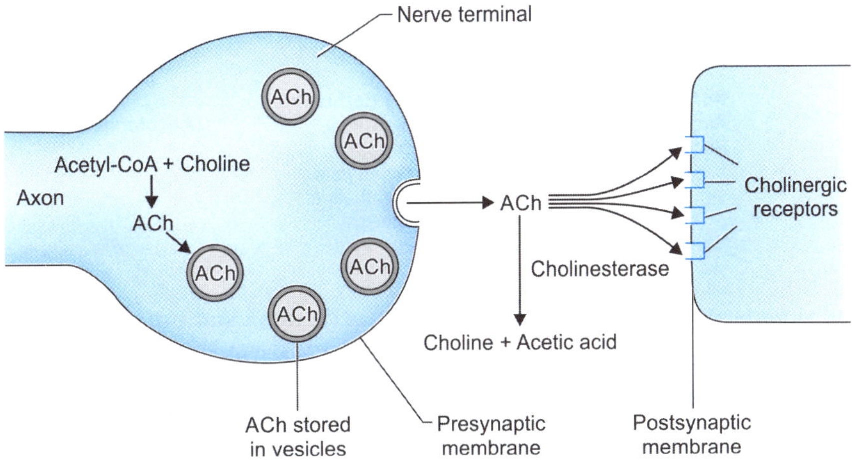

Fig. 2.4: Cholinergic transmission—schematic representation.

therefore called parasympathomimetics or cholinomimetics.

Cholinergic drugs may be classified as:

1. **Directly acting**
   a. **Esters of choline:** Acetylcholine, methacholine, carbachol, bethanechol.
   b. **Cholinomimetic alkaloids:** Pilocarpine, muscarine.
2. **Indirectly acting**
   Anticholinesterases:
   a. **Reversible:** Neostigmine, physostigmine, pyridostigmine, edrophonium
   b. **Irreversible:** Organophosphorus compounds.

Pharmacological Actions of Acetylcholine

Acetylcholine is taken as the prototype of parasympathomimetic drugs. Acetylcholine produces its actions by binding to muscarinic and nicotinic receptors.

Muscarinic Actions

Muscarinic actions resemble the actions of the alkaloid muscarine found in some mushrooms.

1. **Heart:** The action of ACh is similar to that of vagal stimulation. It reduces the heart rate and force of contraction. In larger doses, AV conduction is depressed.

Flowchart 2.3: Drugs acting on parasympathetic nervous system.

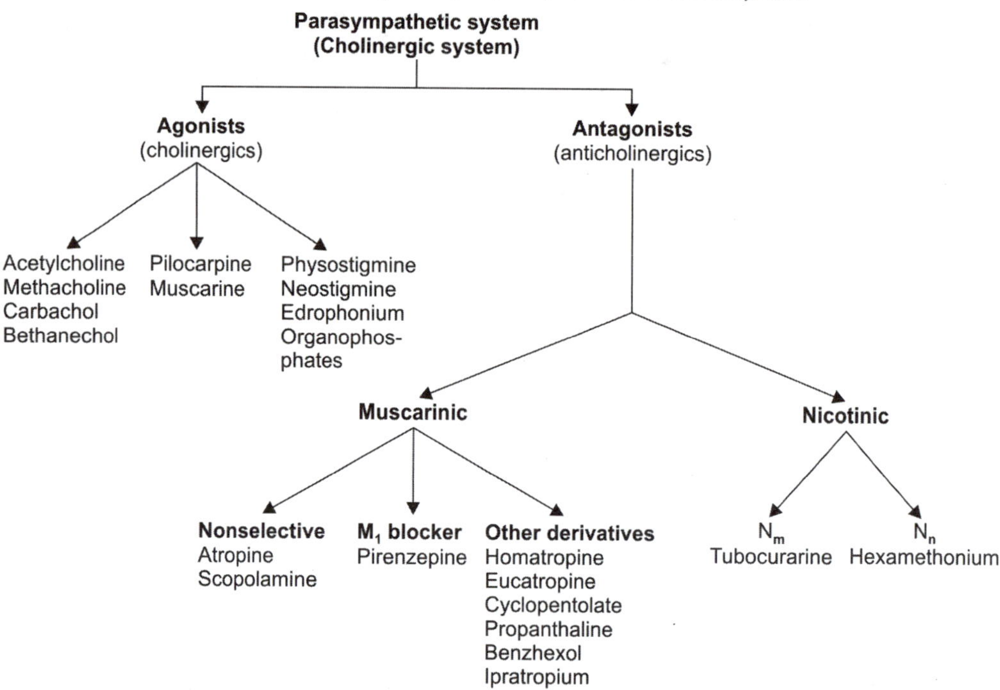

2. **Blood vessels:** ACh relaxes the vascular smooth muscles and dilates the blood vessels of the skin and mucous membrane. The BP falls due to a fall in total peripheral resistance.
3. **Smooth muscle:** ACh increases the tone of all other smooth muscles.
   - **Gastrointestinal tract**—tone and peristalsis is enhanced, sphincters are relaxed, resulting in rapid forward propulsion of intestinal contents.
   - **Urinary bladder**—detrusor contracts and trigonal sphincter relaxes—promotes voiding of urine.
   - **Bronchial smooth muscle**—contracts resulting in bronchospasm.
4. **Secretory glands:** Acetylcholine enhances the secretions of all glands; salivary, lacrimal, nasopharyngeal, tracheobronchial, gastric and intestinal secretions are increased. Sweating is also increased. Enhanced bronchial secretions and bronchospasm result in severe dyspnea.
5. **Eye:** Acetylcholine brings about constriction of pupil (miosis) by contracting the circular muscles (M3 receptors) of the iris. It improves drainage of aqueous humor and reduces intraocular pressure. Ciliary muscle contracts resulting in spasm of accommodation.

Sphincter pupillae contracts

↓

↑Drainage of aqueous humor

↓

↓IOP

Nicotinic Actions

These effects resemble the actions of the alkaloid nicotine.

1. **Neuromuscular junction (NMJ):** ACh brings about contraction of skeletal

Table 2.1: Actions of acetylcholine.

CVS	Vasodilatation, ↓HR ↓BP
Non-vascular smooth muscle	Contraction, ↑ gut peristalsis, promotes urine voiding, bronchospasm
Glands	↑ secretion
Eye	Miosis, spasm of accommodation, ↓ intraocular pressure
NMJ	Muscle contraction
Ganglia	Stimulation

(CVS: cardiovascular system; HR: heart rate; BP: blood pressure; NMJ: neuromuscular junction; IOP: intraocular pressure)

muscles. Large doses cause persistent depolarization of skeletal muscles resulting in paralysis.

2. **Autonomic ganglia:** ACh stimulates sympathetic and parasympathetic ganglia and the adrenal medulla.
3. **CNS:** ACh is a neurotransmitter at several sites in the CNS.

The important actions of acetylcholine are summarized in Table 2.1.

Uses: Acetylcholine is destroyed in the gut when given orally. On intravenous administration, it is rapidly metabolized by pseudocholinesterases in the plasma and by true cholinesterase at the site of action. Therefore it is **not used** therapeutically. Among the choline esters, methacholine is rarely used. Carbachol is used in glaucoma. Bethanechol may be used in some cases of postoperative paralytic ileus and urinary retention.

Cholinomimetic Alkaloids

Pilocarpine is an alkaloid obtained from the leaves of *Pilocarpus microphyllus*. Like ACh it stimulates cholinergic receptors, but its muscarinic actions are prominent.

Its actions on the eye are important—when applied to the eye it causes miosis, spasm of accommodation and a fall in intraocular pressure (IOP). It also increases sweat (diaphoretic) and salivary secretions (sialogogue).

Adverse effects: When used as eye drops, burning senzation and painful spasm of accommodation can occur.

Uses

1. Pilocarpine is used in **glaucoma** (0.5–4% eye drops). Pilocarpine ocusert is a special drug delivery system that can deliver pilocarpine constantly for 7 days.
2. Pilocarpine eye drops are also used alternately with mydriatics like homatropine **to break the adhesions** between the iris and the lens.
3. Pilocarpine can be used to overcome **dryness of mouth** that is seen following radiation of head and neck.
4. **Sjogren's syndrome** characterized by dryness of mouth and lack of tears—pilocarpine is useful.

Cevimeline a derivative of acetylcholine directly stimulates the muscarinic receptors and can be used to increase salivary secretions in Sjogren's syndrome and radiation-induced xerostomia.

Anticholinesterases

Anticholinesterases (antiChEs) or cholinesterase inhibitors are drugs which inhibit the enzyme cholinesterase.

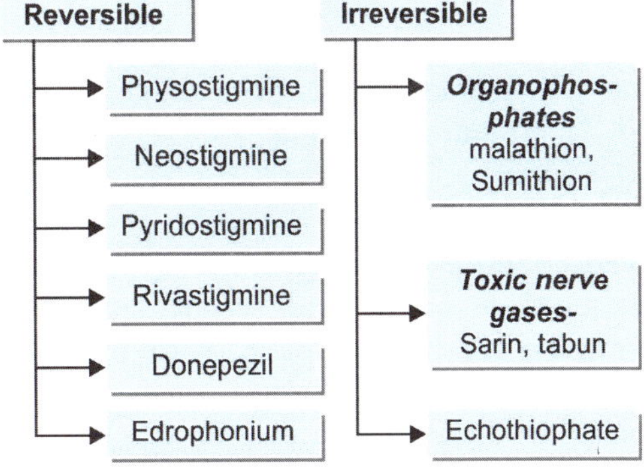

Mechanism of action: As the structures of antiChEs resemble that of ACh, they bind to AChEs and inactivate them.

Acetylcholine
↓ Cholinesterase ←✕— AntiChE
Choline + Acetic acid

Thus ACh is not hydrolyzed and it accumulates. The actions of these drugs are due to this accumulated ACh. Hence the actions are similar to cholinergic agonists. The structure of AChE contains an anionic site and an esteratic site (Fig. 2.5). Reversible anticholinesterases except edrophonium bind to both anionic and esteratic sites. Edrophonium binds only to anionic site and the binding is quickly reversible—hence it is very short acting. Organophosphates (OP) bind only to the esteratic site but the enzyme is phosphorylated (by covalent bonds) and the binding is stable. With some OPs the binding takes many days to be reversed while with others it is not fully reversible at all.

Anticholinesterases are either esters of carbamic acid (carbamates) or phosphoric acid. They may be:

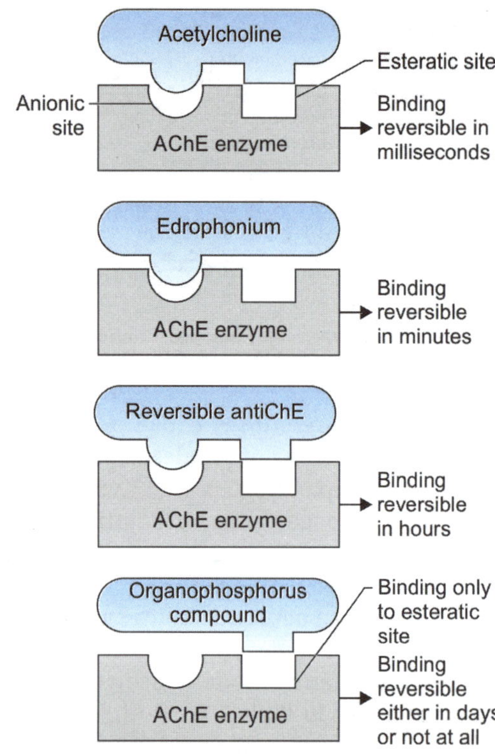

Fig. 2.5: Acetylcholine and reversible anticholinesterases bind to both anionic and esteratic sites of the acetylcholinesterase (AChE) enzyme. Edrophonium binds only the anionic site and is short acting as the binding is rapidly reversible. OP compounds bind only esteratic site but exception is echothiophate which binds both anionic and esteratic sites.

Physostigmine

Physostigmine is an alkaloid obtained from the plant *Physostigma venenosum*. It is a tertiary ammonium compound—hence has better penetration into tissues and also crosses the BBB. It is available as 0.1–1 percent eye drops.

Uses:

- Used in glaucoma as eye drops - it can cause browache, and on long-term use retinal detachment and cataract.
- In atropine poisoning.

Neostigmine

Neostigmine is a synthetic quaternary ammonium compound—poorly absorbed from the gut; it does not cross the BBB. It is used in myasthenia gravis, postoperative paralytic ileus and atony of the urinary bladder.

Pyridostigmine and **ambenonium** are similar to neostigmine but longer acting.

Mnemonic–uses of anticholinesterases

MAAM C CUP
M—Myasthenia gravis
A—Atropine poisoning
A—Alzheimers
M—Miotic
C—Curare poisoning
C—Cobra bite
U—Urinary retension
P—Post operative paralytic ileus

Edrophonium

Edrophonium is rapid and short-acting. It is used in myasthenia gravis, snake bite and in curare poisoning.

Rivastigmine

Rivastigmine is a longer acting carbamate that somewhat selectively binds to the AChE in the brain. Being highly lipid soluble, rivastigmine is rapidly absorbed and reaches the brain and augments cholinergic transmission in the brain. It is used in the treatment of mild to moderate Alzheimer's disease. Dose: 1.5–6 mg BD.

Donepezil

Donepezil is another reversible anticholinesterase with longer duration of action—given once daily. It was shown to produce improvement in the symptoms in Alzheimer's disease. Dose: 5–10 mg OD.

Uses of Reversible Anticholinesterases

1. **As a miotic:** Physostigmine causes miosis, spasm of accommodation and a ↓ IOP. It is used:
   a. In glaucoma—can be used with pilocarpine for better effect.
   b. Alternately with a mydriatic to break the adhesions between the iris and the lens.
   c. To reverse the effects of mydriatics.
2. **Myasthenia gravis:** Anticholinesterases improve muscle strength in myasthenia gravis and are the drugs of choice (*See* page 66).
3. **Poisoning due to anticholinergic drugs:** Physostigmine is used in atropine poisoning and in toxicity due to other drugs with anticholinergic activity like phenothiazines, tricyclic antidepressants and antihistamines. Because physostigmine crosses the BBB, it reverses all the symptoms of atropine poisoning including CNS effects.
4. **Curare poisoning:** Skeletal muscle paralysis caused by curare can be antagonized by AntiChEs. Edrophonium is preferred for its fast action. But, neostigmine has a better capacity to antagonize the effects of curare because of which it is preferred in severe poisoning.
5. **Postoperative paralytic ileus and urinary retention:** Neostigmine may be useful.
6. **Cobra bite:** Cobra venom, a neurotoxin causes skeletal muscle paralysis. Specific treatment is antivenom. Intravenous edrophonium prevents respiratory paralysis.
7. **Alzheimer's disease:** To overcome the deficient cholinergic neurotransmission, rivastigmine and donepezil are tried.

Irreversible Anticholinesterases

Organophosphorus compounds are powerful inhibitors of AChE enzyme; binding with the enzyme is permanent—by covalent bonds. Actions are similar to ACh as ACh accumulates in the tissues. Organophosphates are highly lipid soluble and hence are absorbed from all routes including intact skin. Hence even while spraying insecticides, poisoning can happen.

Uses

Glaucoma—echothiophate eye drops are sometimes used in glaucoma.

Organophosphorus Poisoning

As organophosphates are used as agricultural and domestic insecticides, poisoning from them is quite common. Poisoning may be occupational—as while spraying insecticides, accidental or suicidal. Symptoms include muscarinic, nicotinic and central effects; vomiting, abdominal cramps, diarrhea, miosis, sweating, increased salivary, tracheobronchial and gastric secretions and bronchospasm; hypotension, muscular twitchings, weakness, convulsions and coma. Death is due to respiratory paralysis.

Treatment (Flowchart 2.4)

1. If poisoning is through skin—remove clothing and wash the skin with soap and water; if consumed by oral route—gastric lavage is given.

Flowchart 2.4: Treatment of organophosphorus poisoning.

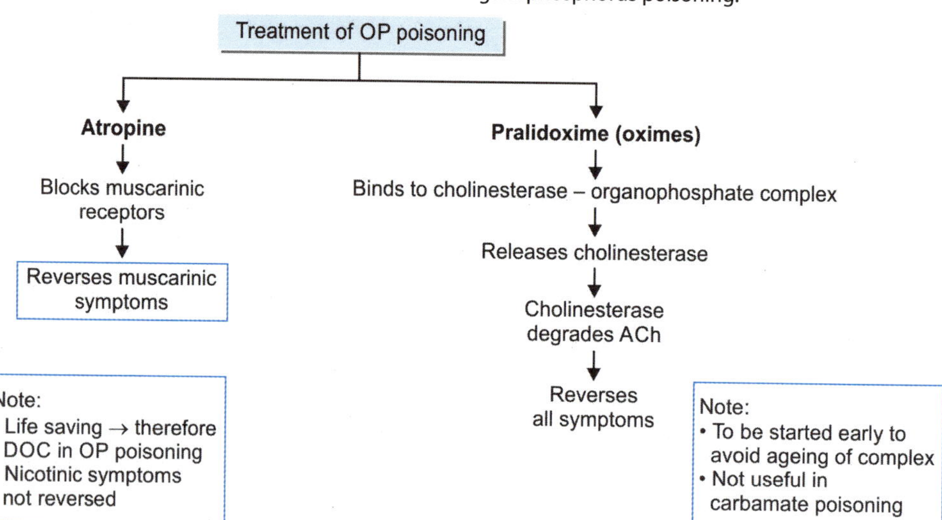

2. Maintain BP and patent airway.
3. Drug of choice is atropine (2 mg IV every 10 minutes till pupil dilates) because it blocks the muscarinic receptors and thereby antagonises the muscarinic effects of organophosphorus compounds.
4. Cholinesterase reactivators—**pralidoxime, obidoxime, diacetyl monoxime.** These compounds combine with cholinesterase organophosphate complex, release the binding and set free AChE enzyme. They should be given within minutes after poisoning, preferably immediately because the complex undergoes '*ageing*' and then the enzyme cannot be released.

Chronic OP Toxicity

Some OP compounds can produce neurotoxicity (polyneuropathy) several days after exposure to the compound. This toxicity came to light when thousands of people developed paralysis in America after consuming 'Jamaica ginger' which contained small amounts of an OP compound (triorthocresylphosphate). The symptoms include weakness, fatigue, ataxia, sensory disturbances, muscle twitching and in severe cases flaccid paralysis—which may last for several years.

ANTICHOLINERGIC DRUGS

Anticholinergic drugs are agents which block the effects of ACh on cholinergic receptors but conventionally antimuscarinic drugs, i.e., drugs which block only muscarinic receptors are referred to as anticholinergic drugs. They are also called cholinergic blocking or parasympatholytic drugs. Drugs that block the nicotinic receptors are ganglion blockers and neuromuscular blockers.

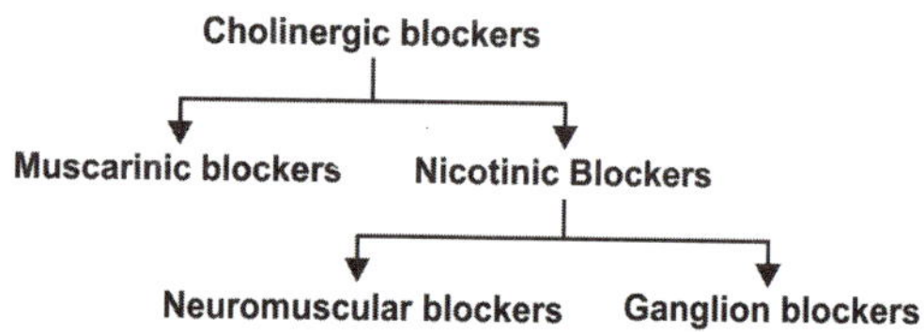

Anticholinergic drugs include atropine and related drugs—atropine is the prototype.

Atropine is obtained from the plant *Atropa belladonna*. Atropine and scopolamine (hyoscine) are the belladonna alkaloids. They compete with acetylcholine for muscarinic receptors and block these receptors—they are muscarinic antagonists.

Classification

1. **Natural alkaloids**
   Atropine, hyoscine (scopolamine)
2. **Semisynthetic derivatives**
   Homatropine, ipratropium bromide, tiotroprium bromide
3. **Synthetic substitutes**
   - **Mydriatics**
     Eucatropine, cyclopentolate, tropicamide
   - **Antispasmodic-antisecretory agents**
     Propantheline, methantheline, dicyclomine, oxyphenonium, glycopyrrolate, telenzepine, tolterodine, propiverine
   - **Antiparkinsonian agents**
     Benzhexol (trihexyphenidyl), benztropine
   - **Vesicoselective (used in urinary disorders)**
     Oxybutynin, tolterodine.

Mechanism of action: Atropine and scopolamine bind to muscarinic receptors and block the effects of acetylcholine (and other cholinergic agonists) on these receptors. These are competitive antagonists and the antagonism is reversible by increasing the concentration of the agonist. Atropine and scopolamine are non-selective antagonists and block all the subtypes (M_1 to M_5) of muscarinic receptors.

Actions

The actions of atropine and scopolamine are similar except that atropine is a CNS stimulant while scopolamine is a CNS depressant and causes sedation.

1. **Cardiovascular system:** Atropine increases heart rate. In large doses, vasodilation and hypotension occurs.
2. **Secretions:** Atropine reduces all secretions except milk. Lacrimal, salivary, nasopharyngeal, tracheobronchial and gastric secretions are decreased. Sweating is also reduced.
3. **Smooth muscle:**
   Gastrointestinal tract (GIT)—↓ tone and motility and relieves spasm → may result in constipation.
   Biliary tract—smooth muscles are relaxed; biliary spasm is relieved.
   Bronchi—atropine causes bronchodilatation.
   Urinary bladder—relaxes urinary bladder and may cause urinary retention.
4. **Eye:** On local instillation, atropine produces mydriasis by blocking the muscarinic receptors in the sphincter pupillae. The ciliary muscle is paralyzed resulting in cycloplegia or paralysis of accommodation. Because of mydriasis, the iris may block the drainage of aqueous humor—IOP increases and may precipitate glaucoma in some patients.
5. **CNS:** In higher doses atropine stimulates the CNS resulting in restlessness, disorientation, hallucinations and delirium. In contrast, scopolamine produces sedation and drowsiness.

Pharmacokinetics: Atropine and hyoscine are well-absorbed, cross the BBB and are metabolized in the liver.

Adverse effects are common but not serious and include blurring of vision, dry mouth, dysphagia, dry skin, fever, constipation and urinary retention. Skin rashes may appear. High doses cause palpitation, flushing, restlessness, delirium, hallucinations, psychosis, convulsions and coma. Poisoning is treated with IV physostigmine.

Uses of Atropine/Belladonna Alkaloids

1. **Antispasmodic:**
   - Atropine, dicyclomine, and propiverine relieve spasm of the gut. In diarrhea and dysentry, they relieve abdominal pain.
   - In renal and biliary colic—atropine is used with morphine because atropine

partly overcomes spasm of the sphincter of Oddi.

2. **Mydriatric and cycloplegic:**
   - **Diagnostic** for testing error of refraction and fundoscopic examination of the eye.
   - **Therapeutic:**
     - To provide rest to the iris in iritis, iridocyclitis and keratitis.
     - Mydriatics are used alternately with miotics to break the adhesions between the iris and the lens.
3. **Preanesthetic medication:** When administered 30 minutes before anesthesia, atropine reduces salivary and respiratory secretions. This will prevent the development of laryngospasm. It also prevents bradycardia during surgery. Its bronchodilator action is of additional value. ***Glycopyrrolate*** an atropine substitute, is most commonly used for this purpose (Flowchart 2.5). Glycopyrrolate reduces salivary secretion and this will prevent the development of laryngospasm and aspiration pneumonia.

Flowchart 2.5: Glycopyrrolate in preanesthetic medication

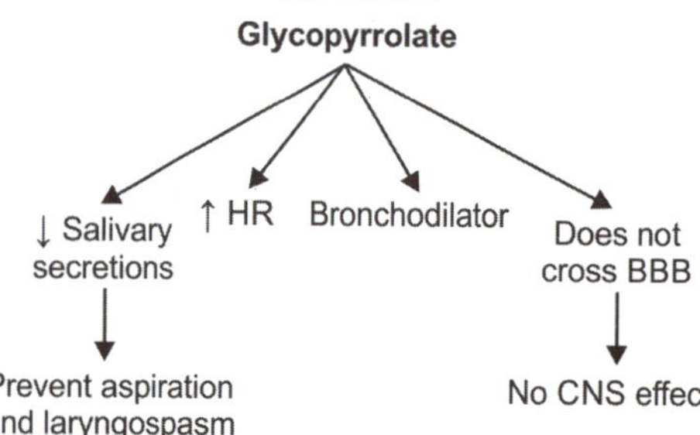

4. **Organophosphorus poisoning (OP):** Atropine is life saving in OP poisoning and is also useful in **mushroom poisoning**.
5. **Heart block:** Atropine produces tachycardia and can be used to overcome bradycardia and partial heart block due to its vagolytic properties.
6. **Bronchial asthma, 7. Peptic ulcer and 8. Parkinsonism:** Atropine derivatives are preferred over atropine.

Mnemonic for Uses of Atropine

HM Maam Beat A PLUMP COP
H—Heart block
M—Motion sickness
M—Mydriatic
B—Bronchial asthma
A—Antispasmodic
P—Peptic ulcer
L—Labor (hyoscine for sedation)
U—Urinary disorder
M—Mushroom poisoning
P—Parkinsonism
C—Curare poisoning (with neostigmine)
O—OP poisoning
P—Preanaesthetic medication

9. **Motion sickness:** Hyoscine given 30 minutes before the journey prevents travelling sickness. Transdermal hyoscine patches are available to be applied behind the ear for a prolonged action.
10. **Urinary disorders:** As muscarinic receptors are present in the urinary tract, atropine derivatives are used in urinary disorders like overactive bladder and urinary incontinence. They reduce urgency, frequency, relieve bladder spasm, improve bladder capacity and reduce involuntary voiding in urinary disorders.

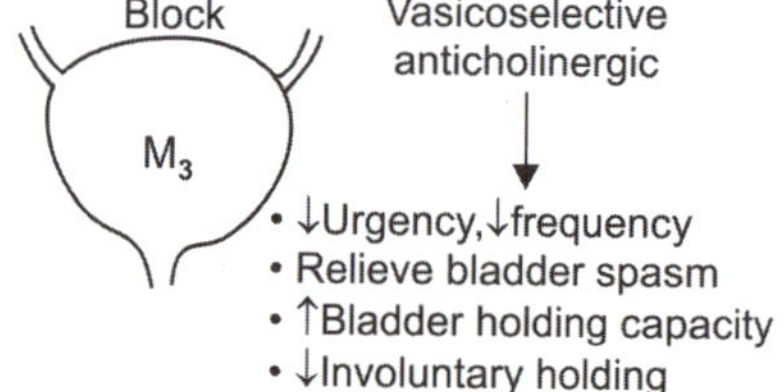

11. **During labor:** Hyoscine can also be used during *labor* to produce sedation and amnesia. It can be used for lie detection because of these properties.
12. **Truth serum:** Hyosine is used in truth serum to obtain information from criminals and suspects and also as a lie detector.

Drug interactions: When anticholinergics are given with other drugs that also have anticholinergic property like antihistaminics, phenothiazines, tricyclic antidepressants—side effects get added up.

Atropine Substitutes/Derivatives

Belladonna alkaloids lack selectivity and exert a wide range of effects—producing many side effects. Hence, several synthetic and semisynthetic derivatives with selective action were introduced (Table 2.2).

ADRENERGIC SYSTEM

The prime function of the adrenergic or sympathetic nervous system is to help the human beings to adjust to stress and prepare the body for fight or flight reactions. When exposed to stress, the heart rate and stroke volume increase with the resultant increase in cardiac output (CO). The blood is shifted from the skin, gut, kidney and glands to the heart, skeletal muscles, brain and lungs, as these organs need more blood during stress. Pupils and bronchi are dilated and sweating is increased. Blood glucose increases by glycogenolysis.

Neurotransmitters of the sympathetic system are noradrenaline (NA, norepinephrine) and dopamine (DA). Adrenaline (epinephrine) is the major hormone secreted by the adrenal medulla.

Synthesis of catecholamines: The 3 catecholamines—NA, adrenaline and DA are synthesized from the amino acid tyrosine (Fig. 2.6).

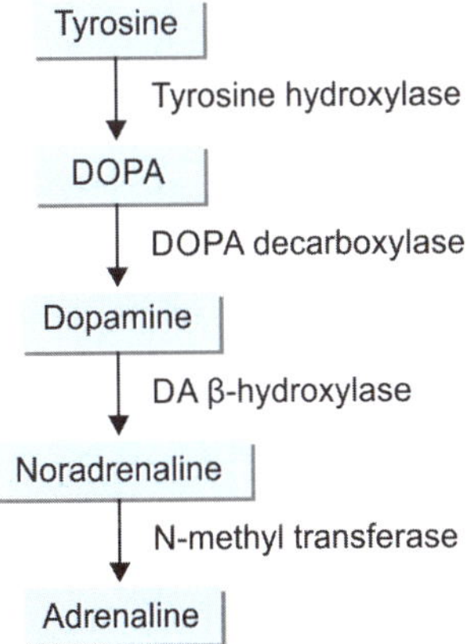

Fig. 2.6: Biosynthesis of catecholamines.

Table 2.2: Atropine substitutes.

• Derivatives used on the eye	Homatropine, eucatropine, cyclopentolate, tropicamide
• Antispasmodics	Dicyclomine, propantheline, methantheline, oxyphenonium, glycopyrrolate
• Derivatives used in peptic ulcer	Pirenzepine, telenzepine
• Derivatives used in bronchial asthma	Ipratropium Tiotropium
• Antiparkinsonian drugs	Benzhexol (trihexyphenidyl), benztropine
• Preanesthetic medication	Glycopyrrolate
• Derivatives used in urinary disorders	Tolterodine, roterodine Trospium, oxyphenonium Solifenacin, flavoxate

The sympathetic postganglionic nerve fibers that synthesize, store and release NA are called **adrenergic.** Noradrenaline is stored in small vesicles in the adrenergic nerve terminals. In response to nerve impulse, NA is released into the synaptic cleft by a process of **exocytosis**. This NA binds to adrenergic receptors located on the postsynaptic membrane to produce the response (Fig. 2.7). A small portion of NA is metabolized by the enzyme catechol-o-methyltransferase (COMT). But a large portion (nearly 80%) is taken back into the nerve terminals by an active transport process termed **uptake 1**, which is responsible for termination of action of NA. Of this, a fraction is metabolized by monoamine oxidase (MAO) and the remaining NA is then transferred to the storage vesicles. Some part of NA released into the synaptic cleft penetrates into the effector cells and is known as **uptake 2**.

Adrenergic receptors Alquist classified adrenergic receptors into 2 types—α and β. With the availability of newer, synthetic, selective drugs, these are further classified into subdivisions. We now know α_1 α_2, β_1, β_2 and β_3 adrenergic receptors.

The stimulation of α receptors mainly produces excitatory effects (exception-GIT);

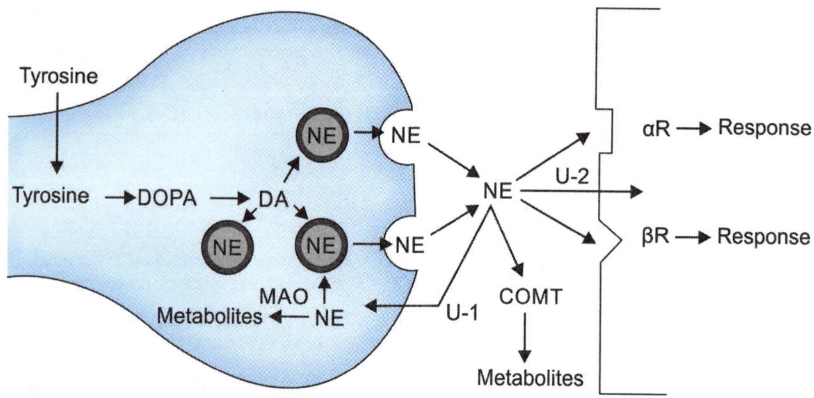

Fig. 2.7: Synthesis, storage, release and metabolism of noradrenaline.

Table 2.3: Characteristics of adrenergic receptors.

Receptor type	*Selective agonist*	*Selective antagonist*	*Location*	*Response*
α_1	Phenylephrine	Prazosin	Vascular smooth muscle Gut Genitourinary smooth muscle	Contraction Relaxation Contraction
α_2	Clonidine	Yohimbine	Pancreatic β cells Platelets Nerve terminals	↓ Insulin release Aggregation ↓ NE release
β_1	Dobutamine	Metoprolol Atenolol	Heart	↑ Force of contraction, heart-rate, AV conduction velocity
β_2	Salbutamol	Butoxamine	Smooth muscle—vascular, bronchial, gut and genitourinary Liver	Relaxation Glycogenolysis
β_3	Mirabegron	Cyanopindolol	Adipose tissue	Lipolysis

β stimulation causes mainly inhibitory effects (exception- heart). The characteristics of these receptors are given in Table 2.3. α_2 receptors are located on the presynaptic membrane. When the concentration of NA reaches adequate levels in the synapse, these presynaptic α_2 receptors are stimulated and inhibit the further release of NA. Thus α_2 receptors exert a negative feedback on NA release. α_2 receptors are also present postsynaptically in pancreatic islets, platelets and brain.

ADRENERGIC DRUGS (SYMPATHOMIMETICS)

Sympathomimetics are drugs whose actions mimic that of sympathetic stimulation (Flowchart 2.6). They may be classified in various ways.

Classification

- **Therapeutic or clinical classification:**
  1. **Vasopressors:**
     - Noradrenaline
     - Dopamine
     - Methoxamine
     - Metaraminol
  2. **Cardiac stimulants:**
     - Adrenaline
     - Dopamine
     - Dobutamine
     - Isoprenaline
     - Ephedrine
  3. **CNS stimulants:**
     - Amphetamine
     - Ephedrine
  4. **Bronchodilators:**
     - Adrenaline

Flowchart 2.6: Drugs acting on sympathetic nervous system.

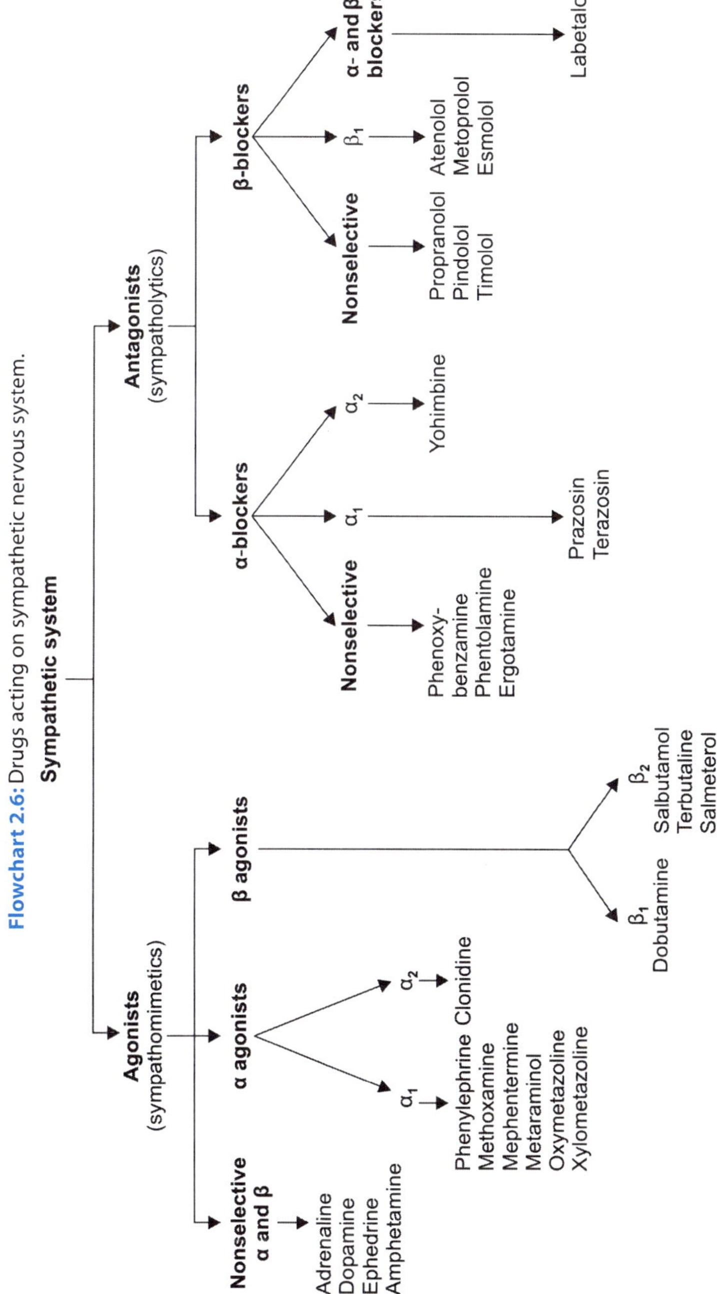

- Isoprenaline
- Salbutamol
- Terbutaline
- Salmeterol

5. **Nasal decongestants:**
   - Ephedrine
   - Pseudoephedrine
   - Phenylephrine
   - Oxymetazoline
   - Xylometazoline
6. **Appetite suppressants (anorectics):**
   - Dexfenfluramine
7. **Uterine relaxants:**
   - Salbutamol
   - Terbutaline
   - Isoxsuprine, ritodrine.

- **Depending on the mode of action:**
  1. **Directly acting sympathomimetics:**
     - By stimulating adrenergic receptors —NA, isoprenaline, dopamine, adrenaline, phenylephrine
  2. **Indirectly acting sympathomimetics:**
     - By releasing NA from nerve terminals—amphetamine, tyramine
  3. **Mixed action amines:**
     - Both direct and indirect actions—ephedrine, methoxamine
- **Chemical classification—based on presence/absence of catechol nucleus:**
  1. **Catecholamines:**
     - Noradrenaline (NA)
     - Adrenaline
     - Dopamine (DA)
     - Isoprenaline (synthetic)
  2. **Non-catecholamines:**
     - Ephedrine
     - Amphetamine

Actions

1. Cardiovascular System

Heart: Adrenaline is a powerful cardiac stimulant. Acting through β_1 receptors, it increases the heart rate, force of contraction, cardiac output and conduction velocity. The work done and the resultant O_2 consumption of the heart is increased.

Blood vessels and BP: Blood vessels of skin and mucous membrane are constricted (α_1) and that of skeletal muscles are dilated (β_2) by adrenaline.

Moderate doses given IV produce a rapid increase in BP followed by a fall—a biphasic response. The rise in BP is due to α_1 mediated vasoconstriction. Action on β receptors is more persistent and as the action on alpha receptors wears off, the action on β receptors gets unmasked resulting in ↓ BP. Sir Henry Dale demonstrated that when α receptors are blocked (with alpha blockers—ergot alkaloids), adrenaline produces only a fall in BP and this is named after him as **Dale's vasomotor reversal** (or Dale's phenomenon).

Noradrenaline is mainly an alpha agonist and brings about a rise in BP.

Other vascular beds: Adrenaline causes renal vasoconstriction resulting in a fall in renal blood flow; it also causes pulmonary and mesenteric vasoconstriction.

Cerebral and coronary blood flow is increased.

2. Smooth Muscles

Bronchi: Adrenaline is a powerful bronchodilator and a weak respiratory stimulant. Pulmonary vasoconstriction relieves bronchial congestion. All these result in an increase in vital capacity.

Bronchodilation + Pulmonary vasoconstriction

↓ Relieve bronchial congestion

↑↑Vital capacity

Uterus: Nonpregnant uterus—contracts

Last month of pregnancy—relaxes.

Gut: Smooth muscle is relaxed—but weak and transient action.

Splenic capsule: Contracts resulting in the release of RBCs into the circulation.

Pilomotor muscles of the hair follicle: Contraction.

Bladder: Detrusor is relaxed while trigonal sphincter is contracted thereby increasing the urine holding capacity of the bladder.

3. Eye

Adrenaline causes mydriasis due to contraction of the radial muscles of the iris (α_1); it also reduces intraocular pressure.

4. Metabolic Effects

Adrenaline increases the blood sugar level by enhancing hepatic glycogenolysis. It also inhibits insulin release. It acts on β_3 receptors in the adipocytes to increase the breakdown of triglycerides.

5. Skeletal Muscles

Catecholamines facilitate neuromuscular transmission by action on both α and β receptors—they enhance the amount of ACh released.

Pharmacokinetics: Because catecholamines are rapidly inactivated in the gut and the liver, they are not given orally. Adrenaline and NA are metabolized by COMT and MAO (Flowchart 2.7).

Flowchart 2.7: Metabolism of catecholamines.

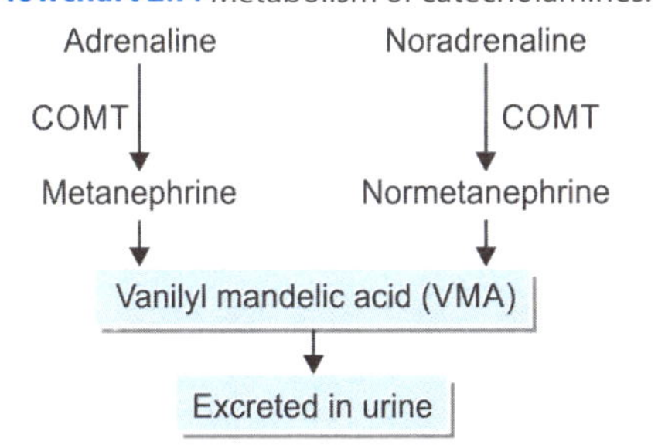

Adverse reactions: Anxiety, palpitation, weakness, tremors, pallor, dizziness, restlessness and throbbing headache may follow adrenaline/NA administration. In patients with ischemic heart disease, both adrenaline and NA can precipitate anginal pain. Rapid IV injection can cause sudden sharp rise in BP which may precipitate arrthythmias, subarachnoid hemorrhage or hemiplegia.

Preparations: Adrenaline 1:1000, 1:10,000 and 1:1,00,000 solutions are available for injection. Adrenaline is given subcutaneous/ intramuscular (SC/IM); intracardiac in emergencies. Adrenaline aerosol for inhalation and 2 percent ophthalmic solution are also available.

Uses of Adrenaline

1. **Anaphylactic shock:** Adrenaline is the drug of choice (0.3–0.5 mL of 1:1000 solution). It promptly reverses hypotension, laryngeal edema and bronchospasm and is life saving in anaphylactic shock. IM route is preferred as absorption by SC route is not reliable in shock (Fig. 2.8).
2. **Cardiac arrest:** Sudden cardiac arrest due to drowning, electrocution, etc. are treated with intracardiac adrenaline.
3. **Control of hemorrhage:** Adrenaline in 1: 10,000 to 1 : 20,000 concentration is used as a topical hemostatic to control bleeding from skin and mucous membrane. Bleeding stops due to vasoconstriction. Adrenaline packs are used.
4. **With local anesthetics (LA):** Injected with LA, adrenaline produces vasoconstriction and reduces the rate of absorption of LA. By this it prolongs the action and reduces

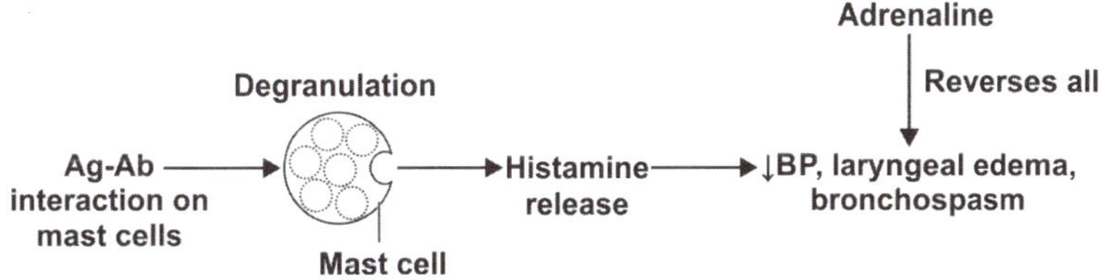

Fig. 2.8: Adrenaline in anaphylactic shock.

systemic toxicity of LA. 1: 10,000 to 1: 2,00,000 adrenaline is used.

5. **Acute bronchial asthma:** SC/inhalation of adrenaline produces bronchodilation.
6. **Glaucoma:** Adrenaline reduces IOP and can be used in glaucoma. It has the disadvantages of being:
   - Poorly absorbed
   - Short acting—as it is quickly metabolized in the eye.

Dipivefrin is a prodrug which gets converted to adrenaline in the eye by the action of corneal esterases. Dipivefrin has good penetrability due to high lipid solubility and is used in glaucoma.

Contraindications: Adrenaline is contra-indicated in patients with angina pectoris, hypertension and in patients on β-blockers.

Other Catecholamines

Noradrenaline: Can be used in shock to increase BP—but it is very rarely used.

Isoprenaline (isoproterenol, isopropyl-arterenol) is a synthetic catecholamine with predominantly β receptor stimulant action and negligible α actions. It has cardiac stimulant and smooth muscle relaxant properties. Due to vasodilation BP falls; it is a potent bronchodilator. Adverse effects include palpitation, angina, headache and flushing.

Isoprenaline is used in heart block and shock for its cardiac stimulant actions. It can be used in bronchial asthma.

Dopamine is the precursor of NA (Flowchart 2.8). It acts on the dopaminergic and adrenergic receptors. It is a central neurotransmitter. Low doses stimulate vascular D_1 receptors in renal, mesenteric and coronary beds causing vasodilatation in these vessels. Higher doses cause cardiac stimulation through β_1 receptors and in high doses α_1 receptors are activated resulting in vasoconstriction and ↑ BP.

Adverse effects: Nausea, vomiting, palpitation, angina, sudden ↑ in BP may occur.

Uses: DA is used in the treatment of shock—cardiogenic, hypovolemic and septic shock. It increases the renal blood flow and also increases the force of contraction of the heart. It is specially useful when there is renal dysfunction and low cardiac output.

Dobutamine a derivative of dopamine, is a relatively selective β_1 agonist. Though it also activates α receptors, in therapeutic doses the only dominant action is an increase in the force of contraction of the heart without a significant increase in the heart rate. Thus, it is used in patients with congestive cardiac failure (CCF) or acute myocardial infarction or following cardiac surgery when there may be heart failure.

Fenoldopam is a selective D_1 agonist which dilates coronary, renal and mesenteric arteries. It is used as an IV infusion in severe hypertension to rapidly reduce the BP.

Non-Catecholamines

Non-catecholamines are devoid of catechol nucleus, they act both by direct stimulation

Flowchart 2.8: Actions of dopamine.

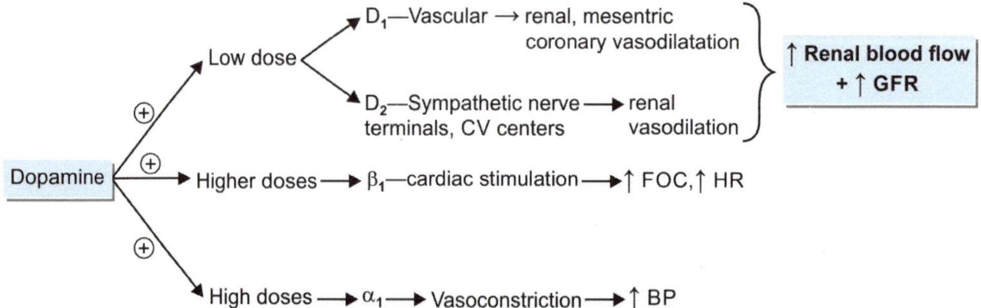

of adrenergic receptors and indirectly by releasing NA. In contrast to catecholamines, they are effective orally, relatively resistant to MAO and therefore are longer-acting; they cross the blood-brain barrier and have CNS effects.

Ephedrine is an alkaloid obtained from the plants of the genus *Ephedra*. It acts by direct stimulation of α and β receptors and indirectly through release of NA. Repeated administration at short intervals result in tachyphylaxis. Ephedrine ↑ BP by peripheral vasoconstriction and by increasing the cardiac output. Like adrenaline it relaxes smooth muscles; it is a CNS stimulant and produces insomnia, restlessness, anxiety, tremors and increased mental activity.

Adverse effects include sleeplessness, tremors and difficulty in micturition.

Uses

Ephedrine is now not preferred as it is nonselective in its actions.

1. **Hypotension:** For prevention and treatment of hypotension during spinal anesthesia—IM ephedrine is used.
2. **Bronchial asthma:** Ephedrine is useful in mild, chronic bronchial asthma but not preferred.
3. **Nasal decongestion:** Pseudoephedrine, an isomer of ephedrine is used orally for decongestion.

Amphetamine is a synthetic compound with actions similar to ephedrine, tachyphylaxis can occur on repeated use. Amphetamine is a potent CNS stimulant; it produces increased mental and physical activity, alertness, increased concentration and attention span, elation, euphoria and increased capacity to work. It also increases initiative and self confidence, postpones fatigue and improves physical performance (temporarily) as seen in athletes. All these properties make amphetamine a drug of dependence and abuse. Higher doses produce confusion, delirium and hallucinations. The effects may be reversed with overdosage.

Respiration: Amphetamine stimulates respiration—analeptic.

Decreased appetite: Acting on the feeding center in the hypothalamus, amphetamine reduces hunger and suppresses appetite.

Amphetamine also has weak anticonvulsant property.

Adverse effects include restlessness, tremors, insomnia, palpitation, anxiety, confusion and hallucinations. Prolonged use may precipitate psychosis.

High doses cause angina, delirium, arrhythmias, hypertension, acute psychosis, coma and death due to convulsions.

Dependence: Amphetamines cause psychologic dependence and **are drug of abuse**. Withdrawal symptoms include weakness, depression, drowsiness, tremors and craving for the drug.

Tolerance develops to its central effects on prolonged use.

Uses

Due to the risk of dependence, amphetamine is not preferred for any of the clinical indications.

1. **Attention deficit hyperactivity disorder (ADHD)** in children is characterized by decreased ability to concentrate and hold attention, aggressive behavior and hyperactivity; Amphetamine increases attention span in such children and improves performance in school. However, due to anorectic effects (which may result in growth retardation) and risk of addiction amphetamine is not used for this.
2. **Narcolepsy:** Amphetamine is effective but **modafinil** a newer psychostimulant is now preferred.

Vasopressors

These are α_1 agonists and include metaraminol, mephentermine, phenylephrine and methoxamine. They increase the BP by increasing total peripheral resistance (TPR) or cardiac output (CO) or both. They are given parenterally with constant monitoring of BP. Tachyphylaxis may develop.

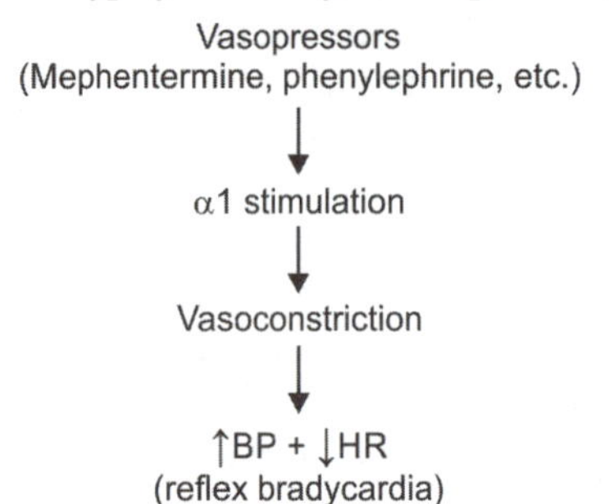

Uses: Vasopressors are used to raise the BP in hypotension as seen in cardiogenic or neurogenic shock and during spinal anesthesia.

Metaraminol is an alpha stimulant and also acts indirectly by NA release. CO is increased. It is also a nasal decongestant.

Mephenteramine acts on both α and β receptors to ↑ TPR, ↑ CO and thereby raises BP. It is orally effective. Pressor effect is accompanied by bradycardia.

Phenylephrine is a selective α_1 stimulant; it is also a nasal decongestant. Reflex bradycardia is prominent. It produces mydriasis without cycloplegia.

Methoxamine has actions similar to phenylephrine.

Nasal Decongestants

Nasal decongestants are α agonists which relieve congestion due to vasoconstriction. They may be used:

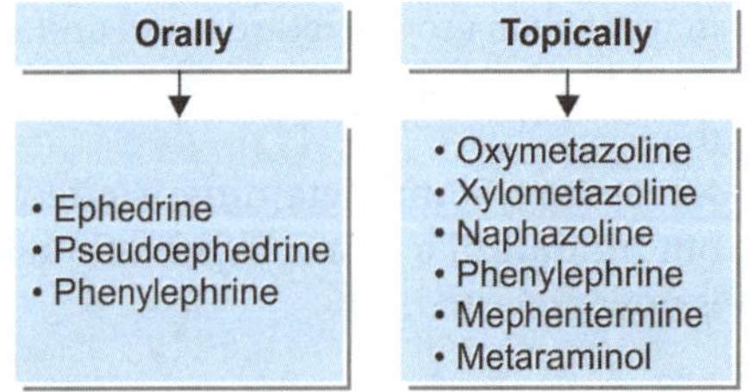

Disadvantages

- Irritation and after congestion
- On prolonged use nasal decongestants may cause atrophy of the mucosa due to intense vasoconstriction.

Uses: Rhinitis in upper respiratory infection, allergic and vasomotor rhinitis, sinusitis and blocked eustachian tubes—nasal decongestants afford symptomatic relief.

Alpha 2 Agonists

Clonidine, apraclonidine and brimonidine are selective alpha 2 agonists. Clonidine is used in hypertension. Apraclonidine and brimonidine are used in glaucoma as they lower intraocular pressure.

Selective β_2 Stimulants

Selective β_2 stimulants include **orciprenaline, salbutamol, terbutaline and salmeterol.** These are smooth muscle relaxants which produce bronchodilatation, vasodilation and uterine relaxation without significant cardiac stimulation. They can be given by inhalation and are used in:

- Bronchial asthma
- As uterine relaxants to delay premature labor.

Side effects include muscle tremors, palpitation and arrhythmias.

Isoxuprine is a selective β rcccptor stimulant used as uterine relaxant in premature labor, threatened abortion and dysmenorrhea.

Anorectic Agents (Anorexiants)

Though amphetamine and amphetamine-like drugs suppress appetite, they are not recommended for the treatment of obesity due to the central stimulant effects.

ADRENERGIC ANTAGONISTS

Adrenergic blockers bind to the adrenergic receptors and prevent the action of adrenergic drugs. They may block alpha or beta receptors or both.

Alpha Adrenergic Blocking Agents

Alpha receptor antagonists block the adrenergic responses mediated through alpha adrenergic receptors. Some of them have selectivity for α_1 or α_2 receptors.

Actions

The important effects of α receptor stimulation are α_1 mediated vasoconstriction and α_2-(presynaptic) receptor mediated inhibition of NA release. The result of blockade of these alpha receptors by α-antagonists is hypotension with tachycardia (Flowchart 2.9). This effect is due to:

- α_1-blockade—inhibits vasoconstriction —leading to vasodilation and thereby ↓ BP. This fall in BP is opposed by the baroreceptor reflexes which increase heart rate and cardiac output.
- α_2-blockade—increases the release of NA which stimulates β receptors (α are already blocked).
- β_1 stimulation in heart results in tachycardia and ↑ cardiac output.

Selective α_1-blockade—results in hypotension without much tachycardia.

Selective α_2-blockade—↑ NA release resulting in hypertension.

α-blockade also results in miosis and nasal stuffiness. α-blockade in the bladder and prostate leads to decreased resistance to the flow of urine.

Adverse effects of α-blockers—postural hypotension, palpitation, nasal stuffiness, miosis and impaired ejaculation which may result in impotence.

Classification (Flowchart 2.10)

Phenoxybenzamine binds covalently to alpha receptors causing irreversible blockade. Given IV, blood pressure gradually falls and is associated with tachycardia. The action lasts for 3–4 days.

Flowchart 2.9: Effects of alpha blockade.

α-blockers ⟶ Vaso dilation (α_1 Blocked) ⟶ ↓BP ↑HR (Reflex tachycardia)

Ergot alkaloids like ergotamine, ergotoxine and their derivatives are competitive α antagonists and the blockade is of short duration.

Phentolamine and tolazoline are imidazoline derivatives. They are competitive α-blockers. In addition they also block 5-HT receptors, stimulate gut motility and ↑ gastric secretion. Hence they can cause vomiting and diarrhea in addition to the effects of α-blockade.

Prazosin

Prazosin is a potent, highly selective, α_1-blocker with 1000 times greater affinity for α_1 receptors. Arterioles are dilated more than veins resulting in hypotension. There is not much tachycardia (as α_2 receptors are spared there is no ↑ in NA release).

It is orally effective and is metabolized in the liver.

Adverse Effects

First dose phenomenon (Flowchart 2.11)—1 hour after the initial dose, marked postural hypotension occurs which may lead to fainting. To avoid this, prazosin should be started with a low dose and taken at bed time.

Flowchart 2.10: Classification of alpha-blockers.

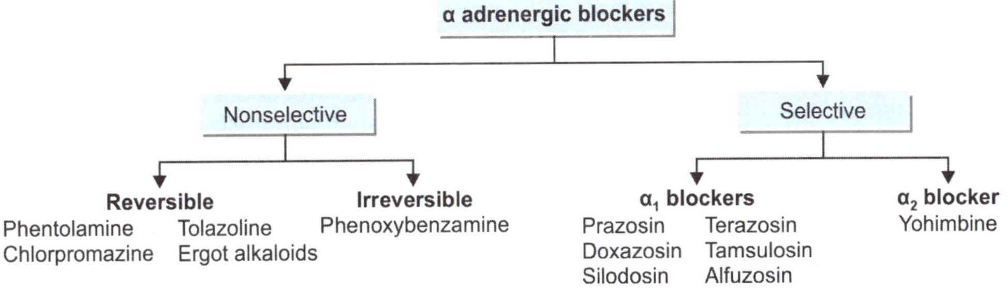

Flowchart 2.11: First dose phenomenon with α-blockers.

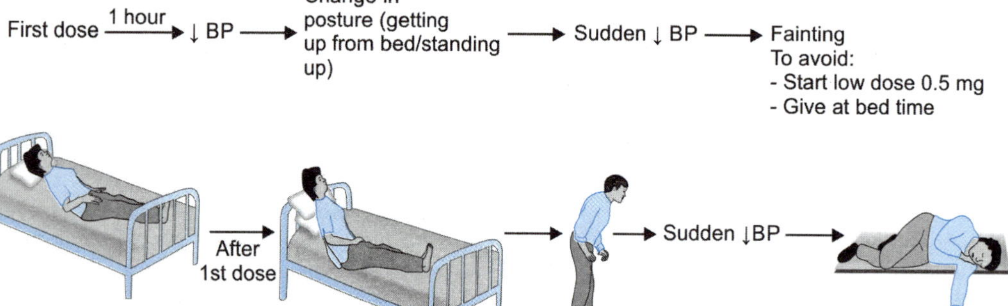

Congeners of prazosin: Include terazosin, doxazosin, alfuzosin, tamsulosin, indoramin and urapidil.

- These congeners are longer acting and can be given once daily
- Highly selective for α_1 receptors
- Postural hypotension is milder than with prazosin
- No significant effect on cardiac function
- ↓LDL and ↑HDL cholesterol
- Tamsulosin has selective activity on α_{1A} receptors in the bladder and prostate while hypotension (mediated by α_{2B}) is mild (Flowchart 2.12). Therefore tamsulosin relieves the symptoms of benign prostatic hypertrophy (BPH) and is used in BPH
- Alfuzosin is also useful in BPH
- Terazosin and doxazosin are used in hypertension
- Urapidil has α_1 and β_1 (weak) blocking properties. It is used in hypertension and BPH.

Yohimbine is a relatively selective α_2-blocker which increases BP and heart rate due to ↑ NA release. It causes congestion of genitals for which it is used to treat psychogenic impotence. It is also claimed to be an aphrodisiac (drug that increases sexual desire) though the effect is only psychological.

Uses of α-blockers

1. **Hypertension:** Selective α_1-blockers like prazosin are used in the treatment of hypertension. Phenoxybenzamine or phentolamine can be used in hypertensive crisis.
2. **Benign prostatic hypertrophy (BPH):** Blockade of α_1 receptors in the bladder, prostate and urethra reduce resistance to urine outflow. Prazosin is useful in patients who cannot be operated upon. Tamsulosin is particularly preferred because of selective action on α_{1A} receptor.

Flowchart 2.12: Tamsulosin in BPH.

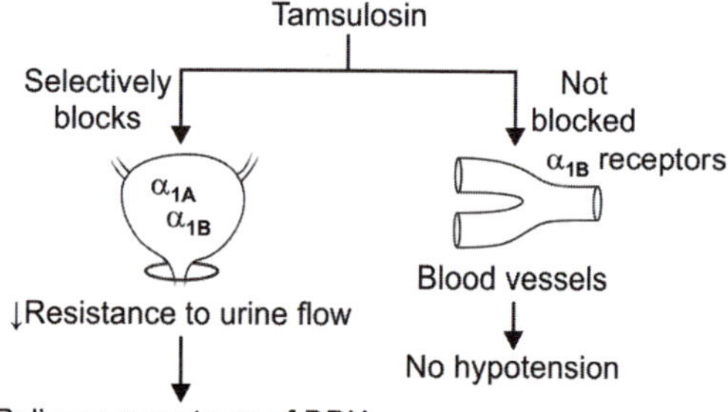

3. **Peripheral vascular diseases** like Raynaud's phenomenon may be benefited by α-blockers which afford symptomatic relief.
4. **Congestive cardiac failure:** Because of its vasodilator action, prazosin is useful in CCF. But angiotensin-converting-enzyme (ACE) inhibitors are preferred.
5. **Pheochromocytoma** is an adrenal medullary tumor which secretes large amounts of catecholamines resulting in hypertension. The tumor has to be

removed surgically. Phenoxybenzamine and phentolamine are used for the preoperative management of the patient and during the operation. Inoperable cases are put on long-term treatment with phenoxybenzamine.

Beta Adrenergic Blocking Agents

β-blockers are drugs that block the actions of catecholamines mediated through the β receptors.

Classification

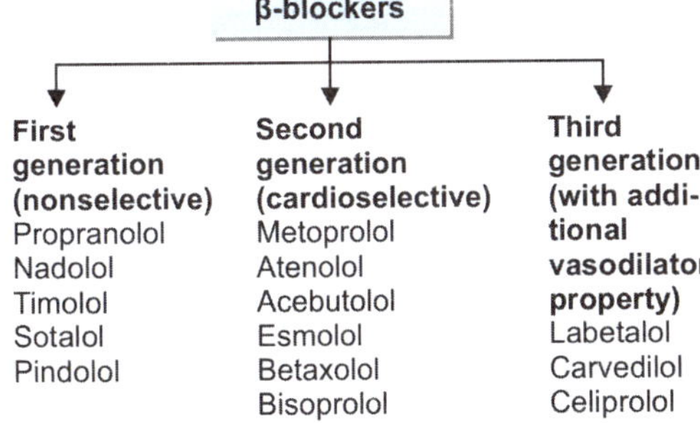

Pharmacological Actions (Flowchart 2.14)

1. **CVS:** β-blockers decrease heart rate, force of contraction and cardiac output. Blood pressure falls. The effect is more pronounced in presence of increased sympathetic tone than in a normal situation. AV conduction is delayed. Myocardial oxygen requirement is reduced due to reduced cardiac work.

High doses produce membrane-stabilizing activity like quinidine, causing direct depression of the heart.

2. **Effects on exercise:** β-blockers prevent the increase in heart rate and force of contraction which are brought about by exercise. β-blockers may also reduce the work capacity. Weakness, fatigue and reduced exercise capacity are common. This could be because of their:

- metabolic effects
- blockade of beta 2 receptors which prevents the increase in blood flow to the skeletal muscles during exercise
- reduced cardiac output (beta 1 blockade)

These effects are less prominent with β_1 selective agents. β-blockers improve exercise tolerance in patients with angina.

Flowchart 2.13: Effects of β-blockers on skeletal muscles/exercise.

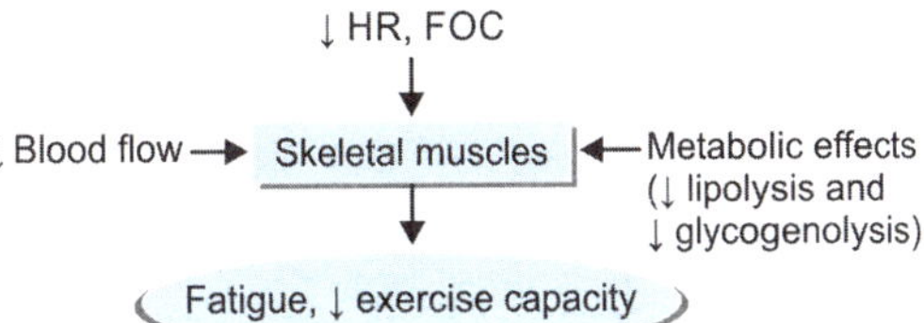

Flowchart 2.14: Actions of β-blockers.

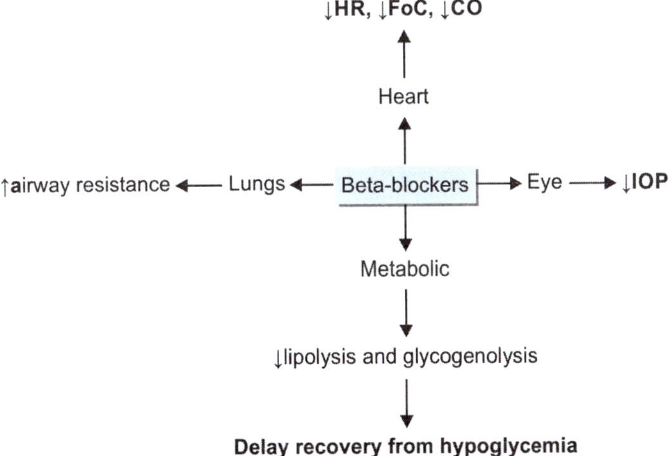

3. **Respiratory tract:** Blockade of β_2 receptors in the bronchial smooth muscle causes increase in airway resistance—may precipitate acute attacks in asthmatics.
4. **Eye:** Many β-blockers reduce intraocular pressure by decreased secretion of aqueous humor.
5. **Metabolic:** β-antagonists block lipolysis and glycogenolysis induced by sympathetic stimulation. Plasma triglycerides may increase and HDL levels decrease in some patients.

Pharmacokinetics

Though well absorbed on oral administration, some β-blockers like propranolol undergo extensive first pass metabolism. Most of them have short t½ and are metabolized in the liver.

Adverse Reactions

1. **Bradycardia** is common: Patients with AV conduction defects may develop arrhythmias and heart block with β-blockers.
2. **Fatigue and weakness:** Reduced blood flow to the muscles during physical activity and reduced cardiac output.
3. **Congestive cardiac failure (CCF):** In patients with impaired cardiac function, sympathetic activity supports the heart. β-blockade eliminates this and may result in CCF.
4. **Cold extremities** may be experienced especially in patients with peripheral vascular disease.
5. **CCF:** When used carefully in selected patients, beta blockers may be beneficial in CCF. They may improve cardiac function, reduce the risk of sudden death and prolong survival.
6. β-blockers can precipitate **acute asthmatic attacks** and are contraindicated in asthmatics.
7. **Central nervous system (CNS):** Insomnia, depression and rarely hallucinations can follow the use of β-blockers.
8. **Metabolic effects:** Weakness and reduced exercise capacity may be seen due to its metabolic effects.
9. Abrupt withdrawal of β-blockers after prolonged use can cause **rebound hypertension** and precipitate anginal attacks. This is due to up-regulation of β receptors. Hence β-blockers should be gradually withdrawn over many weeks.
10. β-blockers can also cause dizziness.
11. **Topical:** Timolol eye drops can cause burning and dryness of the eyes.

Contraindications: Beta-blockers are contraindicated in bradycardia, heart block, asthmatics and chronic obstructive pulmonary disease (COPD).

Some Important Drug Interactions

- Propranolol + insulin—when diabetics on insulin also receive propranolol:
  - β-blockade masks tachycardia which is the first warning signal of hypoglycemia.
  - β-blockade delays the recovery from hypoglycemia by preventing glycogenolysis induced by sympathetic stimulation. This may be avoided by using a β_1-selective blocker.
- Propranolol + verapamil—since both cause myocardiac depression, profound depression may result. Hence the combination should be avoided.

First generation β-blockers like propranolol are non-selective. Propranolol being highly lipid soluble, readily crosses the BBB. Nadolol is long acting. Timolol is used in glaucoma as eye drops.

Second generation β-blockers are **cardioselective β-blockers,** e.g., atenolol, metoprolol, esmolol, e.g., atenolol, metoprolol, esmolol.

These drugs:

- Selectively block β_1 receptors, β_2-blockade is weak
- Bronchospasm is less/negligible
- Inhibition of glycogenolysis is lower—hence safer in diabetics

- Exercise performance impaired to a lesser degree
- Reduced chances of peripheral vascular disease
- Atenolol is long-acting—given once daily
- Esmolol is very short-acting and can be given intravenously in emergencies.

Third generation β-blockers are β-blockers with additional vasodilatory properties. Some of them, viz. celiprolol and nebivolol selectively block cardiac β_1 receptors.

Celiprolol

- β_1-blocker and β_2-agonistic effects
- Safer in asthmatics
- Used in hypertension.

Partial agonists: Some β-blockers like pindolol, oxprenolol have some sympathomimetic activity due to their partial β-agonistic property. As a result, bradycardia and myocardiac depression are less marked. They are therefore preferred in patients with low cardiac reserve or those who are likely to have severe bradycardia.

Uses of β-blockers

1. **Hypertension:** β-blockers are useful in the treatment of mild to moderate hypertension. A β-blocker can be used alone or with other antihypertensives.
2. **Angina pectoris:** β-blockers are useful in the prophylaxis of exertional angina. Both the severity and frequency are reduced.
3. **Cardiac arrhythmias:** β-blockers are useful in the treatment of both ventricular and supraventricular arrhythmias.
4. **Myocardial infarction:** IV β-blockers in acute MI may limit the size of the infarct.

   In patients who have recovered from MI, long-term treatment with β-blockers prolongs survival.
5. **CCF:** When used carefully in selected patients, beta-blockers may be beneficial in CCF. They may improve cardiac function, reduce the risk of sudden death and prolong survival.
6. **Obstructive cardiomyopathy:** β-blockers are found to be beneficial.
7. **Pheochromocytoma:** Propranolol is given with α-blockers before surgery to control hypertension.
8. **Thyrotoxicosis:** Propranolol controls palpitation, tremors and affords symptomatic relief in thyrotoxicosis.
9. **Glaucoma:** Timolol is used topically in open angle glaucoma.
10. **Prophylaxis of migraine:** Propranolol reduces frequency and severity of migraine headache; used for prophylaxis.
11. **Anxiety:** Propranolol prevents the acute panic symptoms seen in public speaking, examination and other such anxiety-provoking situations. Performance in musicians can be improved. Tremors, tachycardia and other symptoms of sympathetic overactivity are alleviated.
12. **Cirrhosis:** β-blockers may help by reducing the portal venous pressure by about 40%.
13. **Alcohol withdrawal:** Beta-blockers help to overcome some of the symptoms of alcohol withdrawal by reducing the central sympathetic over activity.
14. **Esophageal varices:** Beta blockers reduce bleeding in bleeding esophageal varices

Alpha and Beta-adrenergic Blockers

Labetalol: Blocks both α_1 and β (β_1 and β_2) receptors. It is a competitive antagonist. Heart rate, contractility, AV conduction and BP fall. Blood flow to the limbs increases.

Side effects include postural hypotension, GI disturbances and other effects of alpha and β-blockade.

Uses: Labetalol is used in hypertensive emergencies and pheochromocytoma.

Carvedilol and **medroxalol** also block both alpha and beta receptors. They are used in the treatment of hypertension and CCF.

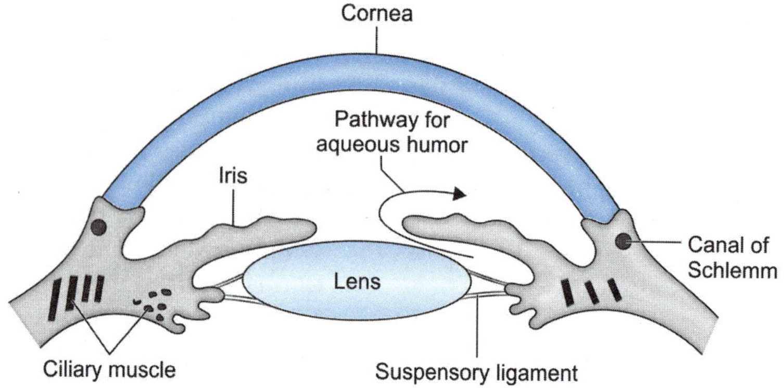

Fig. 2.9: Schematic diagram showing pathway for the drainage of aqueous humor.

Table 2.4: Drugs used in glaucoma.

Drugs	*Routes*	*Mechanisms*
Prostaglandin analogs		
Latanoprost, bimatoprost	Topical	↑ drainage of aqueous humor
Cholinergic drugs		
Pilocarpine, carbachol	Topical	Miosis - ↑ drainage
Physostigmine, echothiophate	Topical	↑ drainage of aqueous humor
Alpha adrenergic agonists		
Adrenaline, Dipivefrin, Apraclonidine, brimonidine	Topical	↑ drainage of aqueous humor
β-blockers		
Timolol, Betaxolol	Topical	↓ aqueous humor secretion
Diuretics		
Acetazolamide, dorzolamide	Oral	↓ aqueous humor secretion
Brinzolamide	Topical	↓ aqueous humor secretion

Drugs used in Glaucoma

Glaucoma is an eye disease characterized by increased intraocular pressure. If untreated, irreversible damage can occur, because optic nerve degenerates due to constant increase in pressure and this leads to permanent blindness. Glaucoma is of two types:

i. Acute congestive/narrow angle glaucoma—In this, iris blocks the drainage of aqueous humor at the canal of Schlemn leading to increased intraocular pressure (Fig. 2.9). It needs immediate treatment.
ii. Chronic simple/open angle glaucoma—onset is slow; needs long-term treatment. Surgery is the preferred option.

Drugs used in glaucoma are summarized in Table 2.4.

3

CHAPTER

Drugs Acting on Musculoskeletal System

CHAPTER HIGHLIGHTS

- Skeletal Muscle Relaxants
- Drugs Used in the Treatment of Local Muscle Spasm
- Drugs Used in Other Musculoskeletal Diseases
- Drugs Used in the Treatment of Immunological and Inflammatory Neuromuscular Diseases
- Agents Affecting Bone Mineral Turnover
- Agents Used in the Prevention and Treatment of Osteoporosis
- Drugs and Exercise

SKELETAL MUSCLE RELAXANTS

Skeletal muscle relaxants (SMR) are drugs that reduce the muscle tone either by acting peripherally at the neuromuscular junction (neuromuscular blockers) or centrally in the cerebrospinal axis or directly on the contractile mechanism. They reduce the spasticity in a variety of neurological conditions and are also useful in surgeries.

Classification

Classification of skeletal muscle relaxants—*see* Flowchart 3.1.

Peripherally Acting Skeletal Muscle Relaxants

Neuromuscular Blockers (NMB)

Competitive Blockers

Curare was used by the South American Indians as arrow poison for hunting wild animals because curare paralyzed the animals. On extensive research, the active principle from curare, **tubocurarine** was identified. d-tubocurarine (d-Tc) is the dextrorotatory

Flowchart 3.1: Classification of skeletal muscle relaxants.

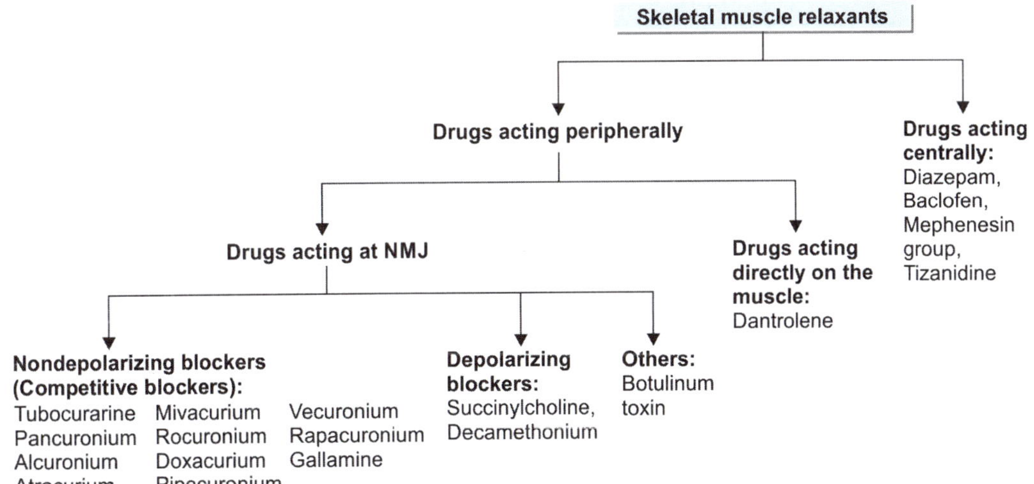

quaternary ammonium alkaloid obtained from the plant *Chondrodendron tomentosum* and plants of the *Strychnos* species (l-tubocurarine is less potent). Several synthetic agents have been developed. All these are quaternary ammonium compounds, because of which they are not well absorbed and are quickly excreted.

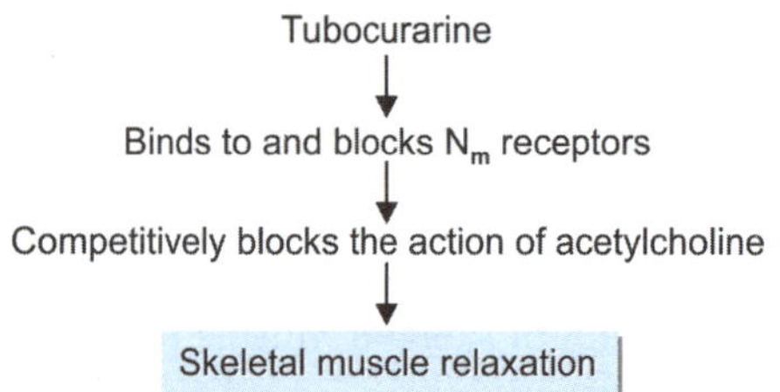

Table 3.1: Duration of action of competitive neuromuscular blockers.

Drug	*Duration (min)*
Tubocurarine	35–60
Gallamine	35–60
Pancuronium	35–80
Doxacurium	90–120
Atracurium	20–35
Vecuronium	20–35
Mivacurium	12–18
Pipecuronium	80–100
Rapacuronium	15–30
Rocuronium	30–60

Mechanism of Action

Non-depolarizing blockers bind to nicotinic receptors on the motor end plate and block the actions of acetylcholine by competitive blockade (Fig. 3.1). These compounds slowly dissociate from the receptors and transmission is gradually restored. Thus, their action is reversible.

Tubocurarine Pharmacological Actions

Skeletal muscle: On parenteral administration, tubocurarine initially causes muscular weakness followed by flaccid paralysis. Small muscles of the eyes and fingers are the first to be affected, followed by those of the limbs, neck and trunk. Later the intercostal muscles and finally the diaphragm are paralyzed and respiration stops. **Consciousness is not affected throughout.** Recovery occurs in the reverse order, i.e., the diaphragm is the first to recover. The effect lasts for 30–60 minutes (Table 3.1).

Autonomic ganglia: In high doses tubocurarine can block autonomic ganglia and adrenal medulla resulting in hypotension.

Histamine release: Tubocurarine can cause histamine release the mast cells from leading to bronchospasm, increased salivary, tracheobronchial and gastric secretions and this also contributes to hypotension.

Pharmacokinetics

Tubocurarine is a quaternary ammonium compound—hence not absorbed orally. It is given either IM or IV.

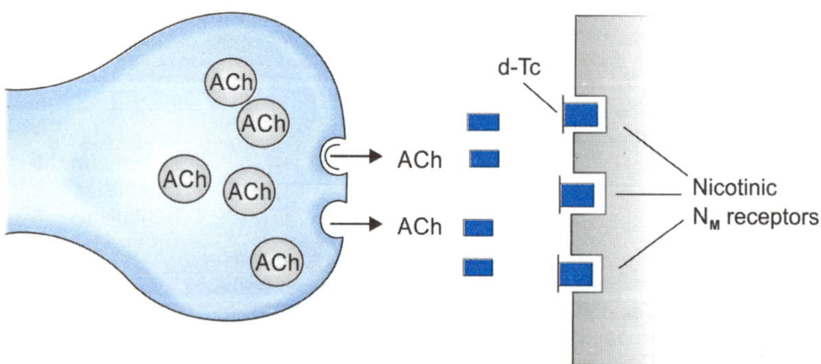

Fig. 3.1: d-Tc molecules bind to nicotinic receptors and prevent the binding of ACh on these receptors

Adverse Reactions

1. Respiratory paralysis and prolonged apnea. It should be treated with artificial ventilation. Neostigmine reverses the skeletal muscle paralysis.
2. Hypotension due to ganglion blockade and histamine release.
3. Flushing and bronchospasm due to histamine release by tubocurarine; this is not seen with newer agents.

Treatment of toxicity: Neostigmine and edrophonium may be used to reverse the skeletal muscle paralysis and are the antidotes in curare poisoning. Antihistamines should be given to counter the effects of histamine.

Sugammadex, a newly introduced antidote binds to rocuronium and reverses its effects. The complex is excreted in the urine. It can also chelate other NMBs like vecuronium and pancuronium.

Synthetic Competitive Blockers

Pancuronium, atracurium, vecuronium, gallamine, doxacurium, mivacurium, pipecuronium, rapacuronium, rocuronium (Table 3.1) are synthetic competitive blockers. The synthetic compounds have the following **advantages over tubocurarine**.

- Less/no histamine release.
- Do not block autonomic ganglia hence cause less hypotension.
- Spontaneous recovery takes place with most of these drugs.
- Some are more potent than tubocurarine.
- **Atracurium** can be safely used in patients with renal impairment because it is degraded by spontaneous rearrangement of the molecule called Hoffmann elimination and also by plasma esterases and therfore does not depend on the kidney for elimination.

  The newer agent **rocuronium** has a rapid onset of action. Hence they can be used as alternative to succinylcholine (SCh) for muscle relaxation before endotracheal intubation. Rocuronium does not cause hypotension,tachycardia and is fast acting. Rapacuronium which is also rapid acting is withdrawn due to severe bronchospasm.
- Tubocurarine, doxacurium and gallamine have a slow onset (4–5 minutes) but long duration of action; pancuronium, vecuronium, atracurium and mivacurium have intermediate onset (2–4 minutes) while rocuronium has fast onset of action (1–2 minutes).
- **Mivacurium** is rapidly metabolized by plasma cholinesterases—hence short acting. It causes significant histamine release.
- Tubocurarine causes histamine release, ganglion blockade (resulting in hypotension) and its muscle relaxant effect needs to be reversed with drugs. Hence **tubocurarine is not used now**. The synthetic compounds are used.

Depolarizing Blockers

Succinylcholine (SCh, Suxamethonium) is a quaternary ammonium compound with the structure **resembling two molecules of acetylcholine joined together**.

Mechanism of Action

The neuromuscular effects of SCh are like those of ACh because of its structure. SCh reacts with nicotinic receptors (Flowchart 3.2) and depolarizes the skeletal muscle membrane. But, unlike ACh, it is destroyed very slowly by pseudocholinesterase. Thus continued presence of the drug causes persistent depolarization resulting in flaccid paralysis. This is phase I block. In high doses SCh produces a dual block—initial depolarizing block followed by non-depolarizing block. The membrane gets slowly repolarized but cannot be depolarized again. The mechanism of this phase II block is not clearly known.

Pharmacological Actions

Skeletal muscle: On intravenous administration onset of action is very rapid—

Flowchart 3.2: Mechanism of action of succinylcholine.

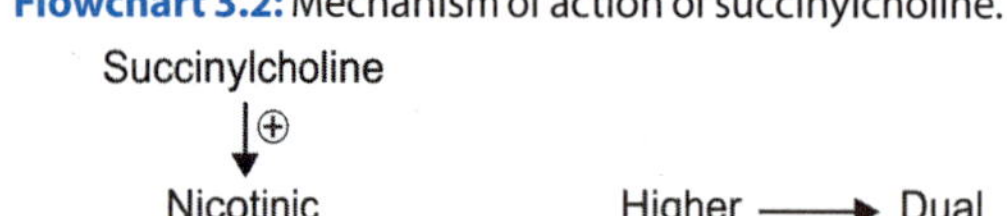

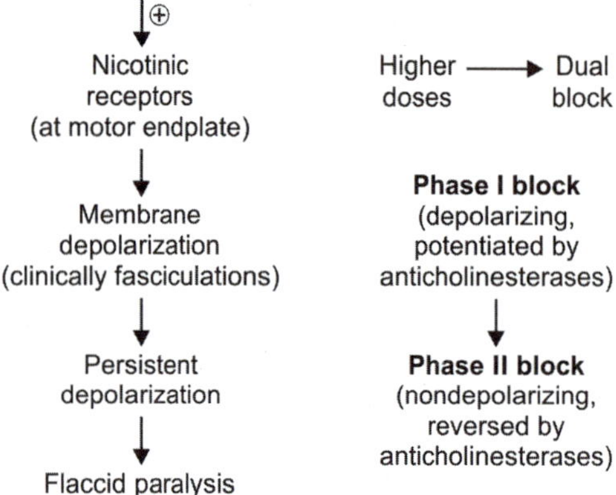

within 1 minute. Initial transient muscular fasciculations and twitchings, mostly in the chest and abdominal regions are followed by skeletal muscle paralysis. The fasciculations are maximum in 2 minutes and subside in 5 minutes. It is due to stimulation of the muscle fibers by a discharge of action potentials in them. SCh is a short-acting muscle relaxant and the effect lasts for 5–10 minutes. Hence it has to be given continuously as an infusion for longer effect.

CVS: Initially hypotension and bradycardia may result from stimulation of the nicotinic receptors in vagal ganglia. This is followed by tachycardia and hypertension due to stimulation of sympathetic ganglia. Higher doses can cause cardiac arrhythmias. SCh can also cause histamine release if injected rapidly.

Other effects: SCh can cause hyperkalemia as it triggers the release of K^+ from the cells by increasing the permeability to cations. It can also cause a transient increase in intraocular pressure.

Pharmacokinetics

SCh is rapidly hydrolyzed by pseudocholinesterases—hence it is short-acting (about 5 minutes). Some people (1 in 2000) have an **abnormal pseudocholinesterase**, a hereditary defect; SCh does not get metabolized and even the usual dose results in **prolonged apnea** and paralysis which may last for several hours. Artificial ventilation and fresh blood transfusion to supply pseudocholinesterase are needed.

Adverse Reactions

1. **Postoperative muscle pain** is a common adverse effect of SCh. It may be due to the damage to muscle fibers that occurs during initial fasciculations.
2. **Hyperkalemia:** This may result in cardiac arrest in patients with burns and nerve injuries.
3. **Cardiac arrhythmias:** SCh can cause cardiac arrhythmias.
4. **Malignant hyperthermia:** It is a rare genetically determined condition where there is a sudden increase in body temperature and severe muscle spasm due to release of intracellular Ca^{++} from the sarcoplasmic reticulum. Certain drugs like halothane, isoflurane and succinylcholine can trigger this process which can be fatal. Combination of halothane and SCh is the most common triggering factor. Intravenous dantrolene is life-saving in malignant hyperthermia. Oxygen inhalation and immediate cooling of the body also help.
5. **Succinylcholine apnea** can be a serious adverse effect in people with atypical/abnormal pseudocholinesterase. People belonging to some particular communities (like vysyas and chettiars) are known to inherit this abnormal pseudocholinesterase.

Drug Interactions

1. General anesthetics augment the action of SMRs.
2. Anticholinesterases like neostigmine—reverse the action of competitive blockers.
3. Aminoglycosides and calcium channel blockers potentiate the action of SMRs.

4. Succinylcholine and halothane given together increase the risk of malignant hyperthermia.

Uses of Peripherally Acting Skeletal Muscle Relaxants

Inappropriate use of peripherally acting SMRs can be fatal. Hence they should be given only by qualified anesthetists or adequately trained doctors.

1. **Adjuvant to anesthesia:** Adequate muscle relaxation is essential during surgeries. Skeletal muscle relaxants are used as adjuvants to general anesthesia. Short-acting SMRs like succinylcholine is used during endotracheal intubation. SMRs are also useful in laryngoscopy, bronchoscopy, esophagoscopy and in orthopedic procedures like reduction of fractures and dislocations.
2. **In electroconvulsive therapy (ECT):** SMRs protect the patient from convulsions and trauma during ECT.
3. **In spastic disorders:** SMRs are used to overcome the spasm of tetanus, athetosis and status epilepticus.
4. **In minor procedures:** SMRs are also useful in laryngoscopy, bronchoscopy, esophagoscopy, tracheal intubation and in orthopedic procedures like reduction of fractures and dislocations.
5. **In status epilepticus:** When convulsions cannot be controlled by anticonvulsants alone, sometimes a neuromuscular blocker (NMB) is used to control the muscular component of convulsions. However, they do not cross the blood brain barrier (BBB) and have no central effects.
6. **Patients on ventilator:** To reduce the resistance of the chest wall and enhance thoracic compliance and to facilitate artificial ventilation, NMBs are used in intensive care units.

Directly Acting Muscle Relaxants

Dantrolene directly affects the skeletal muscle contractile mechanism. It inhibits the muscle contraction by preventing the calcium release from the sarcoplasmic reticulum.

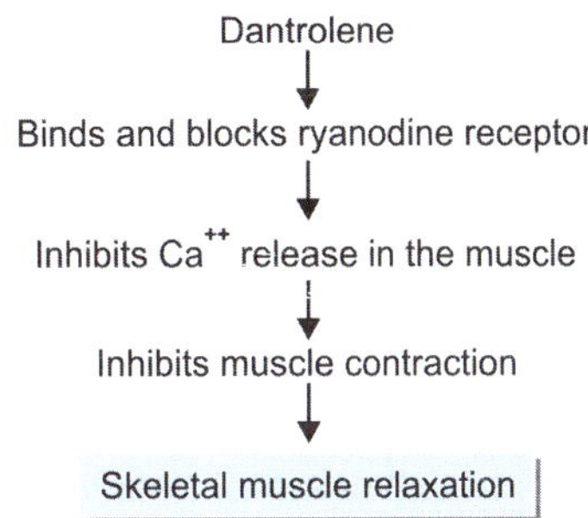

Adverse effects include drowsiness, dizziness, fatigue, muscle weakness, diarrhea and rarely hepatotoxicity. Liver function tests should be done to look for hepatotoxicity.

Uses

1. **Spastic disorders:** Dantrolene is used in spastic disorders like hemiplegia, paraplegia, spinal injuries, multiple sclerosis and cerebral palsy.
2. **Malignant hyperthermia:** Dantrolene is the drug of choice in malignant hyperthermia which is due to excessive release of calcium from the sarcoplasmic reticulum. Dantrolene blocks the release of Ca^{++} from the sarcoplasmic reticulum and relieves muscle spasm in malignant hyperthermia.
3. **Malignant neuroleptic syndrome**—dantrolene is found to be useful.

Quinine: The antimalarial quinine is a skeletal muscle relaxant. It is a sodium channel blocker, it reduces the excitability of the motor end plate. Quinine is used in myotonia congenita and in nocturnal muscle cramps.

Botulinum toxin (BOTOX) is produced by the anerobic bacterium *Clostridium botulinum.* The toxin inhibits the release of acetylcholine at the cholinergic synapses resulting in flaccid paralysis of skeletal muscles.

Botulinum toxin is useful (local injection) in the treatment of dystonias, including sports or writer's cramps, muscle spasms, tremors, cerebral palsy and in rigidity seen in extrapyramidal disorders. It is commonly used to relieve blepharospasm. Botulinum toxin is also popular in cosmetic therapy to remove facial lines by local injection.

Centrally Acting Muscle Relaxants

These drugs act on higher centers and cause muscle relaxation without loss of consciousness. They also have sedative properties. Drugs in this category are:

- **$GABA_A$ agonists:** Benzodiazepines like diazepam
- **$GABA_B$ agonist:** Baclofen
- **Central alpha-2 agonist:** Tizanidine
- **Others:** Mephenesin, carisoprodol, methocarbamol, thiocolchicoside, riluzole, gabapentin, progabide.

Mechanism of action: Centrally acting muscle relaxants depress the spinal polysynaptic reflexes. These reflexes maintain the muscle tone. By depressing these spinal reflexes, centrally acting SMRs reduce the muscle tone.

Central muscle relaxants
↓
Depress spinal polysynaptic reflexes
↓
Decrease muscle tone

Centrally acting muscle relaxants include:

Benzodiazepenes like diazepam have useful antispastic activity. They can be used in relieving muscle spasm of almost any origin including local muscle trauma (*See* page 151).

Baclofen is an analog of the inhibitory neurotransmitter GABA. It is a GABA agonist—it depresses the monosynaptic and polysynaptic reflexes in the spinal cord. It relieves painful spasms including flexor and extensor spasms and may also improve bladder and bowel functions in patients with spinal lesions. Normal tendon reflexes and voluntary muscle power are not affected. Baclofen is generally given orally.

Baclofen is also useful in reducing craving in deaddiction of chronic alcoholics.

Baclofen ($GABA_B$ agonist)
↓
Activates $GABA_B$ receptors
↓
Depresses monosynaptic and polysnaptic reflexes in the spinal cord
↓
Muscle relaxation

Side effects are drowsiness, weakness and ataxia. Baclofen should be gradually withdrawn after prolonged use because abrupt withdrawal can cause anxiety, palpitations and hallucinations.

Mephenesin is not preferred due to its side effects. A number of related drugs like **carisoprodol, methocarbamol, chlorzoxazone** are used in acute muscle spasm caused by local trauma. All of them also cause sedation.

Tizanidine is a congener of clonidine. It is a central α_2 agonist like clonidine. It increases presynaptic inhibition of motor neurons and reduces muscle spasms. Adverse effects include drowsiness, weakness, hypotension and dry mouth. Tizanidine is used in the treatment of spasticity due to stroke, multiple sclerosis and amyotropic lateral sclerosis.

Other centrally acting spasmolytic agents include **riluzole, gabapentin** and **progabide**. Riluzole has both presynaptic and postsynaptic effects. It inhibits glutamate release in the CNS. It is well tolerated with minor adverse effects like nausea and diarrhea. It is used to reduce spasticity in amyotropic lateral sclerosis.

Uses of Centrally Acting Muscle Relaxants

1. **Musculoskeletal disorders** like muscle strains, sprains, myalgias, torticollis, cervical root syndromes, herniated disc syndromes, low backache, dislocations, arthritis, fibrositis and bursitis all cause painful muscle spasms. Muscle relaxants are used with analgesics in these.
2. **Spastic neurological disorders** like cerebral palsy, multiple sclerosis, poliomyelitis, hemiplegia and quadriplegia are treated with diazepam or baclofen.

3. **Tetanus:** Diazepam is given IV.
4. **ECT:** Diazepam is given along with peripherally acting SMRs.
5. **Orthopedic procedures** like fracture reduction may be done after administering diazepam.

DRUGS USED IN THE TREATMENT OF LOCAL MUSCLE SPASM

Several agents are used for the treatment of local muscle spasms which may result from injury or strain. They are:

- Cyclobenzaprine
- Metaxalone
- Carisoprodol
- Chlorzoxazone
- Meprobamate
- Methocarbamol.

They have the following common features:

- All these drugs act by depressing spinal polysynaptic reflexes.
- Common adverse reactions include drowsiness and dizziness.
- Cyclobenzaprine has anticholinergic effects and can therefore cause dryness of mouth, drowsiness and dizziness.
- Many of them are available in combination with NSAIDs.
- NSAIDs are also effective in relieving muscle spasms.

DRUGS USED IN OTHER MUSCULOSKELETAL DISEASES

1. **Osteomalacia and rickets:** Vitamin D deficiency results in osteomalacia. Vitamin D (*See* page 73) is used for the prevention and treatment of osteomalacia.
2. **Paget's disease:** It is due to abnormal osteoclastic activity which results in altered bone architecture. NSAIDs, calcitonin and bisphosphonates are used. Analgesics reduce pain while calcitonin and bisphosphonates reduce bone resorption.
3. **Osteoarthritis:** NSAIDs and glucocorticoids are used.
4. **Drugs used in spasticity:** Spasticity is due to hypertonic contraction of the skeletal muscles. Spasticity is seen in cerebral palsy, stroke and multiple sclerosis. Drugs used in spasticity include baclofen, diazepam and dantrolene.
5. **Amyotropic lateral sclerosis:** Amyotropic lateral sclerosis is a rapidly progressive motor neuron disorder that is characterized by damage to motor neurons of the ventral horn of the spinal cord that control the voluntary muscles. Manifestations include progressive muscle weakness, atrophy, fasciculations and spasticity. Both upper and lower motor neurons are affected. Till now, it was treated symptomatically—for example, muscle relaxants, like baclofen, are used for spasticity. The only drug that was recently made available for the treatment of ALS in riluzole.

   Riluzole blocks the sodium channels and calcium channels. It is an NMDA/glutamate receptor antagonist. It has been shown to increase survival in ALS patients. It is orally effective, highly protein bound and given 50 mg BD. It is well-tolerated. Nausea, diarrhea and rarely hepatotoxicity are noted.

   Ginkgo biloba: An extract of the Chinese plant contains ginkgoflavon glycosides. It is thought to act as a PAF antagonist and decreases the production of TXA and inhibits platelet aggregation. It has been used as a cognition enhancer—but the benefits have yet to be proved.

   Ginkocer, ginkoba 40 mg tab.
6. **Other muscular disorders:** Some muscular disorders like congenital myotonia, Lambert-Eaton syndrome, McCardle syndrome and tetany are due to impaired neuromuscular transmission.
   - **Congenital myotonia** is characterized by violent muscle spasm, which results from irritability of the muscle fiber membrane. Membrane stabilizing

agents like phenytoin and quinine are found to be useful in this condition.

- **Lambert-Eaton syndrome** is characterized by muscular weakness and easy fatiguability. It is associated with some cancers like lung cancer. Physical exercise and calcium are found to be useful in improving muscle power.
- **McCardle syndrome** in some people, glycogen cannot be converted to glucose in the muscle due to an enzyme deficiency. Hence after some exercise such persons develop severe muscle weakness, stiffness and pain. It can be treated with large doses of glucose or by adrenaline injection, which releases glucose from the liver.
- **Tetany:** Hypocalcemia results in tetany and increased neuromuscular excitability. Calcium salts should be given orally or in more severe cases intravenously (*See* page 71).

DRUGS USED IN THE TREATMENT OF IMMUNOLOGICAL AND INFLAMMATORY NEUROMUSCULAR DISEASES

1. Myasthenia Gravis

Myasthenia gravis is a chronic autoimmune disease characterized by progressive weakness with rapid and easy fatiguability of the skeletal muscles. Anticholinesterases improve muscle strength by enhancing the amount of ACh released during each nerve impulse. Antibodies to nicotinic receptors are formed which destroy these receptors, resulting in a decrease in the number of these receptors at the neuromuscular junction (NMJ).

Treatment

Edrophonium is used IV for the diagnosis. Treatment with anticholinesterases bring about improvement in muscle strength. Neostigmine (15 mg tab 6 hourly) or pyridostigmine or a combination of these two may be given. AntiChEs increase ACh levels at the NMJ by preventing the destruction of ACh. They thus increase the force of contraction and improve muscle power by more frequent activation of the existing nicotinic receptors.

Neostigmine in Myasthenia gravis

- By AntiChE activity, it increases ACh levels at the NMJ.
- In addition, neostigmine directly stimulates the nicotinic receptors
- It also increases the amount of ACh released during each nerve impulse.

In advanced disease, anticholinesterases are not effective because the available nicotinic receptors are very few.

Factors like infection, surgery and stress can result in severe muscle weakness called– **myasthenic crisis**. But severe weakness may also result from an excess dose of an anticholinesterase drug (flaccid paralysis due to more of acetylcholine) called **'cholinergic crisis'**. These two crises can be differentiated by 2 mg IV edrophonium—the patient immediately improves if it is myasthenic crisis but the weakness worsens if it is cholinergic crisis. Treatment of cholinergic crisis is with atropine while myasthenic crisis requires a higher dose of an alternative anticholinergic drug.

Other drugs used in myasthenia gravis are:

- **Glucocorticoids:** They inhibit the production of antibodies to the nicotinic receptors. These are used when anticholinesterases alone are not adequate.
- **Immunosuppressants:** Azathioprine and cyclosporine can be used as alternatives to prednisolone in advanced myasthenia gravis. They inhibit the production of antinicotinic receptor antibodies.

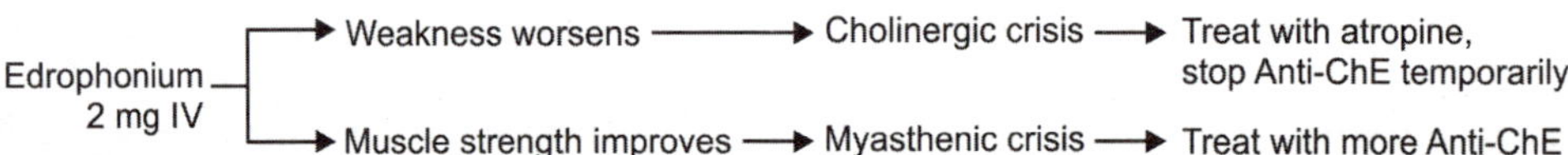

2. Idiopathic Inflammatory Myopathies

Inflammatory myopathies (IM) are inflammatory disorders of the skeletal muscle characterized by symmetric muscle weakness of proximal muscles of the limbs and rarely neck and pharyngeal muscles. These could be accompanied by polymyositis and dermatomyositis. The etiology is not known but toxins and infections may be involved. Inclusion body myositis is a type of inflammatory myopathy with frequent episodes of distal muscle weakness. In biopsy of the muscle, unique inclusions are seen in the muscle.

Treatment is to suppress inflammation.

Drugs used are:

- Glucocorticoids
- Immunosuppressive agents
- Hormone replacement therapy in postmenopausal women
- Physiotherapy.

Glucocorticoids are the first line drugs because they suppress inflammation. Prednisolone is started in the dose of 1–2 mg/kg/day in 2–3 divided doses. A gradual improvement in grip strength may be noticed. However, this condition is slow to respond and some may take as long as 3 months. Once the response is established, a lower maintenance dose is effective to prevent steroid-induced osteoporosis. Daily dietary supplements of calcium and vitamin D should be given, guided by screening of bone mineral density.

Immunosuppressive agents: Patients who do not respond to steroids or poorly tolerate steroids may be put on immunosuppressive agents. Azathioprine, methotrexate, mercaptopurine, cyclophosphamide and cyclosporin are all found to be effective. Immunoglobulins given intravenously appear to be useful in patients not responding to the above measures.

Hormone replacement therapy: Postmenopausal women may need hormone replacement therapy.

Physiotherapy plays a vital role in the treatment. Patients should be advised bed rest during periods of active inflammation. A daily exercise program should be designed to include passive stretching. This avoids muscle contractures. Reasonable active exercises should be encouraged. Training the use of inspiratory muscles can be of benefit for patients with inspiratory muscle weakness.

Other facilitatory measures like grip bars, raised toilet seats, walking aids can also be of help.

3. Demyelinating Disease

Demyelinating disease could be acute inflammatory demyelinating polyneuropathy [Guillain-Barré (GB) syndrome] or chronic inflammatory demyelinating disease.

Acute demyelinating disease is a motor neuropathy which develops over 1–4 weeks after respiratory infection or diarrhea. Microorganisms commonly involved are *Campylobacter jejunum* and cytomegalovirus. Cell mediated immune response is directed at the myelin protein of the spinal roots and cranial nerves. This results in the release of inflammatory mediators viz cytokines which block nerve conduction and complement mediated destruction of the myelin sheath and associated axon.

Clinical features include prodromal symptoms with headache, vomiting, fever, pain in the back and limbs. After a few days, the stage of paralysis begins with distal paresthesias, rapidly ascending muscle weakness, facial and bulbar weakness, (ophthalmoplegia) and in some patients weakness of the respiratory muscles. Involvement of head and neck muscles causes dysphagia. Sensory symptoms with pain, tingling and numbness of the limbs, tenderness in the muscles, cranial nerve paralysis, depressed or loss of reflexes and sometimes urinary retention are also seen.

Nerve conduction studies done in the first few days show prolonged distal motor latencies in the limbs, prolonged F wave latencies and action potential amplitudes are small. Later stages show slowing of nerve conduction which indicates demyelination.

By about 3 weeks, quadriparesis and respiratory paralysis may develop. However majority recover with minor residual neurological symptoms.

Treatment

- Analgesics like paracetamol or ibuprofen and hot packs for pain.
- Regular respiratory monitoring-assisted respiration if required.
- Glucocorticoids may be tried in patients with severe weakness or bulbar involvement—but not shown to be useful by studies.
- Physiotherapy—early active and passive movements.
- In more severe cases plasma exchange may be needed.
- Intravenous immunoglobulin therapy may be given to shorten the course of illness.

Acute axonal polyneuropathy: It is an axonal variant of GB syndrome with antibodies to peripheral nerve gangliosides. It could also result from exposure to certain drugs and toxins.

Miller-Fisher syndrome: It is a variant of Guillain-Barré syndrome with ataxia, areflexia and ophthalmoplegia.

Chronic inflammatory demyelinating polyneuropathy: It develops over months (usually two months) or years. It could be due to an aberrant immune response leading to chronic GB syndrome or hereditary type. Several abnormal gene types have been shown to result in hereditary demyelinating peripheral neuropathies (known as Charcot-Marie-Tooth (CMT) disease). This condition is characterized by distal wasting, i.e., the legs resemble an inverted champagne bottle or the legs of a 'stork'.

Chronic inflammatory demyelinating peripheral neuropathy manifests as progressive generalized neuropathy with predominantly motor symptoms. Treatment is with immunosuppressants, plasma exchange and immunoglobulins.

Chronic axonal polyneuropathy may be caused by drugs and toxins.

4. Osteoarthritis

Osteoarthritis (OA, osteoarthrosis) is a degenerative joint disease characterized by degeneration of articular cartilage and simultaneous proliferation of new bone. Pain is due to low grade inflammation of the joints resulting from abnormal wearing out of the cartilage and a decrease in synovial fluid. The word osteoarthritis is derived from the Greek words 'osteo' meaning 'of the bone' and 'arthritis' meaning joint. However, inflammatory changes in the synovium are usually minor. Though both men and women are affected, OA is more severe in older women. Osteoarthritis with no known etiology is called primary and when the cause for degenerative joint changes can be identified, it is known as secondary osteoarthritis. Genetic predisposition is known particularly in primary osteoarthritis.

Symptoms: Pain in the joints is the most common symptom. The joints affected may be those of the spine, hip, knees and hand—usually only one of these joints is involved. Onset of symptoms is gradual with sharp pain with the use of the joint. As the disease progresses, the joint movement becomes restricted, joints become stiff and the associated muscles go into spasm. There may be effusions into the joint, the surrounding muscles atrophy and the related ligaments may become lax. This associated muscle wasting is an important indicator of the duration and progress of the disease. 'Crepitus' may be felt or heard when the joint is touched or moved.

Treatment: The pathological changes in the joint are largely irreversible. Hence the aim of treatment is to reduce the pain and improve joint function. Analgesics like paracetamol help most patients. If the pain is severe, antiinflammatory doses of NSAIDs like ibuprofen, diclofenac or piroxicam may be needed. However, these are not to be used for long periods because of the risk of gastric ulceration, renal impairment and fluid retention.

Local: Intra-articular or periarticular injection of a glucocorticoid can relieve pain particularly in the knee. Intra-articular injection of hyaluronan or a local anesthetic like lignocaine can also afford temporary symptomatic relief. Local application of a gel of a NSAID like diclofenac or ibuprofen gel may be helpful and safe in most patients. Though drugs like tramadol and opioids may relieve pain in severe OA, they should be avoided for the risk of dependence. Their use must be restricted only to patients with severely painful joints and debilitating disease.

Other Drug Supplements

Several drugs have been tried:

a. **Glucosaminoglycan, pentosan polyphosphate and hyaluronan** - are shown to have a chondroprotective effect in the animals and in 'in vitro' experiments. Glucosamine is the precursor of glucosaminoglycan and chondroitin is the most abundant glucosaminoglycan in the cartilage. They help in the process of cartilage formation and repair. Dietary supplements of glucosamine and chondroitin sulfate have been tried in patients with OA. They are thought to improve the symptoms and delay the disease progression. However, clinical trials have not shown the combination of glucosamine and chondroitin to be anyway better than just placebo.
b. **Omega-3-fatty acids:** Dietary supplements of omega-3-fatty acids from certain marine fish have been tried in order to subdue the inflammatory process.
c. **Antioxidants:** Dietary supplements containing vitamin E are given for their antioxidant properties.
d. **Vitamin D:** Supplementation is recommended since many patients with OA have vitamin D deficiency.

Non-pharmacological Measures

Lifestyle modification to bring about a reduction in weight, regular exercises and rest to the affected joints, appropriate physiotherapy, relaxation techniques, mechanical devices to support the joint (like knee braces when knee is affected)—all these help in reducing morbidity to a large extent.

Surgery: If medical line of treatment is ineffective, surgery to remove the damaged fragments or in some cases joint replacement may be needed.

5. Systemic Lupus Erythematosus

Systemic lupus erythematosus (SLE) is a chronic autoimmune disease involving connective tissue characterized by the presence of antibodies leading to widespread tissue damage. Systemic lupus erythematosus is particularly common among Americans of African origin with a higher incidence in women (9:1).

The immune system regulation is impaired and the autoantibodies attack the host cells and tissue resulting in inflammation and tissue damage. Though not clear, the etiology of immunologically mediated tissue damage could be multifactorial including genetic, environmental (like Sunrays) hormones and drugs. SLE is a multi-system connective tissue disease affecting joints, skin, lungs, liver, heart, kidneys, blood vessels and nervous system.

Mucocutaneous manifestations include skin rashes (classic malar rash or butterfly rash), alopecia, livido reticularis, ulcers in the nose, mouth and vagina. Most patients experience joints pain with chronic inflammatory arthritis involving small joints of the hand and wrist though other joints may also be affected. However joint destruction is milder when compared to other types of arthritis. Migratory arthalgia with mild morning stiffness and tenosynovitis may be misdiagnosed as rheumatoid arthritis. However, unlike rheumatoid arthritis, joint deformities are rare in SLE.

Other features include anemia, lupus glomerulonephritis with hematuria and proteinuria; cardiorespiratory manifestations resulting from inflammation of various parts leading to pericarditis, endocarditis, myocarditis, atherosclerosis, fibrosing alveolitis, lupus pneumonitis, pulmonary hypertension and progressive dyspnea.

SLE can also manifest with esophagitis with pain during swallowing, malabsorption, lupus gastroenteritis, pancreatitis, hepatitis, cystitis and systemic vasculitis.

Treatment

Most patients have mild disease and would respond to NSAIDs. Hydroxychloroquine, glucocorticoids, immunosuppressants like methotrexate, azathioprine and cyclophosphamide may be needed for more severe cases.

Patients must be advised to avoid exposure to direct sun light, use sun protective clothing and sun block lotions containing sun protection factor 25–50. Weight reduction is recommended in overweight subjects. Patients who had earlier episodes of thrombosis should be put on life long warfarin.

6. Systemic Sclerosis (Scleroderma)

Systemic sclerosis is a chronic connective tissue disorder affecting the skin, internal organs and vasculature with excessive deposits of collagen in the skin or other organs. It was earlier called scleroderma. The characteristic clinical features include sclerodactyly with Raynaud's phenomenon. It is of two types:

1. **Systemic type:** The diffuse cutaneous systemic sclerosis which is the severe form.
2. **Localized type:** Limited cutaneous systemic sclerosis which is the localized type of the disease.

In the systemic form, most patients have vascular symptoms—**Raynaud's phenomenon** can lead to painful ulcers on the fingers and toes known as digital ulcers. Calcinosis near the elbows, knees and joints may restrict joint mobility particularly of the small joints. Arthralgia, morning stiffness, weakness and discomfort in the muscles and flexor tenosynovitis are the common musculoskeletal manifestations. It may be associated with pulmonary, gastrointestinal, renal and other complications.

Decreased gastric motility, gastric ulcers, upper gastrointestinal bleeding, scleroderma renal crisis with malignant hypertension, high renin levels, hematuria and proteinuria, pulmonary manifestations with pulmonary hypertension and in later stages pulmonary hemorrhage and pneumothorax can be seen.

Treatment

Depending on the organ/system involved, treatment is initiated to control the symptoms.

- Raynaud's phenomenon is treated with vasodilators (*See* page 134). Joints pain and myositis may be alleviated with NSAIDs.
- Infected ulcers need antibiotics. Poor penetration of drugs through skin lesions makes it necessary for drugs to be given in higher doses and for longer periods. Patients with severe ischemia and ulceration of the digits may be benefited by prostaglandin analogs epoprostenol or iloprost.
- Alveolitis, myositis and severe manifestations requiring immunosuppression may be treated with methotrexate, cyclosporine, cyclophosphamide or glucocorticoids. Scleroderma renal crisis with acute renal failure and severe hypertension can be given an ACE inhibitor like enalapril.

- Maintenance of core body temperature is important to avoid Raynaud's phenomenon.

AGENTS AFFECTING BONE MINERAL TURNOVER

Calcium and phosphorus are the most important minerals of the bone with 1–2 kg of calcium and 1 kg of phosphorus stored in it. Calcium and phosphorus metabolism are chiefly regulated by vitamin D and parathormone and also by calcitonin. Vitamin D and parathormone increase plasma calcium levels but calcitonin reduces it. Other hormones that also influence calcium and phosphorus metabolism are growth hormone, insulin, thyroid hormone, prolactin, glucocorticoids and sex hormones.

Calcium

Calcium is essential for:

- Tissue excitability,
- Muscular excitation-contraction coupling,
- Secretion from glands,
- Myocardial contractility and
- Formation of bone and teeth.

It also maintains the integrity of mucous membranes and cell membrane.

Calcium is essential for normal blood coagulation.

Calcium is absorbed from the small intestine by a carrier mediated active transport. Normally about 30 percent of the dietary calcium is absorbed, while in Ca^{++} deficiency, the absorption increases under the control of vitamin D (Fig. 3.2). The normal plasma calcium level is 9–11 mg/dL. It is excreted in feces, urine and sweat.

Some preparations of calcium

Salt	Formulation	Dose
Calcium gluconate	10% inj—given IV 500 mg, 1 g tablets	10–20 mL
Calcium chloride	5–10% solution IV	5–10 mL

Adverse effects: Oral calcium can produce constipation.

Uses

- To prevent and treat calcium deficiency, calcium supplements are given orally in children, pregnant and lactating women and in postmenopausal osteoporosis to prevent calcium deficiency.

Tetany: 5–10 mL IV calcium gluconate followed by 50–100 mL slow IV infusion

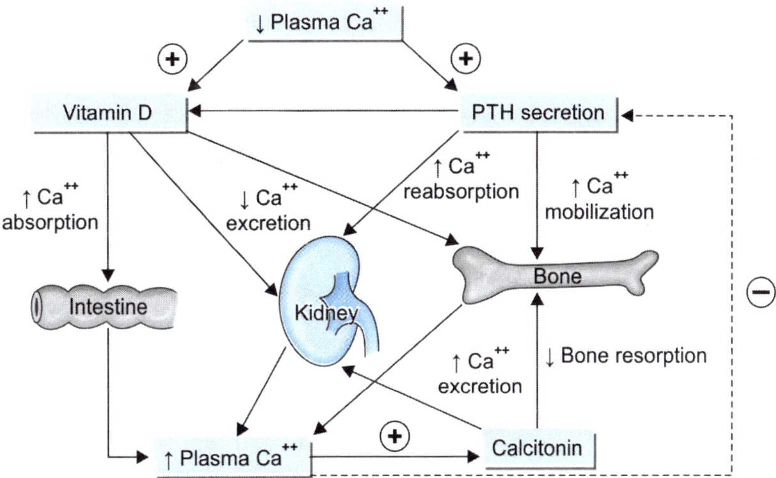

Fig. 3.2: Regulation of plasma calcium level

promptly reverses the muscular spasm. The injection produces a sense of warmth. This is followed by oral calcium 1.5 g daily for several weeks.

- Vitamin D deficiency rickets—calcium is given along with vitamin D.
- As an antacid—calcium carbonate is used.
- For placebo effect—intravenous calcium is used in weakness, pruritus and some dermatoses. The feeling of warmth produced by the injection could afford psychological benefit.

Phosphorus

Phosphorus is present in many food items—including milk, cereals, fish, meat, pulses and nuts.

Daily requirement of phosphorus is about 900 to 1,000 mg in adults. Human body contains about 500-600 g of phosphorus of which 75% is present in bones. In bones and teeth, phosphorus is in the form of orthophosphates while in soft tissues it is in the form of organic esters. When plasma phosphate is measured it is nothing but the plasma inorganic phosphate measured. Phosphorus is absorbed by the small intestine. Excretion of phosphorus is under the control of parathormone. The renal excretion of phosphorus is increased by parathormone.

Physiological Function

1. Phosphorus is necessary for the formation of bones and teeth.
2. Phosphorus is essential for phosphorylation reactions.
3. Phosphorus is present in the nuclei and cytoplasm.
4. Phosphorus is important in maintaining the acid-base balance in the plasma and the cells— phosphates are buffers.
5. Phosphates play a vital role in various enzymatic reactions and are important for the structure and function of the cells.

Hypophosphatemia

Causes

1. Dietary phosphorus deficiency
2. Long-term intake of aluminum containing antacids
3. Vitamin D deficiency
4. Hyperparathyroidism
5. Chronic alcoholism
6. Diabetic ketoacidosis

Signs and symptoms: Anorexia, muscular weakness and pain, abnormal bone mineralization, hemolysis, decreased myocardial contractility and respiratory failure.

Hyperphosphatemia

Causes: Hypoparathyroidism, acromegaly and renal failure.

Clinical features: Hypocalcemia, bone resorption and calcification of soft tissues.

Uses of Phosphorus

1. Phosphorus deficiency
2. Chronic hypercalcemia (without hyperphosphatemia).

Parathyroid Hormone (Parathormone, PTH)

Parathormone is a peptide secreted by the parathyroid gland. Secretion of PTH is regulated by plasma Ca^{++} concentration—low plasma Ca^{++} stimulates PTH release, while high levels inhibit secretion (Fig. 3.2). Parathormone maintains plasma calcium concentration by mobilizing calcium from the bone, promoting reabsorption of Ca^{++} from the kidneys and by stimulating the synthesis of calcitriol which in turn enhances calcium absorption from the intestines. PTH also promotes phosphate excretion.

Hypoparathyroidism is characterized by low plasma calcium levels with its associated manifestations. Hyperparathyroidism which is most commonly due to parathyroid tumor produces hypercalcemia and deformities of the bone.

PTH is not therapeutically used. It is used for the diagnosis of pseudohypoparathyroidism.

Hormones that influence bone metabolism

- Vitamin D
- Parathormone
- Calcitonin
- Glucocorticoids
- Estrogens

Vitamin D

Vitamin D a fat-soluble vitamin, is a prehormone produced in the skin from 7-dehydrocholesterol under the influence of ultraviolet rays. It is converted to active metabolites in the body which regulate plasma calcium levels and various functions of the cells.

Source

- Diet—as ergocalciferol (vitamin D_2) from plants.
- Cholecalciferol (vitamin D_3) is synthesized in the skin from 7-dehydrocholesterol.

Cholecalciferol (vitamin D_3) is converted to 25-OHD_3 (calcifediol) in the liver (Fig. 3.3) which is in turn converted to 1,25-dihydroxycholecalciferol (calcitriol) in the kidneys. Calcitriol is the active form of vit D while calcifediol is the main metabolite in circulation. Convertion of calcifediol to calcitriol is influenced by PTH and plasma phosphate concentration.

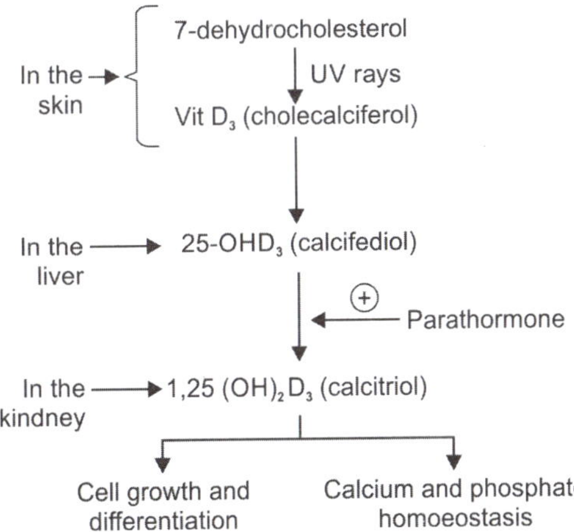

Fig. 3.3: Synthesis and functions of vitamin D

Mechanism of Action

Mechanism of action of vitamin D is similar to glucocorticoids–it binds to the vitamin D receptors, the drug-receptor complex moves to the nucleus where it directs the synthesis of proteins needed for its actions.

Actions

The chief actions of calcitriol are:

- It stimulates calcium and phosphate absorption in the intestine. Calcitriol enhances the synthesis of calcium channels and the calcium binding protein called 'Calbindin' in the gut which is a carrier protein for calcium. Calcitriol may also act directly on the gut mucosa to enhance calcium uptake from the gut.
- Mobilizes calcium from bone by promoting osteoclastic activity.
- Increases reabsorption of Ca^{++} and phosphate from the kidney tubules.

Calcitriol is essential for normal bone mineralization for skeletal muscles as well as cellular growth and differentiation.

Vitamin D deficiency results in low plasma calcium and phosphate levels with abnormal mineralization of the bone; causes rickets in children and osteomalacia in adults.

Daily requirement: 400 IU (10 mg).

Pharmacokinetics

Given orally, vitamin D is well-absorbed from the small intestines in the presence of bile salts. It is converted to 25-OHD_3 in the liver and circulates in the plasma, bound to a protein and is stored in the adipose tissue. Vitamin D is also degraded in the liver and the metabolites are excreted in the bile.

Preparations

- Calciferol capsules 25000; 50,000 IU.
- Cholecalciferol granules—oral 60,000 IU in Ig; 3,00,000 IU/mL; 6,00,000 IU/mL inj.

- Shark liver oil with vit D—1000 IU/mL, vit A—6000 IU/mL.

Adverse Reactions

High doses of vitamin D used for long periods result in hypervitaminosis D manifesting as generalized decalcification of the bones, hypercalcemia, hyperphosphatemia resulting in weakness, drowsiness, nausea, abdominal pain, thirst, renal stones and hypertension. Hypervitaminosis D in children is most often due to unnecessary vit D supplementation by parents.

Uses

1. **Prophylaxis:** 400 IU daily or 3,00,000 IU every 3–6 months IM prevents vit D deficiency. Adequate dietary calcium and phosphate intake is necessary. In the breastfed infants, from the first month onwards oral vit D supplements are needed. In obstructive jaundice, prophylactic 6,00,000 units vit D given IM prevents deficiency.
2. **Nutritional rickets and osteomalacia:** 6,00,000 units IM repeated after 4–6 weeks is needed in rickets and osteomalacia along with calcium supplements.
3. **Vitamin D resistant rickets:** It is a hereditary disorder with abnormality in renal phosphate reabsorption. Phosphate with vitamin D is found to be useful.
4. **Vitamin D dependent rickets:** It is due to calcitriol deficiency (inability to convert calcifediol to calcitriol) and is treated with calcitriol.
5. **Senile osteoporosis:** Oral vitamin D supplements with calcium may be tried.
6. **Hypoparathyroidism:** Calcitriol with Ca^{++} supplements are beneficial.

Calcitonin

Calcitonin is a peptide hormone secreted by the parafollicular 'C' cells of the thyroid gland. Secretion is regulated by plasma Ca^{++} concentration, i.e., high plasma Ca^{++} stimulates calcitonin release.

Actions

The chief effects of calcitonin are to lower serum calcium and phosphate by its actions on the bone and kidney. It inhibits osteoclastic bone resorption and in the kidney, it reduces both calcium and phosphate reabsorption.

In general the effects are opposite to that of PTH. Calcitonin is used to control hypercalcemia, Paget's disease, metastatic bone cancer and osteoporosis and to increase bone mineral density.

Other hormones that regulate bone turnover are glucocorticoids and estrogens. Glucocorticoids antagonize vitamin D stimulated intestinal calcium absorption and enhance renal Ca^{++} excretion. Estrogens reduce bone resorption by PTH and also enhance calcitriol levels. Estrogen receptors are found in bone which suggests that they may also have a direct effect on bone remodeling.

Bisphosphonates

Bisphosphonates are analogs of pyrophosphate; they inhibit bone resorption.

Classification

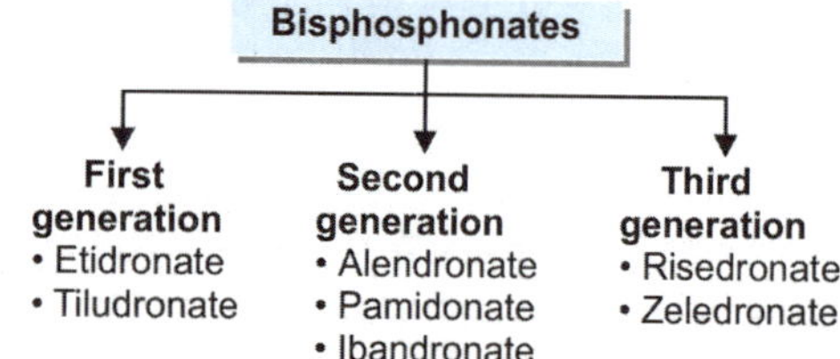

Mechanism of action: Bisphosphonates have a high affinity for calcium, are taken up into bone matrix, are imbibed by osteoclasts and then incapacitate the osteoclasts resulting in reduced bone resorption. They also slow the formation and dissolution of hydroxyapatite crystals.

The most common adverse effect is gastroesophagitis due to irritation. It should always be taken along with a full glass of water. The patient should be in sitting position and not lie down for at least an hour after swallowing the tablet. Fever and hypocalcemia can occur. Long-term use can lead to osteomalacia due to inhibition of bone mineralization. Higher doses can rarely cause osteonecrosis of the jaw.

Uses

1. **Osteoporosis:** Alendronate, residronate and ibandronate are **used along with calcium and vitamin D** for the prevention and treatment of osteoporosis in men and postmenopausal women.
2. **Pagets disease of the bone:** Bisphosphonates relieve pain and induce remission.
3. **Hypercalcemia in malignancies:** Some malignancies are associated with hypercalcemia and some of them may result in severe hypercalcemia which needs to be treated as an emergency. Intravenous infusion of palmidronate 60–90 mg over 2–3 hours (or zoledronate) along with IV fluids and frusemide promote excretion of calcium in a few hours.

AGENTS USED IN THE PREVENTION AND TREATMENT OF OSTEOPOROSIS

Drugs may be used either to prevent bone resorption or promote bone formation or a combination of both in the prevention and treatment of osteoporosis. These agents reduce the risk of fractures in patients with osteoporosis.

Drugs that prevent bone resorption are:

1. Calcium [↑ bone mineral density (BMD)]
2. Vitamin D (↑absorption of calcium)
3. Estrogens (prevent osteoporosis)
4. Raloxifene (selective estrogen receptor modulator - SERM - ↑BMD).
5. Calcitonin (prevents bone resorption, ↑BMD)
6. Bisphosphonates (↓bone resorption, ↑BMD)

Drugs that promote bone formation:

1. Fluoride in small doses ↑osteoblastic activity →↑bone mass — but generally not preferred
2. Testosterone - in hypogonadal men
3. Anabolic steroids in postmenopausal women
4. Parathormone (PTH) analogs are used.

Bisphosphonates are used to inhibit bone resorption.

Raloxifene acts as an estrogen receptor agonist in the bone. In women with postmenopausal osteoporosis, raloxifene has antiresorptive effects on the bone. It reduces bone loss and may even help to gain bone mass. Raloxifene also lowers LDL. It acts as an estrogen antagonist in the breast cancer. Raloxifene does not stimulate the uterine endometrial proliferation.

Adverse effects include hot flushes, leg cramps and an increased risk of deep vein thrombosis and pulmonary embolism. Raloxifene is indicated for the prevention of post-menopausal osteoporosis.

DRUGS AND EXERCISE

Effect of Exercise on the Cardiorespiratory Function

During exercise, oxygen consumption of the skeletal muscle increases. Hence it requires more oxygen supply. In order to meet this increased demand, various changes take place in the cardiovascular and respiratory system. The heart rate, force of contraction and thereby the cardiac output increase; the respiratory rate, depth and thereby tidal volume increase. The blood vessels of skeletal muscles are dilated which increases blood supply as well as washes away the metabolites formed.

Drugs that Influence Exercise

Drugs like amphetamines, anabolic steroids, methylxanthines and cocaine improve exercise performance while β-blockers decrease exercise tolerance.

Amphetamine: Improves both mental and physical performance (*See* page 51). It improves alertness and performance even in highly tiring conditions. It postpones fatigue and brings about a significant improvement in athletic performance in sportsmen.

Amphetamines are banned in sports. Amphetamine is also a drug of dependence.

Cocaine: Like amphetamine, cocaine is a psychomotor stimulant. It produces euphoria and increased motor activity. It inhibits the uptake of catecholamines in the nerve terminals resulting in increased sympathetic activity. Cocaine is a drug of dependence and its long-term use results in various adverse effects.

Anabolic steroids are androgens with selective anabolic effects and lesser degree of androgenic effects. Anabolic steroids improve muscle strength. They are misused by athletes and are now banned in them. Androgens can cause various side effects if used over a long-time including reduced sperm production and decreased fertility. Some cause gynecomastia, hepatotoxicity, an increase in serum cholesterol and psychological disorders. Androgens cause virilization in women.

Bronchodilators: Methylxanthines are bronchodilators. The main compounds are theophylline and caffeine. They are present in coffee, tea and cocoa. Methylxanthines are CNS stimulants. They reduce fatigue, improve alertness and physical performance. They are mild psychomotor stimulants. They also bring about bronchodilation and cardiac stimulation which add to their beneficial effects on exercise.

β-adrenergic agonists: Adrenaline and selective β_2-agonists like salbutamol, terbutaline and salmeterol are bronchodilators. Though their bronchodilator effect may help better oxygenation during respiration, these drugs cause skeletal muscle tremors. The exact mechanism is not known but they may act through β-receptors to increase the discharge of muscle spindles. *Clenbuterol* is a β_2-agonist used by sportsmen for its anabolic effects.

Drugs that Decrease Exercise Tolerance

β-adrenergic blockers prevent the exercise induced increase in heart rate and force of contraction. β-blockers reduce the work capacity and impair exercise performance. The increase in blood flow to the skeletal muscle during exercise is reduced by β_2 blockade. They also prevent the rise in blood glucose level brought about by catecholamines. They may also increase airway resistance. By all these effects, β-blockers reduce exercise tolerance.

SPORTS MEDICINE AND DRUG ABUSE IN SPORTS

Drugs are used in sports to treat sports ailments. Unfortunately many drugs are also abused in sports.

Drugs of Abuse in Sports

Several drugs like anabolic steroids and growth hormone, are used by sports persons for improving performance in competitions. However, such use of performance-enhancing drugs is officially prohibited. **World Anti-Doping Agency (WADA)** has defined doping as the occurrence of one or more of the anti **doping** rule violations mentioned in the WADA code. Tests are done to detect such drugs or their metabolites in the urine or blood samples. If an athlete tests positive for any of the banned drugs, he/she is disqualified from an athletic event, suspended for a particular period or banned for life from competitions.

Sports persons as well as their coaches should be aware of the rules and harmful effects of such drugs.

Prohibited Substances

Anabolic agents are used by athletes and body builders with the hope of increasing muscle mass, lean body mass, strength and thereby improve performance. They reduce catabolic effects on muscles and promote muscle building if combined with adequate 'work out' and the required high protein diet. They could also instill the 'aggressive tempo'. They are available as tablets, injections, nasal sprays and gels/ creams for local application. Though use of anabolic steroids could bring about some increase in muscle mass, there is no evidence that they improve athletic performance. They could cause serious adverse effects and are not medically recommended. Anabolic steroids can cause acne, fluid retention, hepatotoxicity (17-alpha methylated steroids) and masculinizing effects in women. Large doses taken for long periods can cause decreased spermatogenesis, testicular atrophy, gynecomastia, hypertension and abnormalities of lipid metabolism with increased risk of atherosclerosis. Such doses can also cause psychiatric disturbances.

Other Banned Substances

1. **Erythropoietin** stimulates the synthesis of erythrocytes leading to increased oxygen carrying capacity with increased oxygen supply to the tissues and thereby improved performance. Erythropoietin can increase blood viscosity, hypertension and increase the risk of stroke and coronary thrombosis.
2. **Insulin-like growth factors** influence skeletal muscle growth when infused into target muscles.
3. **Chorionic gonadotrophin and luteinizing hormone in males and corticotrophins:** HCG enhances the production of testosterone by stimulating the Leydig cells of the testis.
4. **Growth hormone:** Parenteral administration of human growth hormone promotes muscle development, increases lean body mass and reduces body fat. It also stimulates the secretion of insulin like growth factors which could promote bone and muscle growth, enhance muscle mass and produce a feeling of well-being. However, it can cause gigantism, acromegaly, cardiac hypertrophy and cardiomyopathy.
5. **Beta-2 adrenergic agonists** like salbutamol used by athletes to produce bronchodilation and cardiac stimulation with the intention of improving performance is prohibited except in patients with exercise-induced asthma.
6. **Hormones**, aromatase inhibitors (e.g., anastrozole), SERMs, other anti-estrogenic and metabolic modulators like peroxisome proliferator activated receptor d (PPARd) agonists are banned by WADA.
7. **Various CNS stimulants** like ephedrine, amphetamines and other sympathomimetics, nikethamide, caffeine and cocaine, have shown to improve performance in some of the sports like weight lifting. Use of all stimulants is banned except some of them for topical use. Local administration (e.g., nasal, ophthalmologic) of adrenaline or co-administration with local anesthetic agents is not prohibited.

   Narcotics (opioids) used as protection against pain from injuries in sports and cannabinoids are prohibited substances.

   Glucocorticoids: Used for their anti-inflammatory and euphoric effects are banned except when medically indicated.
8. **Diuretics, and other masking agents:** Diuretics are used for rapid weight reduction so that they could fit into lower weight categories. Diuretics also counter the fluid retention brought about by anabolic and other steroids. Moreover, as diuretics modify the urinary excretion of drugs including banned drugs, they could **mask** their presence in the urine. Therefore, diuretics are abused in sports for multiple reasons but such use is prohibited.

   Other drugs used as masking agents include epitestosterone (mask testosterone in urine samples), alpha reductase inhibitors like finasteride (mask steroid excretion), probenecid (alters excretion of acidic drugs), plasma expanders (mask erythropoietin use) and desmopressin.

Prohibited Methods

1. **Enhancement of oxygen transfer Blood doping:** Athletes get IV infusion of RBCs, RBC products in order to increase the oxygen delivery to the tissues particularly muscles. This is associated with the risk of thrombosis due to increased viscosity of the blood. Plasma expanders, hemoglobin-based oxygen carriers and perfluorocarbons are also used for the same purpose.
2. **Chemical and physical manipulation:** Tampering or attempting to tamper samples collected during doping control.
3. **Gene doping** is the transfer of nucleic acids or use of genetically modified cells.

Substances Prohibited in Particular Sports

Alcohol: Consumption of alcohol is prohibited in aeronautic events, archery, automobile competitions, karate, motorcycling, power-boating.

Beta blockers: Beta adrenergic blockers, like propranolol, are used to overcome anxiety and its associated symptoms in some sports like shooting which may be affected by anxiety. They also reduce benign essential tremors. In most other sports, they could impair performance and are neither abused nor banned in them. Thus, use of β blockers is restricted in some sports like archery, billiards, golf, shooting and aeronautic events.

Drugs used for the Treatment of Ailments Related to Sports

- Analgesics-sprays for muscle catches may be needed for quick relief
- Rehydration with water
- Electrolytes to replace lost electrolytes during the sports events
- Glucose supplementation for energy

Minor injuries, strains, sprains, muscle catches and such similar conditions may be treated. However, major accidents, injuries and emergencies in sports are treated in hospitals.

4

CHAPTER

Anti-inflammatory Drugs and Immunopharmacology

Chapter Highlights

- Nonsteroidal Anti-inflammatory Drugs (NSAIDs)
- Corticosteroids
- Drugs used in Treatment of Rheumatoid Arthritis
- Treatment of Gout
- Immunosuppressants and Immunostimulants

Inflammation is the primary pathology behind most painful conditions. Two major classes of anti-inflammatory drugs are available to suppress inflammation *viz*:

- Corticosteroids (glucocorticoids)
- Non-steroidal anti-inflammatory drugs.

Both are discussed in this section.

Pain or algesia is an unpleasant sensation. It cannot be easily defined. Pain is a warning signal and indicates that there is some impairment in the body. It is the most important symptom that brings the patient to the doctor or physiotherapist and demands immediate relief. Prompt relief of pain instills enormous confidence in the patient regarding the doctors treating ability.

Pain arising from the skin and integumental structures, muscles, bones and joints is known as **somatic pain**. It is usually caused by inflammation and is well-defined or sharp pain.

Pain arising from the viscera is vague, dull-aching type, difficult to pinpoint to one site and is known as **visceral pain**. It may be accompanied by autonomic responses like sweating, nausea and hypotension. It may be due to spasm, ischemia or inflammation.

When pain is referred to a cutaneous area which receives nerve supply from the same spinal segment as that of the affected viscera, it is known as **referred pain**, e.g., cardiac pain referred to the left arm.

Pain consists of two components—the original 'sensation' and the 'reaction' to it. The original sensation is carried by the afferent nerve fibers and is the same in all. The reaction component differs widely from one person to another.

Analgesic is a drug which relieves pain without loss of consciousness. Analgesics only afford symptomatic relief from pain without affecting the cause.

Analgesics are of two classes:

1. Opioid or morphine type of analgesics (narcotic analgesics) (*See* page 163).
2. Non-opioid or aspirin type of analgesics.

NONSTEROIDAL ANTI-INFLAMMATORY DRUGS

Nonsteroidal anti-inflammatory drugs (NSAIDs) are aspirin-type or non-opioid analgesics. In addition they have anti-inflammatory, antipyretic and uricosuric properties—without addiction liability.

The medicinal effects of the bark of the willow tree has been known since centuries. The active principle 'salicin' was isolated from the willow bark. This salicin is converted to glucose and salicylic acid in the body. In 1875, sodium salicylate was first used in the treatment of rheumatic fever. After its anti-inflammatory and uricosuric properties were established, efforts were made to synthesize derivatives which were less expensive. Now they have replaced the natural ones for clinical use.

Mechanism of Action

During inflammation, arachidonic acid liberated from membrane phospholipids is converted to prostaglandins (PGs), catalyzed by the enzyme cyclo-oxygenase. These prostaglandins produce hyperalgesia—they sensitize the nerve endings to pain and other mediators of inflammation like bradykinin and histamine.

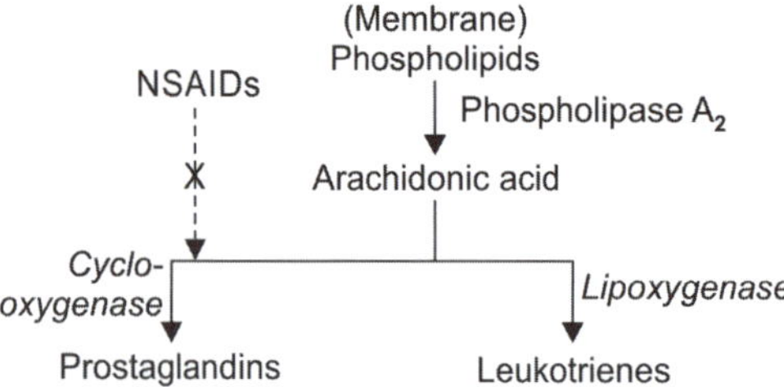

NSAIDs inhibit the PG synthesis by inhibiting the enzyme cyclo-oxygenase. There are two forms of cyclooxygenase, viz. COX-1 and COX-2. COX-1 is found in most of the normal cells (constitutive) and is involved in maintaining normal tissue function. COX-2 is produced in inflammatory cells during inflammation. This COX-2 catalyzes the synthesis of prostanoids which are the mediators of inflammation. Most NSAIDs inhibit both COX-1 and COX-2 while some newer ones, such as celecoxib selectively inhibit only COX-2.

Classification

I. *Nonselective COX Inhibitors*

Mnemonic for classification groups

She's Pretty Priyanka A fantastic POP singer
S—Salicylates
P—Para-aminophenol derivatives
P—Propionic acid derivatives
A—Acetic acid derivatives
F—Fenamates (Anthranilic acids)
P—Pyrazolone derivative
O—Oxicams (Enolic acid derivatives)
P—Preferential COX 2 inhibitors
S—Selective COX 2 inhibitors

1. **Salicylates**
   Aspirin
2. **Para-aminophenol derivatives**
   Paracetamol
3. **Propionic acid derivatives**
   Ibuprofen, fenoprofen, carprofen, naproxen, ketoprofen, flurbiprofen
4. **Acetic acid derivatives**
   Ketorolac, tolmetin, indomethacin, sulindac, nabumatone
5. **Fenamates**
   Mefenamic acid, meclofenamic acid
6. **Pyrazolone derivatives**
   Phenylbutazone, azapropazone
7. **Oxicams (Enolic acid derivatives)**
   Piroxicam, tenoxicam.

II. *Preferential COX-2 Inhibitors*

Diclofenac, aceclofenac, etodolac, meloxicam, nimesulide.

III. *Selective COX-2 Inhibitors*

Celecoxib, parecoxib, etoricoxib.

I. NONSELECTIVE COX INHIBITORS

1. Salicylates

Salicylates are salts of salicylic acid, e.g., methyl salicylate, sodium salicylate, acetyl salicylic acid (aspirin). Aspirin is taken as the prototype.

Pharmacological Actions

1. **Analgesia:** Aspirin is a good analgesic and relieves pain of inflammatory origin without euphoria. Pain originating from the integumental structures like muscles, bones, joints, and pain in connective tissues is relieved. But in vague visceral pain, aspirin is relatively ineffective.

The pain is relieved without euphoria and hypnosis. Hence there is no development of dependance. But aspirin is weaker analgesic when compared to morphine.

2. **Antipyretic action:** In fever, salicylates bring down the temperature to normal level. But, in normal individuals, there is no change in temperature.

In fever, pyrogen—a protein, circulates in the body and this increases the synthesis of PGs in the hypothalamus, thereby raising its temperature set point. The thermostatic mechanism in the hypothalamus is thus disturbed. Aspirin inhibits PG synthesis in the hypothalamus and resets the thermostat at the normal level bringing down the temperature.

Increased sweating and cutaneous vasodilatation promote heat loss and assist in the antipyretic action.

3. **Anti-inflammatory action:** At higher doses of 4-6 g/day, aspirin acts as an anti-inflammatory agent. Signs of inflammation like tenderness, swelling, erythema and pain are all reduced or suppressed. But, the progression of the disease in rheumatoid arthritis, rheumatic fever or osteoarthritis is not affected.

Once again the mechanism of action is PG synthesis inhibition—PGs present in inflammatory tissue are responsible for edema, erythema and pain. In addition, aspirin also interferes with the formation of chemical mediators of the kallikrein system. As a result, it decreases the adherence of granulocytes to the damaged vessels, stabilizes lysomes and decreases the migration of the polymorphonuclear leukocytes and macrophages into the site of inflammation.

4. **Respiration:** In therapeutic doses of 4-6 g/day—salicylates increase consumption of oxygen by skeletal muscles. As a result there is ↑CO_2 production. The ↑CO_2 stimulates respiratory center. Salicylates also directly stimulate the medullary respiratory center. Both these actions increase the rate and depth of respiration. These effects are dose dependent.

As a result of this stimulation of respiration, plasma CO_2 is washed out leading to respiratory alkalosis. With toxic doses, the respiratory center is depressed leading to respiratory failure.

5. **Acid-base and electrolyte balance:** In anti-inflammatory doses, salicylates produce significant respiratory stimulation so that CO_2 is washed out resulting in respiratory alkalosis; pH becomes alkaline. This is compensated by increased excretion of HCO_3^- in urine.

With toxic doses, salicylates depress the respiratory center directly. As a result, CO_2 accumulates, plasma CO_2 level rises and pH decreases, i.e., there is acidosis.

Toxic doses also depress vasomotor center. This vasomotor depression impairs renal function resulting in accumulation of strong acids of metabolic origin like lactic, pyruvic and acetoacetic acids produced in the body.

The above effects are accompanied by dehydration due to:

- Water lost in urine with HCO_3^-, Na^+ and K^+
- Increased sweating
- Water lost during hyperventilation.

Thus high doses cause severe dehydration with acidosis.

6. **Metabolic effects:** Salicylates increase the cellular metabolism. More of O_2 is used and more CO_2 is produced, especially in skeletal muscles—leading to increased heat production. Glucose utilization is increased leading to mild hypoglycemia.

In toxic doses, hyperpyrexia, increased protein catabolism, negative nitrogen balance and hyperglycemia (due to central sympathetic stimulation which increases adrenaline levels) can occur.

7. **Gastrointestinal (GI) tract:** Aspirin is a gastric irritant. Irritation of the gastric mucosa by drug particles leads to epigastric distress, nausea and vomiting. Aspirin also stimulates the chemoreceptor trigger zone (CTZ) to produce vomiting.

Gastric erosion, ulceration and GI bleeding can occur particularly in higher doses.

Salicylates increase gastric acid secretion and suppress the protective effect of prostaglandins by inhibiting their synthesis (we know that PGs increase mucous production in the stomach and protect from ulceration).

In addition aspirin decreases platelet aggregation which also increases the tendency to bleed.

8. **CVS:** In therapeutic doses no significant cardiovascular effects are seen. In toxic doses it depresses the vasomotor center (VMC) and thus depresses the circulation.

9. **Immunological effects:** In higher doses, salicylates suppress several antigen-antibody reactions. It inhibits antibody production, antigen-antibody (Ag-Ab) aggregation and antigen induced release of histamine. These effects might also help in rheumatic fever.

10. **Effects on kidneys:**

a. **Uric acid excretion:** Uric acid is excreted by secretion from the distal tubules. In a dose of 1–2 g/day, aspirin increases plasma urate levels because it inhibits urate secretion by the distal tubules.

Large doses of > 5 g/day increase urate excretion because it inhibits reabsorption of urate by the proximal tubule causing uricosuria. But, its uricosuric effect cannot be used for treatment of gout because high doses are required and such doses result in many adverse effects.

b. **Renal function:** Prostaglandins are released in the kidneys in response to reduced renal blood flow and sodium loss as in hypovolemia. They enhance renal blood flow by renal vasodilation. Inhibition of PG synthesis by NSAIDs reduces renal blood flow and thereby GFR and promote salt and water retention.

Long-term use can result in renal papillary necrosis, all leading to significant impairment of renal function.

11. **Blood:** Even in small doses aspirin inhibits TXA_2 synthesis by platelets. It therefore interferes with platelet aggregation and prolongs the bleeding time. Even a single dose can irreversibly inhibit TXA_2 synthesis in the platelets. Because platelets have no nuclei, they cannot synthesize cyclo-oxygenase and fresh platelets have to be formed to restore TXA_2 activity.

12. **Local effects**: Salicylic acid when applied locally is a keratolytic. It also has mild antiseptic and fungistatic properties. Salicylic acid is also an irritant for the broken skin.

Pharmacokinetics

Salicylates are absorbed from the stomach and the upper small intestine. But aspirin as such is poorly soluble, hence not well-absorbed. When administered as microfine particles, absorption increases. Thus particle size, pH of the GIT, solubility of the preparation and presence of food in the stomach influence the absorption.

Salicylic acid and methyl salicylate are absorbed from the intact skin. They are extensively bound to plasma proteins. Aspirin is broken down in the liver, plasma and other tissues to release salicylic acid which is the active form. Plasma t½ of aspirin is 3–5 hours. Salicylates are excreted in the urine.

Adverse Effects

1. **GIT:** Nausea, epigastric distress, vomiting, gastritis, peptic ulcer, increased (occult) blood loss in stools are common.

2. **Allergic reactions:** Are manifested as rashes, urticaria, angioedema, and asthma especially in those with a history of allergies.

3. **Hemolysis:** Salicylates can cause hemolysis in patients with G_6PD deficiency.

4. **Nephrotoxicity:** Almost all NSAIDs can cause nephrotoxicity after long-term use. Salt and water retention and impaired renal function are seen.

5. **Hepatotoxicity** can occur when high doses are given over long periods.

6. **Respiratory system:** As aspirin inhibits only cyclo-oxygenase pathway, arachidonic acid is available for conversion by lipoxygenase pathway into leukotrienes. Leukotrienes are powerful bronchoconstrictors. Hence, aspirin can precipitate bronchial asthma in some individuals. Of the currently available NSAIDs, diclofenac and indomethacin inhibit the synthesis of both PGs and LTs.

7. **Reye's syndrome:** Seen in children is a form of hepatic dysfunction which may be fatal. It develops a few days after a viral infection especially influenza and varicella.

An increased incidence of this syndrome has been noted when aspirin is used to treat fever. Hence aspirin is contraindicated in children with viral fever. Hence paracetamol should be used to treat fever in such children.

8. **Pregnancy and infancy:** Aspirin when taken in full term pregnancy delays the onset of labor due to inhibition of PG synthesis (PGs play an important role in the initiation of labor).

Premature closure of ductus arteriosus may occur in the fetus resulting in portal hypertension. It can also increase post-partum bleeding due to inhibition of platelet aggregation.

9. **Salicylism:** Prolonged administration of salicylates as in the treatment of rheumatoid arthritis may lead to chronic salicylate intoxication termed 'Salicylism'. The syndrome is characterized by headache, vertigo, dizziness, tinnitus, vomiting, mental confusion, diarrhea, sweating, difficulty in hearing, thirst and dehydration. These symptoms are reversible on withdrawal of salicylates.

Acute salicylate poisoning: Poisoning may be accidental or suicidal. It is more common in children, 15–30 g is the fatal dose of aspirin.

Signs and symptoms: Dehydration, hyperpyrexia, GI irritation, vomiting, sometimes hematemesis, acid-base imbalance, restlessness, delirium, hallucinations, metabolic acidosis, tremors, convulsions, coma and death due to respiratory failure and cardiovascular collapse.

Treatment is symptomatic and includes:

- Stomach wash to remove unabsorbed drugs.
- IV fluids to correct acid-base imbalance and dehydration.
- Temperature is brought down by external cooling with alcohol or cold water sponges.
- If there is bleeding, blood transfusion and vitamin K are needed.
- The IV fluids should contain Na^+, K^+, HCO_3^- and glucose (to treat hypokalemia and acidosis).
- In severe cases, forced alkaline diuresis with sodium bicarbonate and a diuretic like frusemide is given along with IV fluids. Sodium bicarbonate make salicylates water soluble and increases their excretion through kidneys.

Precautions and Contraindications

Peptic ulcer, liver diseases, bleeding tendencies and children suffering from viral fever are contraindications for the use of salicylates. Treatment with NSAIDs should be stopped one week before any surgery.

In pregnancy - aspirin can cause premature closure of ductus arteriosus - hence should be avoided.

Preparations

Preparations and dosage of salicylates (Tables 4.1 and 4.2).

Uses

1. **As analgesic** for headache, backache, myalgias, arthralgias, neuralgias, toothache and dysmenorrhea. The NSAIDs are beneficial in a variety of painful conditions of integumental origin.
2. **Fever:** NSAIDs are useful for the symptomatic relief of fever.
3. **For inflammatory conditions:** Aspirin is effective in a number of inflammatory conditions such as arthritis and fibromyositis.
4. **Acute rheumatic fever:** In a dose of 4–6 g/day, aspirin brings about a dramatic relief of signs and symptoms in 24 to 48 hr. The dose is reduced after 4–7 days and maintenance doses of 2–3 g/day are given for 2–3 weeks.
5. **Rheumatoid arthritis:** Aspirin relieves pain, reduces swelling and redness of joints in rheumatoid arthritis. Joint mobility improves, fever subsides, and there is a reduction in morning stiffness. But NSAIDs do not alter the progress of the disease. The relief is only symptomatic.
   Dose: 4–6 g/day in 4–6 divided doses.

Table 4.1: Preparations and dosage of salicylates.

Drug	*Preparation*	*Dose*
Aspirin	300, 350 tab (Asabuf); Disprin (Aspirin 350 mg and calcium carbonate 105 mg)	Analgesic—300–600 mg every 6–8 hours Anti-inflammatory—4–6 g/day Antiplatelet effects—75–300 mg/day
Sodium salicylate	325, 650 mg tablets	325–650 mg every 4–8 hours
Salicylic acid	2 percent ointment; Whitfield's ointment: • Salicylic acid 3 percent • Benzoic acid 6 percent	For topical use
Methyl salicylate (Oil of wintergreen)	Ointment/liniment for topical use	As counter irritant
Diflunisal	250, 500 mg tab (Dolobid)	250 mg every 8–12 hours

Table 4.2: Topical preparations of NSAIDs.

NSAID	*Preparation*	*Brand name*
Salicylic acid	6% w/w oint 3% oint 2.2% eardrops	KERALIN with acetate and benzoic acid hydrocortisone and menthol MYCODERM with benzoic acid methazil with 6% methanol
Diclofenac diethyl ammonium	1.16% gel	VOVERAN emulgel, RELAXYL gel, INAC gel
Piroxicam	0.5% gel	DOLONEX gel, PIROX gel
Ibuprofen	50 mg gel	ACKS gel with mephenisin, methyl salicylate and menthol
Flurbiprofen	0.03% w/v eyedrops	OCUFLUR
Indomethacin	1% w/v eyedrops	INDOCAP ophthalmic drops
Naproxen	10% gel	XENOLID gel
Ketorolac tromethamine	0.5% w/v eyedrops	KETANOV eyedrops KETLUR
Nimesulide	10 mg gel	NIZU gel with menthol 50 mg and methyl salicylate 100 mg
Rofecoxib	1% gel	ROFIZ gel

6. **Osteoarthritis:** It provides symptomatic relief in osteoarthritis.
7. **Postmyocardial infarction and post-stroke:** Aspirin in a low dose inhibits platelet aggregation and by this it may prevent reinfarction. It also decreases the incidence of transient ischemic attacks (TIA) and stroke in such patients.
8. **Miscellaneous uses:**
   - **To delay labor:** Since PGs are involved in the initiation of labor, aspirin delays labor due to PG synthesis inhibition.
   - **Patent ductus arteriosus:** Aspirin may bring about closure of PDA in the newborn.
9. **Local:** Salicylic acid is used as a keratolytic, fungistatic and mild antiseptic. Methyl salicylate is a counter-irritant used in myalgias.

Drug Interactions

- Salicylates compete for protein binding sites and displace other drugs resulting in toxicity with warfarin, heparin, naproxen, phenytoin and sulfonylureas.
- Inhibition of platelet aggregation may increase the risk of bleeding with oral anticoagulants.

Diflunisal is a derivative of salicylic acid. Diflunisal is 3–4 times more potent than aspirin as an anti-inflammatory agent but is a poor antipyretic due to poor penetration into CNS. Gastrointestinal and antiplatelet effects are less intense than aspirin. Side effects are fewer.

Uses: Osteoarthritis, strain and sprains. Initial dose 500–1000 mg followed by 250 mg twice or thrice daily.

2. Para-aminophenol Derivatives

Paracetamol (Acetaminophen)

Phenacetin was the first drug used in this group. But, due to severe adverse effects it is now banned.

Paracetamol, a metabolite of phenacetin is found to be safer and effective.

Actions: Paracetamol has analgesic, good antipyretic and weak anti-inflammatory properties. Due to weak PG inhibitory activity in the periphery, it has poor anti-inflammatory actions.

Paracetamol is active on cyclo-oxygenase in the brain because of which it acts as an antipyretic. In the presence of peroxides which are present at the site of inflammation, paracetamol has poor ability to inhibit cyclo-oxygenase. It is therefore a poor anti-inflammatory agent. It does not stimulate respiration, has no actions on acid-base balance, cellular metabolism, cardiovascular system and platelet function; it is not an uricosuric agent and gastric irritation is mild.

Pharmacokinetics: Paracetamol is well-absorbed orally, 30 percent protein bound; metabolized by the hepatic microsomal enzymes: by glucuronide and glutathione conjugation.

Adverse effects: In antipyretic doses, paracetamol is safe and well-tolerated. Nausea and rashes may occur. When large doses are taken, *acute paracetamol poisoning* results. Children are more susceptible because their ability to conjugate by glucuronidation is poor. 10–15 g in adults cause serious toxicity. Symptoms are—nausea, vomiting, anorexia and abdominal pain during first 24 hours. Nephrotoxicity may result in acute renal failure in some. Paracetamol is **hepatotoxic** and causes severe hepatic damage. Manifestations are seen within 2–4 days and include increased serum transaminases, jaundice, liver tenderness and prolonged prothrombin time which may progress to liver failure in some patients. Hepatic lesions are reversible when promptly treated.

Mechanism: A small portion of paracetamol is metabolized to a toxic compound—N-acetyl-benzoquinone-imine which is destroyed generally by conjugation with glutathione. However, when large doses of paracetamol are taken, hepatic glutathione gets used up and the levels of toxic compound increase. It causes hepatic necrosis.

Chronic alcoholics and infants are more prone to hepatotoxicity.

Treatment: Stomach wash is given. Activated charcoal prevents further absorption. Antidote is N-acetylcysteine which is more effective when given early.

Uses

- Paracetamol is used as an analgesic in painful conditions like toothache, headache and myalgia.
- As an antipyretic in fevers.

3. Propionic Acid Derivatives

Ibuprofen is better tolerated than aspirin. Analgesic, antipyretic and anti-inflammatory efficacy is slightly lower than aspirin. It is 99 percent bound to plasma proteins.

Adverse effects are milder and the incidence is lower. Nausea, vomiting, gastric discomfort, CNS effects, hypersensitivity reactions, fluid retention are all similar but **less severe**.

Dose: Ibuprofen—400–800 mg TDS (Brufen); Ibuprofen + paracetamol (Combiflam).

Uses

- As an analgesic in painful conditions.
- In fever.
- Soft tissue injuries, fractures, following tooth extraction, to relieve postoperative pain, dysmenorrhea and osteoarthritis.
- Gout.

Other propionic acid derivatives like fenoprofen, ketoprofen, carprofen and naproxen are similar to ibuprofen in actions. Oxaprozin is long acting and given once daily.

4. Acetic Acid Derivatives

Ketorolac: Another PG synthesis inhibitor having good analgesic and anti-inflammatory properties. It is used to relieve postoperative pain. It is mostly used parenterally though it can also be given orally.

Indomethacin is a potent anti-inflammatory agent, antipyretic and good analgesic. It is well-absorbed, 90% bound to plasma proteins; t½—4-6 hours.

Dose: 25-50 mg BD-TDS.

Adverse effects are high: Gastrointestinal irritation with nausea, gastrointestinal bleeding, vomiting, diarrhea and peptic ulcers can occur.

CNS effects include headache, dizziness, ataxia, confusion, hallucinations, depression and psychosis.

Hypersensitivity reactions like skin rashes, leukopenia, and asthma are common. It can also cause bleeding due to decreased platelet aggregation and edema due to salt and water retention.

Drug interactions: Indomethacin blunts the diuretic action of furosemide and the antihypertensive action of thiazides, furosemide, β-blockers and ACE inhibitors by causing salt and water retention.

Uses (Table 4.3)

1. Because of the adverse effects, indomethacin is a reserve drug in rheumatoid

Table 4.3: Properties of some commonly used NSAIDs.

NSAIDs	*Properties*	*Advantages*	*Uses*
Aspirin	Good analgesic, antipyretic, anti-inflammatory and uricosuric agent	• Antiplatelet activity even in low doses • Powerful anti-inflammatory activity	As analgesic-headache, backache, neuralgias, dysmenorrhea; pyrexia, rheumatic fever, rheumatic, psoriatic and osteoarthritis, for antiplatelet activity in post-stroke and post-MI; closure of PDA; to delay labor
Paracetamol	Good analgesic, antipyretic but poor anti-inflammatory	Less gastric irritation	As analgesic in fever
Diclofenac	Analgesic, antipyretic, anti-inflammatory	• Good concentration in synovial fluid • Adverse effects mild	Chronic inflammatory conditions; rheumatoid arthritis, osteoarthritis, acute musculoskeletal pain and postoperative pain; acute pulpitis and acute periapical abscess
Piroxicam	Analgesic, antipyretic, anti-inflammatory	• Long-acting (given once a day) • Less ulcerogenic • Better tolerated	Arthritis, musculoskeletal pain, postoperative pain
Phenylbutazone	Good anti-inflammatory; poor analgesic, antipyretic; salt and water retention causes edema; more toxic than aspirin	Powerful anti-inflammatory agent	Rheumatoid and osteoarthritis; gout, ankylosing spondylitis–however, withdrawn due to toxicity
Indomethacin	Good analgesic, anti-inflammatory and antipyretic but toxicity is high	Potent anti-inflammatory and analgesic	Rheumatoid, psoriatic and osteoarthritis, gout, ankylosing spondylitis, closure of PDA
Ibuprofen	Analgesic, anti-inflammatory, antipyretic all actions milder than aspirin	Adverse effects milder therefore better tolerated	As analgesic in painful conditions, antipyretic, soft tissue injuries, fractures, postoperative pain, arthritis and gout; chronic pulpitis, periodontal abscess, gingival abscess

arthritis, gout, ankylosing spondylitis and psoriatic arthritis.
2. For closure of patent ductus arteriosus.
3. Epidural indomethacin is tried for pain relief in patients who have undergone laminectomy.
4. Topical:
   - Eye drops in inflammation
   - As mouth rinse—to suppress gingival inflammation.

Sulindac has weaker analgesic, antipyretic and anti-inflammatory actions but is less toxic. Does not antagonize the diuretic and antihypertensive actions of thiazides. It may be used as an alternative drug for inflammatory conditions.

Nabumetone is an anti-inflammatory agent with significant efficacy in rheumatoid arthritis and osteoarthritis. It has a relatively low incidence of side effects, it is comparatively less ulcerogenic. Nabumetone is a prodrug and also selectively inhibits COX-2 → due to these reasons nabumetone causes less gastric irritation.

It is used in rheumatoid and osteo-arthritis.

5. Fenamates

Fenamates are analgesic, antipyretic, anti-inflammatory drugs with less efficacy, and are more toxic; contraindicated in children. They should not be used for more than one week. Though they can be used as analgesics they are not preferred.

6. Oxicams

Piroxicam is an oxicam derivative. It is long-acting, has good anti-inflammatory, analgesic and antipyretic activity. No clinically significant drug interactions are seen; better tolerated as it is less ulcerogenic. Dose 20 mg OD. It is **long-acting.** Piroxicam is used for rheumatoid arthritis, osteo-arthritis, ankylosing spondylitis, acute musculoskeletal pain and postoperative pain.

Pivoxicam and **tenoxicam** are other oxicams with action and adverse effects similar to piroxicam.

7. Pyrazolon Derivatives

Phenylbutazone has good anti-inflammatory activity, but has poorer analgesic and antipyretic effects. It is an uricosuric agent.

- Phenylbutazone however is more toxic than aspirin and is poorly tolerated—it can cause GI side effects, edema and CCF.
- Hypersensitivity reactions include serious hematological complications such as bone marrow depression, aplastic anemia, agranulocytosis and thrombocytopenia.
- Hypothyroidism and goiter on long-term use.
- CNS adverse effects are also expected.

Because of its toxicity, phenylbutazone is **withdrawn from the market** in most countries.

Azapropazone is structurally related to phenylbutazone but is less likely to cause agranulocytosis; t½ is 12–16 hours.

Metamizol is a potent analgesic and antipyretic, but poor anti-inflammatory agent and has no uricosuric properties (Analgin, Novalgin) 500 mg 3–4 times a day. It offers no advantages over aspirin. Not recommended in children up to 6 years.

Propiphenazone is similar to metamizol.

Dose: 300–600 mg 3–4 times a day (Saridon).

II. PREFERENTIAL COX-2 INHIBITORS

Diclofenac is an analgesic, antipyretic and anti-inflammatory agent. Its tissue penetrability is good and attains good concentration in synovial fluid which is maintained for a long time. Adverse effects are mild.

Dose: 50 mg BD-TDS. Gel is available for topical application (INAC GEL). Ophthalmic preparation is available for use in postoperative pain.

Uses

- Treatment of chronic inflammatory conditions like rheumatoid arthritis and osteoarthritis.
- Acute musculoskeletal pain.
- Postoperatively for relief of pain and inflammation.

Aceclofenac is more gastric-friendly as it is somewhat COX-2 selective and is also **longer acting**. Hence, it is now largely preferred over diclofenac.

Dose: 100 mg BD (Dolowin 100 mg tab).

Uses

- Treatment of chronic inflammatory conditions like rheumatoid arthritis and osteoarthritis
- Acute musculoskeletal pain, painful dental lesions
- Postoperatively for relief of pain and inflammation
- Eye—to reduce ocular inflammation.

Meloxicam an oxicam is also a preferential COX-2 inhibitor. It causes less gastric irritation and is better tolerated.

Etodolac is similar to diclofenac and is used for its analgesic and anti-inflammatory properties.

Nimesulide a sulfonamide compound is a weak inhibitor of PG synthesis with a higher affinity for COX-2 than COX-1. It inhibits leukocyte function, prevents the release of mediators and in addition has antihistaminic and antiallergic properties. Nimesulide has analgesic, antipyretic and anti-inflammatory actions like other NSAIDs.

Though nimesulide can be used as an analgesic, antipyretic and anti-inflammatory agent and is beneficial in patients who develop bronchospasm with other NSAIDs, **because of the risk of hepatotoxicity, nimesulide is now banned.**

III. SELECTIVE COX-2 INHIBITORS

Coxibs

Though NSAIDs are extremely useful drugs, they are poorly tolerated particularly when they are used for long periods. Gastric irritation is the common side effect which limits their use. Selective inhibition of COX-2 was found to be advantageous because COX-2 is involved in inflammation and COX-1 which is protective on gastroduodenal mucosa is spared (Flowchart 4.1). Highly selective COX-2 inhibitors have been synthesized—such as the coxibs—**celecoxib, parecoxib, etoricoxib** and **valdecoxib**. These drugs have analgesic, anti-inflammatory and antipyretic effects, such as the non-selective NSAIDs but with much less gastric ulcerogenic effects. They also do not inhibit platelet aggregation because COX-1 is involved in platelet function.

Disadvantages

Studies have shown that use of selective COX-2 inhibitors increases the risk of cardiovascular and cerebrovascular thrombotic events—may increase the risk of myocardial infarction and stroke. Hence most of them including rofecoxib and valdecoxib are **withdrawn from the market** and the others are under supervision. They are indicated only in patients who cannot tolerate NSAIDs and are at a high-risk of developing peptic ulcer.

Celecoxib is a highly selective COX-2 inhibitor. It has good anti-inflammatory, analgesic and antipyretic properties but does not affect platelet aggregation.

Flowchart 4.1: Cyclooxygenase activity.

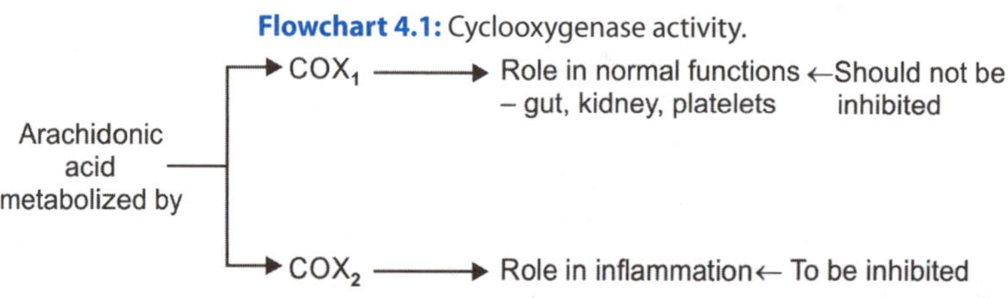

Compare and Contrast
Aspirin and celecoxib (nonselective and selective COX-2 inhibitors)

Features	*Aspirin*	*Celecoxib*
Chemistry	Salicylic acid derivative	Sulfonamide derivatives
COX inhibition	Nonselective (COX-1, COX-2)	Selective COX-2 inhibitors
Ulcerogenic effect on gastric mucosa	+++ (significant)	+ (mild)
t½	Short (2–3 hours)	Long (6–12 hours)
Effect on platelet function	Inhibits platelet aggregation	Does not
Risk of Reye's syndrome in children	Present	Nil
Risk of thrombosis, atherogenesis	Nil	Present
Cardiovascular toxicity	No significant effect	Risk of MI
Cerebrovascular toxicity	No significant effect	Risk of stroke
Use in post-MI patients	Recommended	Contraindicated
Prominent action	Analgesic, antipyretic, anti-inflammatory	Analgesic, antipyretic, anti-inflammatory
PG synthesis	Inhibited	Inhibited

It is better tolerated because of milder gastric irritation (due to COX-2 selectivity)-but more long-term studies are needed. Celecoxib can cause hypertension and edema which can be troublesome in patients with cardiovascular problems. It can be used in acute painful conditions like postoperative pain, dysmenorrhea and dental pain as well as in osteoarthritis and rheumatoid arthritis.

Dose: 100–200 mg once or twice daily.

Etoricoxib is highly selective for COX-2 and long acting to be given once daily. It is better tolerated than other selective COX-2 inhibitors.

Dose: ETOXIB 60, 90, 120 mg tab. HICOX 90, 120 mg tab.

Parecoxib a prodrug of valdecoxib can be given parenterally.

Adverse effects are nausea, epigastric pain, rashes, drowsiness, dizziness and nephrotoxicity. Long-term use can cause **hepatotoxicity**.

Topical NSAID Preparations

Some of the NSAIDs like diclofenac, ibuprofen and paracetamol are available for topical use as ointments and transdermal patch. They may be applied to the site of pain to avoid systemic toxicity. Some systemic absorption occurs but efficacy of these is low. Many NSAIDs are also available as eye drops.

Atypical NSAID

Diacerin has been found to have useful activity in osteoarthritis patients. It inhibits interleukin-1 beta (IL-1 beta) which is involved in the inflammation as well as destruction of the joint cartilage in patients with osteoarthritis. It is well tolerated with minor adverse effects like mild diarrhea which could subside on continued use. It colors the urine a deep yellow. Diacerin is used for long-term generally 6–8 months in osteoarthritis.

CORTICOSTEROIDS

Corticosteroids are hormones produced in the cortex of the adrenal gland. They are **glucocorticoids, mineralocorticoids** and a small amount of **androgens**. Cortisol is the major glucocorticoid while aldosterone is the major mineralocorticoid. The secretion of adrenal cortex is under the control of adrenocorticotropic hormone (ACTH) secreted by the anterior pituitary and this is in turn regulated by corticotropin-releasing factor (CRF). This is termed hypothalamic-pituitary-adrenal axis (Fig. 4.1).

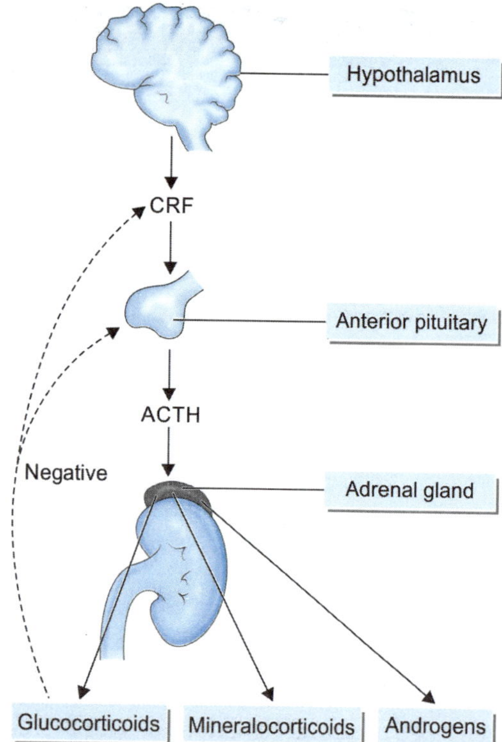

Fig. 4.1: Hypothalamopituitary-adrenal axis; regulation of synthesis and secretion of adrenal corticosteroids.

Structure and Synthesis

The corticosteroids have a steroid (cyclopentanoperhydrophenanthrene) ring. They are synthesized in the adrenal cortex from cholesterol (Flowchart 4.2) under the influence of ACTH.

Every day about 10–20 mg of hydrocortisone (maximum in the early morning) and 0.125 mg of aldosterone are secreted. They are also released in response to stress.

GLUCOCORTICOIDS

Actions

A. *Glucocorticoid Actions*

1. **Metabolic effects:** *Carbohydrate, protein and fat metabolism*—Glucocorticoids promote gluconeogenesis and glycogen deposition in the liver and inhibit peripheral utilization of glucose resulting in increased blood glucose levels. They increase protein breakdown and nitrogen is excreted leading to negative nitrogen balance. Glucocorticoids are catabolic hormones.

They promote lipolysis and redistribution of fat takes place—fat is mobilized from extremities and deposited over the face, neck and shoulder and excess glucocorticoid activity results in symptoms which are described as 'moon face', 'fish mouth' and 'buffalo hump'.

2. **Anti-inflammatory and immunosuppressive effects:** Glucocorticoids have very powerful anti-inflammatory properties

Flowchart 4.2: Synthesis of adrenal steroids.

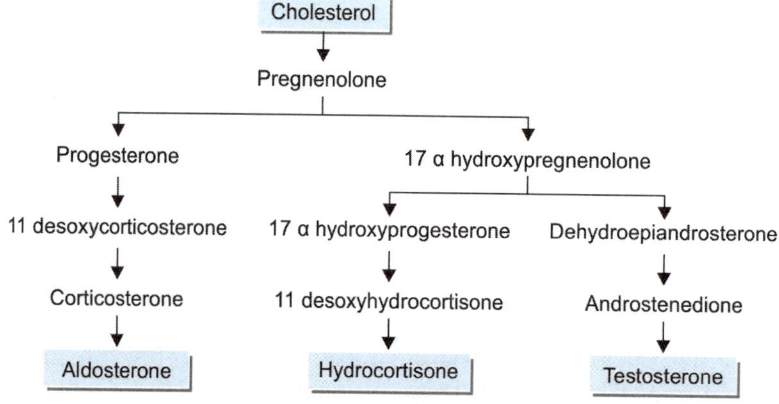

because of which they are used in several conditions. They also have immunosuppressive actions

- Glucocorticoids suppress the development of inflammatory response to all types of stimuli.
- They inhibit both early and late manifestations of inflammation. Inhibition of late response like capillary proliferation, collagen deposition, fibroblastic activity and scar formation may delay wound healing.
- They inhibit migration and depress the function of the leukocytes and macrophages including the release of chemical mediators. The ability of these cells to respond to antigens is decreased.
- In addition glucocorticoids also reduce the synthesis of prostaglandins and leukotrienes by inhibiting phospholipase A2.

Immunosuppressant effects: Glucocorticoids bring about a decrease in the number of WBCs. Glucocorticoids thus suppress cell-mediated immunity, prevent manifestations of allergy and prevent homograft rejection. Large doses also inhibit antibody production.

3. **Other actions:**
   - **Cardiovascular system (CVS):** Glucocorticoids reduce capillary permeability, maintain the tone of arterioles and have a positive inotropic effect. Prolonged use can cause hypertension.
   - **Skeletal muscles:** They are essential for normal muscular activity.
   - **CNS:** They are required for normal functioning of the central nervous system. Deficiency results in apathy and depression while large doses result in restlessness, anxiety and sometimes psychosis.
   - **GIT:** Glucocorticoids enhance the secretion of gastric acid and pepsin in the stomach.
   - **Calcium metabolism:** Glucocorticoids inhibit absorption and increase the renal excretion of calcium—they antagonize the effect of vitamin D on calcium absorption. Bone resorption takes place.
   - **Formed elements of blood:** Glucocorticoids have a lympholytic effect and this effect is very prominent in lymphomas. They also increase the number of platelets and RBCs.
   - **Kidney:** They are essential for maintaining normal GFR.

B. *Mineralocorticoid Action*

Glucocorticoids have a weak mineralocorticoid action—cause some salt and water retention and potassium excretion. Some synthetic glucocorticoids do not have this activity (Table 4.4).

Mechanism of Action

Corticosteroids bind to specific receptors in the cytoplasm, the drug-receptor complex moves into the nucleus where it binds to specific sites on DNA and regulates the synthesis of new proteins that bring about the effects of glucocorticoids. Because of their mechanism of action, steroids are slow acting drugs.

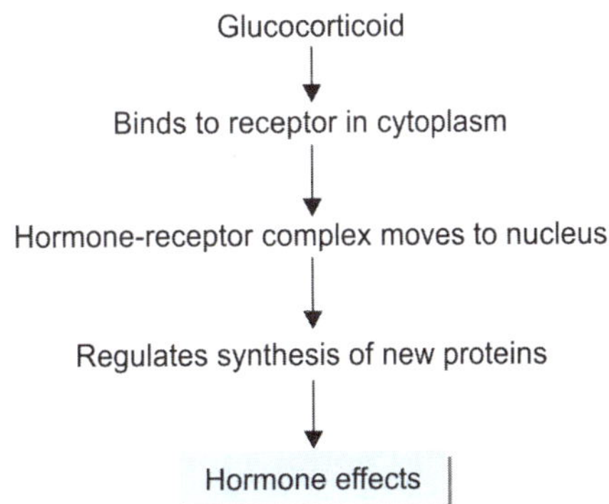

Pharmacokinetics

Most glucocorticoids are well-absorbed orally. Hydrocortisone undergoes high first pass metabolism. It is 95% bound to plasma proteins—transcortin. Glucocorticoids are metabolized by microsomal enzymes in the

Table 4.4: Relative potency of some corticosteroids.

Drug	*Glucocorticoid activity*	*Mineralocorticoid activity*	*Equivalent dose*
Short-acting (8–12 hours)			
Hydrocortisone	1	1	20 mg
Cortisone	0.8	0.8	25 mg
Intermediate-acting (18–36 hours)			
Prednisolone	4	0.8	5 mg
Methylprednisolone	5	0.5	4 mg
Triamcinolone	5	0	4 mg
Fludrocortisone	10	125	2 mg
Long-acting (36–54 hours)			
Paramethasone	10	0	2 mg
Dexamethasone	25	0	0.75 mg
Betamethasone	30	0	0.6 mg
Fludrocortisone	10	125	

liver and are excreted by the kidneys. The t½ varies with each agent and we have short, intermediate and long-acting agents (Table 4.5).

Preparations of glucocorticoids: Glucocorticoids are given by many routes - orally, parenterally, topically, by inhalation and nasal spray (Table 4.6). They may also be injected intra-articularly. The synthetic componds are more potent than hydrocortisone and have less or no mineralocorticoid activity

- **Hydrocortisone**, the chief natural glucocorticoid is used orally and parenterally; in emergencies it is used intravenously.
- **Prednisolone** has potent glucocorticoid with mild mineralocorticoid activity. It is the most commonly used preparation.
- **Prednisone** is a prodrug converted to prednisolone in the liver.
- **Methylprednisolone** is similar to prednisolone and is used as retention enema and for high dose pulse therapy.
- **Triamcinolone, dexamethasone, betamethasone** have no mineralocorticoid activity and have selective, potent glucocorticoid effects.
- **Deflazacort** is a newer glucocorticoid with no mineralocorticoid activity and is particularly suitable for children.

Table 4.5: Preparations and dose of some commonly used glucocorticoids.

Glucocorticoid	*Daily dose*
Hydrocortisone hemisuccinate	30–100 mg IV, IM inj
Prednisolone	5–60 mg oral, 10–40 mg IM
Methylprednisolone acetate	4–32 mg
Triamcinolone	4–20 mg
Dexamethasone	0.5–5 mg oral, 4–20 mg IV/IM
Betamethasone	0.5–5 mg oral, 4–20 mg IM/IV

Table 4.6: Some topical glucocorticoid preparations.

Hydrocortisone (Lycortin oint)	1%
Triamcinolone (Ledercort acetonide oint)	0.1%
Dexamethasone (Decadron cream)	0.1%
Flucinolone acetamide (Flucort oint)	0.025%
Betamethasone (Betnovate oint, cream)	0.025%
Beclomethasone dipropionate (Beclate cream)	0.025%
Clobetasol propionate (Tenovate cream)	0.05%

- **Inhalation:** Beclomethasone, budesonide, fluticasone, mometasone are avilable for inhalation.
- **Nasal spray:** Beclomethasone, budesonide, flunisolide and mometosone are available as nasal spray for allergic rhinitis.

Inhalation steroids	
Beclomethasone (Beclate inhaler)	50 µg, 100 µg 200 µg/metered dose
Budesonide (Budecort)	200 µg/metered dose
Fluticasone (Flohale)	25, 50, 150 µg/metered dose

Topical preparations: Several glucocorticoid preparations are available for topical use as creams, ointments, nasal and eye drops. Some of them also contain antibiotics. The potencies of the preparations vary from mild to very potent. Topical glucocorticoids are used in several inflammatory skin disorders. Topical preparations are more effective when applied under an occlusive dressing, however, such use also increases systemic absorption. Long term use of topical glucocorticooids will result in local thinning and atrophy of the skin and delay wound healing. The area of application also becomes susceptible to infections.

Adverse effects of glucocorticoids: Adverse effects of glucocorticoids (Fig. 4.2) are dependent on the dose, duration of therapy and the relative potency of additional mineralocorticoid effects. Whenever possible, they should be used topically to avoid systemic effects. Single doses are harmless while short courses are well-tolerated. Prolonged use is associated with toxicity. Adverse effects include:

1. **Cushing's syndrome** with characteristic appearance of moon face, buffalo hump, **truncal obesity**, muscle wasting, thinning of the limbs and skin, easy bruising, purple striae and acne.
2. **Hyperglycemia** and sometimes diabetes mellitus may be precipitated.
3. **Increased risk of (susceptibility to) infection:** Risk and severity of any infection may be more because of immunosuppression. Opportunistic infections may occur. Previously inactive tuberculosis may become active.

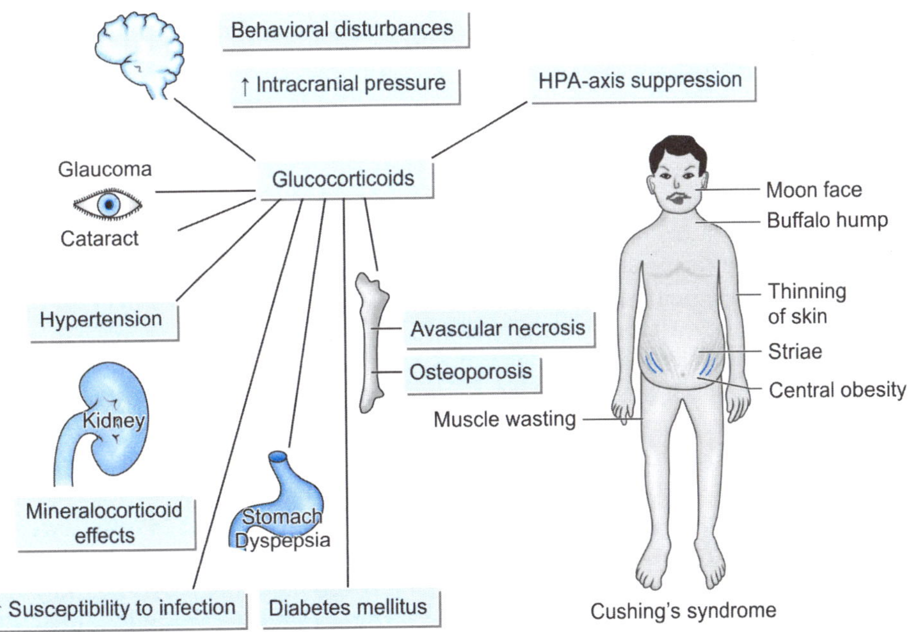

Fig. 4.2: Adverse effects of glucocorticoids.

4. **Osteoporosis** especially of the vertebrae is more common in the elderly.
5. **Avascular necrosis** of the bone due to restriction of blood flow through bone capillaries may cause pain and restriction of movement. Growth in children may be suppressed.
6. **Peptic ulceration** may occur on prolonged therapy especially when other ulcergenic drugs (e.g. NSAIDs) are used together.

Glucocorticoids

↑ gastric acid and pepsin secretion

↓ mucus production → weaken mucosal defense

7. **Mental disturbances** like euphoria, psychosis or depression can occur with high doses.
8. **Cataract** and glaucoma may follow long-term use of glucocorticoids even as eyedrops.
9. **Delayed wound healing:** Steroids may delay wound healing.
10. **Other effects** include raized intracranial pressure, convulsions, hypercoagulability of the blood and menstrual disorders.
11. **Hypothalamic-pituitary-adrenal (HPA) axis suppression:** After prolonged steroid therapy, adrenal cortex gradually atrophies due to feedback inhibition. If steroid administration is suddenly stopped, acute adrenal insufficiency results. Hence after prolonged administration, steroids should be tapered before withdrawal to allow HPA axis to recover. Prior to surgery or general anesthesia, it is advisable to elicit proper drug history. HPA axis suppression depends on the dose, duration and time of administration. If the patient has received long-term steroids within previous six months, prophylactic hydrocortisone should be administered to avoid shock. Two weeks of use of > 20 mg hydrocortisone/day needs tapering of the dose.

In order to minimize HPA axis suppression, (i) **lowest effective** dose of a glucocorticoid for the **shortest possible** *period* should be used, (ii) the drug should be given in a **single morning dose**, (iii) administration on **alternate days** is found to be associated with least/no HPA axis suppression and whenever possible this measure should be followed, especially when long-term steroids are needed.

Mnemonic for Adverse effects

MOM IS DOC AT PHC
M—Mental disturbances
O—Osteoporosis
M—Mineralocorticoid effects
I—↑Intracranial tension
S—Salt and water retention
D—Delayed wound healing
O—Others—convulsions, menstrual disorders
C—Cushing's syndrome
A—HPA axis suppression
T—Truncal obesity
P—Peptic ulceration
H—Hyperglycemia
C—Cataract

12. **Mineralocorticoid effects** including salt and water retention, edema, hypokalemia and hypertension are rare with selective glucocorticoids.

Uses

A. *Replacement Therapy*

1. **Acute adrenal insufficiency** is an emergency condition that could be precipitated by an infection or sudden withdrawal of steroids. Intravenous hydrocortisone hemisuccinate 100 mg bolus followed by infusion is given immediately. Correction of fluid and electrolyte balance are important.
2. **Chronic adrenal insufficiency** (Addison's disease). Oral hydrocortisone 20–40 mg daily is given. Some patients may need additional fludrocortisone (a mineralocorticoid).

B. *Pharmacotherapy*

Glucocorticoids have been used in a variety of nonendocrine conditions where they may even be life saving.

1. **Rheumatoid arthritis:** In progressive disease steroids are given with NSAIDs. If 1–2 joints are involved, intraarticular injections are preferred. They suppress inflammation and benefit such patients.
2. **Osteoarthritis:** Steroids are given as intra-articular injections. A minimum of 3 months interval should be given between two injections of steroids into the joint. Repeated injections can result in joint destruction.
3. **Rheumatic carditis:** Severely ill-patients with fever and carditis but not responding adequately to NSAIDs require glucocorticoids.
4. **Acute gout:** When treatment with NSAIDs have not been successful, prednisolone is used as an adjuvant.
5. **Allergic conditions** like angioneurotic edema, hay fever, serum sickness, contact dermatitis, urticaria, drug reactions and anaphylaxis—steroids are indicated. Steroids are slow acting and in less severe cases, antihistamines should be preferred.

COMPARE AND CONTRAST
Hydrocortisone and dexamethasone

Features	*Hydrocortisone*	*Dexamethasone*
Source	Natural	Synthetic
Mineralocorticoid activity	Present	Absent
Potency	Less potent	More potent
Equivalent dose	20 mg	0.75 mg
Plasma t½	8–12 hours	36–54 hours
Duration of action	Short	Long
Production in the body	Produced (endogenous)	Not produced (exogenous administration)

6. **Bronchial asthma**
   - Acute exacerbations—a short course of prednisolone for 5 days is effective.
   - Status asthmaticus—intravenous hydrocortisone hemisuccinate.
   - Chronic asthma—steroids are used as supplement to bronchodilators. Inhalational steroids are used and in more severe cases low dose oral prednisolone is indicated.
7. **Collagen diseases** like polyarthritis nodosa, lupus erythematosus, polymyositis, Wegener's granulomatosis and other rheumatoid disorders respond to glucocorticoids.
8. **Eye diseases:** Allergic conjunctivitis, uveitis, optic neuritis and other inflammatory conditions are treated with steroids. In ocular infections, steroids are contraindicated.
9. **Renal diseases** like nephrotic syndrome are treated with steroids.
10. **Skin diseases:** Atopic dermatitis, seborrheic dermatitis, inflammatory dermatoses and other local skin conditions are treated with topical steroids. Systemic steroids are *life saving* in pemphigus.
11. **Gastrointestinal diseases:** Mild inflammatory bowel diseases like ulcerative colitis are treated with steroid enema while severe cases need oral prednisolone.
12. **Liver diseases:** Steroids are useful in conditions like chronic active hepatitis and alcoholic hepatitis.
13. **Hematologic disorders** like purpura and hemolytic anemia having immunological etiology respond to steroids.
14. **Cerebral edema:** Large doses of dexamethasone is given.
15. **Malignancies:** Because of their lympholytic effects, steroids are used in the treatment of acute lymphocytic leukemia and lymphomas—as a component of combination chemotherapy. Steroids are used for rapid symptomatic relief in other cancers like breast cancer.
16. **Lung diseases:** Apart from bronchial asthma, steroids are used in other diseases like aspiration pneumonia and

prevention of infant respiratory distress syndrome.

17. **Organ transplantation:** For prevention and treatment of graft rejection, high doses of prednisolone are started at the time of surgery with immunosuppressive agents.
18. **Thyroid storm:** Glucocorticoids inhibit the peripheral conversion of T4 to T3 and may be of additional value.
19. **Autoimmune hemolytic anemia:** Glucocorticoids reduce destruction of RBCs.
20. **Sarcoidosis:** Responds to glucocorticoids.

Contraindications to glucocorticoid therapy	
Steroids should be used with caution in:	
• Peptic ulcer	• Psychoses
• Hypertension	• Epilepsy
• Infections	• CCF
• Diabetes mellitus	• Glaucoma
• Osteoporosis	• Renal failure

Mineralocorticoids

The most important natural mineralocorticoid is aldosterone which is synthesized in zona glomerulosa of the adrenal cortex. Small amounts of desoxycorticosterone is also released.

Actions: Mineralocorticoids promote sodium and water retention by distal renal tubules with loss of potassium. They act by binding to the mineralocorticoid receptor.

Adverse effects: Include weight gain, edema, hypertension and hypokalemia.

Fludrocortisone: Has predominantly mineralocorticoid properties and is used for replacement therapy in aldosterone deficiency as in Addison's disease. Although aldosterone is the principle natural mineralocorticoid, it is not used therapeutically since it is not effective orally.

DRUGS USED IN TREATMENT OF RHEUMATOID ARTHRITIS

Rheumatoid arthritis (RA) is a chronic, progressive, autoimmune, inflammatory disease, mainly affecting the joints and the periarticular tissues. Antigen–antibody complexes trigger the pathological process.

Mediators of inflammation released in the joints initiate the inflammatory process. The earliest lesion is vasculitis, followed by synovial edema and infiltration with inflammatory cells. There is local synthesis of prostaglandins and leukotrienes. Prostaglandins cause vasodilation and pain. The inflammatory cells release lysosomal enzymes which cause damage to bones and cartilage. Drugs used in the treatment of RA are:

I. **NSAIDs**

II. **Glucocorticoids**

III. **Disease modifying anti-rheumatic drugs (DMARDs)**

1. ***Immunosuppressants:*** Methotrexate, cyclophosphamide, azathioprine, cyclosporine, leflunomide, chloroquine, hydroxychloroquine
2. ***Biological agents:***
   a. *Tumor necrosis factor (TNF)-alpha blockers:* Etanercept, infliximab, adalimumab, certolizumab, golimumab
   b. *Other biologicals:* Abatacept, Anakinra, Rituximab, Kanakinumab, Tocilizumab
3. ***Miscellaneous:*** Gold salts, penicillamine, sulphasalazine

Nonsteroidal Anti-inflammatory Drugs

Nonsteroidal anti-inflammatory drugs are the first-line drugs in RA. NSAIDs only **provide symptomatic relief** but do not modify the course of the disease. Long-term use of these drugs is associated with significant toxicity; higher doses are required for anti-inflammatory activity. Aspirin, ibuprofen, diclofenac, naproxen, and piroxicam are commonly used. Many of the selective COX-2 inhibitors are now banned due to toxicity.

Glucocorticoids

Glucocorticoids have anti-inflammatory and immunosuppressant activity. They produce prompt and dramatic relief of symptoms but do not arrest the progress of the disease. However, long-term use of these drugs leads to several adverse effects. Moreover, on withdrawal of glucocorticoids, there may be an exacerbation of the disease.

Therefore, glucocorticoids are used only as adjuvants. They may be used to treat exacerbations. Low dose long-term treatment with prednisolone (5–10 mg/day) or IM depot methylpredinsolone 80–160 mg are used in some patients. Intra-articular corticosteroids are helpful to relieve pain in severely inflamed joints.

Disease Modifying Anti-rheumatic Drugs

Disease modifying antirheumatic drugs (DMARDs) are reserved for patients with progressive disease who do not obtain satisfactory relief from NSAIDs. They are capable of arresting the progress of the disease and inducing remission in these patients.

Recent studies have shown that RA causes significant systemic effects that shorten life expectancy. This has renewed interest in the use of DMARDs in RA. The effects of these drugs may take 6 weeks to 6 months to become evident and are, therefore, also called slow acting anti-rheumatic drugs (SAARDs).

Immunosuppressants

Methotrexate, cyclophosphamide, azathioprine and leflunomide are the immunosuppressants used in RA. They are cytotoxic drugs and are reserved for patients with severe disease with reversible lesions. Among the immunosuppressants, methotrexate is the best tolerated.

Methotrexate: Methotrexate is a commonly used anticancer drug which, in lower doses than that used in cancers, provides significant benefit in patients with RA.

Mechanism of action: Methotrexate is a folic acid antagonist. It inhibits the enzyme dihydrofolate reductase and prevents the synthesis of tetrahydrofolate (THF). This tetrahydrofolate is essential for several reactions in DNA, RNA and protein synthesis. Thus, THF deficiency results in inhibition of protein synthesis. Mechanism of action of methotrexate in RA is probably that:

- It increases adenosine levels which is a potent inhibitor of inflammation.
- Methotrexate also inhibits cytokines, directly suppresses the cells involved in inflammation and immunological diseases and stimulates apoptosis of these cells.
- Inhibition of DHFR could influence macrophage and lymphocyte function.

Methotrexate is now the **most commonly used drug** in autoimmune disorders.

Adverse effects include nausea, vomiting, diarrhea, mucosal ulcers, bone marrow suppression, loss of hair, dermatitis, nephrotoxicity and hepatotoxicity. Weekly regimens of low oral doses are better tolerated.

Folinic acid (or leucovorin) rescue may be given to reduce toxicity with higher doses of methotrexate. Folinic acid gets converted to a form of tetrahydrofolate that can be utilized by the cells.

Azathioprine, a purine analog, is a prodrug converted to 6-thioguanine in the body. It suppresses the cell-mediated immunity and inhibits T and B cell function. It is used as an alternative to methotrexate. **Dose:** 25 mg OD.

Cyclophosphamide, an alkylating agent, also inhibits T cell and B cell function. It is given orally in RA and other autoimmune disorders.

Leflunomide is a prodrug. The active metabolite inhibits autoimmune T cell proliferation and production of auto-antibodies by B cells. Leflunomide is orally effective, undergoes enterohepatic circulation and has a long t½ of 5–40 days.

Adverse effects include diarrhea and raised hepatic enzymes. It can also cause weight gain, hypertension and sometimes alopecia.

Uses: Leflunomide is used with methotrexate in rheumatoid arthritis patients not responding to methotrexate alone.
Dose: Initially 100 mg daily for 3 days followed by 20 mg OD.

Cyclosporine is an immunosuppressant that has now been approved for use in RA, SLE, psoriasis and polymyositis. It is given orally 2–5 mg/kg/day and the dose is gradually increased.

Mycophenolate mofetil has been occasionally used in RA but its efficacy is yet to be established.

Hydroxychloroquine and chloroquine: These antimalarial drugs (*See* page 275) are found to be useful in mild non-erosive rheumatoid arthritis. They induce remission in 50% of patients. Mechanism of action is not exactly understood but they are known to depress cell-mediated immunity.

Adverse effects: Chloroquine and hydroxychloroquine accumulate in tissues leading to toxicity.

The most significant adverse effect is the retinal toxicity on long-term use. This toxicity is less common and reversible with **hydroxychloroquine which is, therefore, preferred over chloroquine in rheumatoid arthritis.**

Every 3 months eyes should be tested. Other adverse effects include myopathy, neuropathy and irritable bowel syndrome.

Hydroxychloroquine: Dose: 400 mg/day for 4–6 weeks; maintenance dose—200 mg/day.

Biological Agents

TNF-α Blocking Agents

Cytokines, particularly tumor necrosis factor (TNF-α) plays an important role in the process of inflammation. TNF-α produced by macrophages and activated T cells, acts through TNF-α receptors to stimulate the release of other cytokines. TNF-α blocking drugs infliximab, etanercept and adalimumab, are found to be useful in RA.

Infliximab is a monoclonal antibody which specifically binds with high affinity to human TNF-α. When given in combination with methotrexate, it slows the progression of RA. It is given intravenously as an infusion 3–5 mg/kg every 8 hour. It has a long t½ of 9–12 days. Adverse effects of the combination include increased susceptibility to upper respiratory infections, dormant tuberculosis may become active. Nausea, headache, cough, sinusitis, skin rashes and allergic reactions can occur. Rarely hepatitis and activation of viral hepatitis have been reported. Antinuclear and anti-DNA antibodies may develop and this can be largely avoided by giving methotrexate along with infliximab.

Dose: 3–5 mg/kg 8 hourly.

Uses: Infliximab can be used in many conditions of autoimmune etiology like ankylosing spondylitis, Crohn's disease, psoriasis, ulcerative colitis and sarcoidosis.

Infliximab is used in RA along with methotrexate or one of the other DMARDs.

Etanercept is a recombinant fusion protein that binds to TNF-α molecules. It is given subcutaneously and is found to slow the progression of the disease in RA patients. It is also found to be useful in psoriatic and juvenile arthritis. Etanercept is also given with methotrexate and the combination has a higher efficacy.

Pain, itching and allergic reactions at the site of injection, anti-etanercept antibodies and anti-DNA antibodies have been detected.

Dose: 50 mg weekly SC.

Adalimumab is an anti-TNF monoclonal antibody which acts similar to infliximab but is less immunogenic. It is given SC 40 mg/week. It is used along with methotrexate for better efficacy.

Certolizumab is an anti TNF-α antibody which neutralizes TNF-α. It is given subcutaneously every 2–4 weeks in moderate to severe RA as monotherapy with other DMARDs.

Golimumab: Another anti TNF-α antibody used SC with methotrexate every 4 weeks in moderate to severe RA.

Other Biologicals

Abatacept inhibits the activation of T cells. It has a long t½ of 13–16 days. Given as IV infusion 800–1000 mg and repeated after 2 and 4 weeks brings about a symptomatic improvement. The infusion is then repeated at monthly intervals. It is well-tolerated, may cause hypersensitivity reactions on infusion. Abatacept may increase the risk of upper respiratory infections particularly if combined with TNF-α blockers and the combination should be avoided.

Rituximab is a monoclonal **antibody against B cells** and is used in lymphomas. Reduction in B cells suppresses the inflammatory process, inhibits the release of cytokines. It has been approved for use in moderate to severe active RA along with methotrexate.

Anakinra is a recombinant **IL-1 receptor antagonist** tried in patients not responding to other DMARDs.

Tocilizumab: IL-6, a proinflammatory cytokine is produced by most inflammatory cells including T cells and B cells. Tocilizumab is an **IL-6 antibody** which binds to IL-6 receptors and blocks its action. Tocilizumab may be used (IV once in 4 weeks) as monotherapy or with a DMARD in moderate to severe RA who have failed to respond to other DMARDs. Increased susceptibility to infection is a limiting factor.

Other Anti-rheumatic Drugs

Gold salts are **no more preferred** because of their toxicity and the availability of safer agents. Gold salts - aurothiamalate and auranofin, depress cell mediated immunity.

Adverse effects: Treatment with gold is associated with **several adverse effects.**

Dermatitis, hepatotoxicity, nephrotoxicity, encephalitis, peripheral neuritis, pulmonary fibrosis and bone marrow suppression can occur.

D-Penicillamine, is a metabolite of penicillin, a chelating agent that chelates copper. Its actions and toxicities are similar to gold and hence it is **not preferred**.

Sulphasalazine is a compound of sulphapyridine and 5-amino salicylic acid. In the colon, sulphasalazine is split by the bacterial action and sulphapyridine gets absorbed. This has anti-inflammatory actions though the mechanism is not known. Adverse effects include GI upset and skin rashes. **Dose:** 500–1000 mg BD-TDS.

Immunoadsorption apheresis: Extracorporeal immunoadsorption of plasma for the removal of IgG containing immunocomplexes has been approved for the treatment of moderate to severe rheumatoid arthritis. The duration of benefit varies from a few months to several years. Adverse effects are mild and tolerable.

Diet and inflammation: Clinical studies have shown that when patients of RA are given a diet rich in unsaturated fatty acids (such as marine fish), there is a decrease in morning stiffness, pain and swelling of the joints. Mediators of inflammation like prostaglandins and leukotrienes are products of arachidonic acid metabolism. Unsaturated fatty acids compete with arachidonic acid for uptake and metabolism. Moreover, the metabolic products of unsaturated fatty acids are only weak inflammatory mediators when compared to the products of arachidonic acid metabolism. Adequate consumption of marine fish should be recommended. For people who do not eat fish, eicosapentaenoic acid 1–4 g/day may be given as tablets. It serves as an adjuvant.

TREATMENT OF GOUT

Gout is a familial metabolic disorder characterized by recurrent episodes of acute arthritis due to deposits of monosodium urate in the joints and cartilage. There is an inherent abnormality of purine metabolism resulting in overproduction of uric acid—a major end product of purine metabolism. As uric acid is poorly water-soluble, it gets recipitated—especially at low pH and deposited in the cartilages of joints and ears, subcutaneous tissues, bursae and sometimes in kidneys. An acute attack of gout occurs as an inflammatory reaction to crystals of sodium urate deposited in the joint tissue. There is infiltration of granulocytes which phagocytize the urate crystals and release a glycoprotein that causes joint destruction. The joint becomes red, swollen, tender and extremely painful.

Secondary hyperuricemia may be drug induced or may occur in lymphomas, leukemias and polycythemia. Chemotherapy and radiation could also result in hyperuricemia due to increased metabolism of nucleic acids and thereby increased production of uric acid. Several drugs can also induce hyperuricemia. Gout may also be due to decreased excretion of uric acid. Strategy in the treatment of gout is either to decrease the biosynthesis of uric acid or increase its excretion.

Drugs Used in Gout

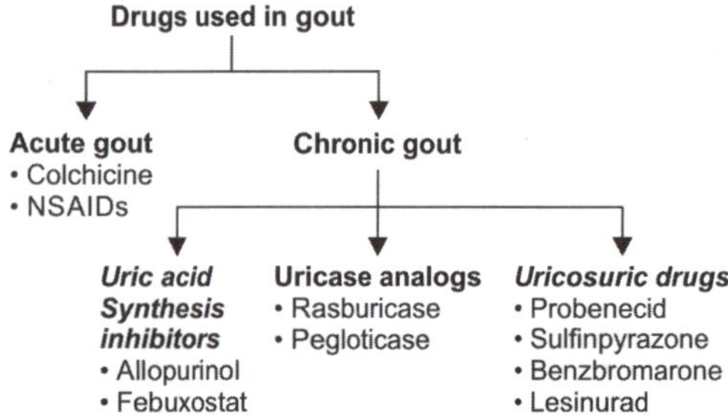

Colchicine is an alkaloid of *Colchicum autumnale.* It is a unique anti-inflammatory agent effective only against gouty arthritis. It is not an analgesic and also does not alter the production of uric acid.

Arrests cell division in metaphase

Colchicine → Binds to tubulin and prevents formation of microtubules

Inhibits migration of leukocytes into inflamed area.
Inhibits release of glycoprotein by leukocytes

Actions: In gout, colchicine is highly effective in acute attacks and it dramatically relieves pain within a few hours.

Mechanism of action: Colchicine inhibits the migration of granulocytes into the inflamed area and the release of glycoprotein by them. It binds to the protein tubulin and prevents its conversion into microtubules and inhibits the migration of leukocytes and also their phagocytosis.

Colchicine also binds to microtubules and arrests cell division in metaphase.

Other actions: It increases gut motility by neurogenic stimulation and causes diarrhea.

Pharmacokinetics: Colchicine is rapidly absorbed orally, metabolized in the liver and undergoes enterohepatic circulation.

Adverse effects are dose related. Nausea, vomiting, diarrhea and abdominal pain are the earliest side effects. Though these may be avoided by giving colchicine intravenously, it can cause serious toxicity and hence IV colchicine should be avoided. Anemia, leukopenia and alopecia may be seen. In high doses, hemorrhagic gastroenteritis, nephrotoxicity, muscular paralysis, acute renal failure, respiratory failure, shock and fatal CNS depression can occur.

Uses

1. **Acute gout:** Colchicine 1 mg orally initially, followed by 0.5 mg every 2–3 hours relieves pain and swelling within 12 hours. But diarrhea limits its use.
2. **Prophylaxis:** Colchicine may also be used for the prophylaxis of recurrent episodes of gouty arthritis 0.6 mg OD-TDS.

NSAIDs provide symptomatic relief in the treatment of gout due to their anti-inflammatory activity.

Indomethacin, piroxicam, naproxen, and diclofenac can be used. They relieve an acute attack in 12–24 hours and are better tolerated than colchicine. They can be given in lower doses for 2–4 weeks. NSAIDs are not recommended for long-term use due to their toxicity.

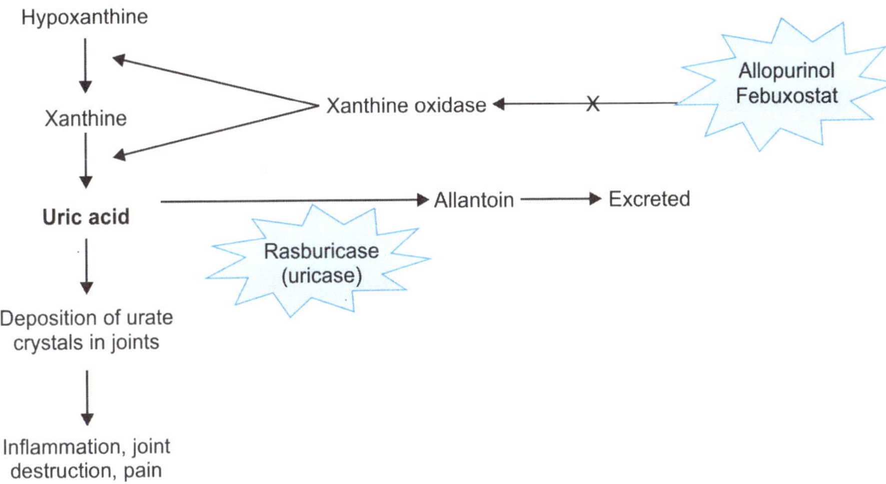

Fig. 4.3: Sites of action of drugs in gout.

Allopurinol is an analog of hypoxanthine and inhibits the biosynthesis of uric acid.

Mechanism of action: Purine nucleotides are degraded to hypoxanthine. Uric acid is produced from hypoxanthine as shown in Figures 4.3 and 4.4. Allopurinol and its metabolite alloxanthine both inhibit the enzyme xanthine oxidase and thereby prevent the synthesis of uric acid. The plasma concentration of uric acid is reduced.

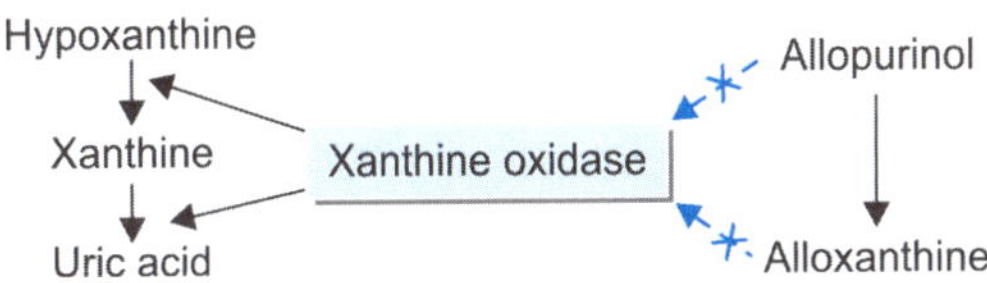

Fig. 4.4: Biosynthesis of uric acid. Both allopurinol and alloxanthine suppress the enzyme xanthine oxidase

Pharmacokinetics: Allopurinol is 80% absorbed orally; t½ of allopurinol is 2–3 hour; and t½ of alloxanthine, 24 hour.

Adverse effects are mild. Hypersensitivity reactions include fever and rashes. GI irritation, headache, nausea and dizziness may occur.

Attacks of acute gouty arthritis may be seen frequently during the initial months of treatment with allopurinol.

Drug interactions: The anticancer drugs, 6-mercaptopurine and azathioprine, are metabolized by xanthine oxidase. Hence when allopurinol is used concurrently, the dose of these anti-cancer drugs should be reduced.

Uses: Allopurinol is used in chronic gout and secondary hyperuricemia. Initial dose is 100 mg/day and may be gradually increased to 300 mg/day depending on the response.

Colchicine or an NSAID should be given during the first few weeks of allopurinol therapy to prevent the acute attacks of gouty arthritis. On treatment with allopurinol, tophi are gradually resorbed and the formation of renal stones is prevented. In patients with large tophaceous deposits, both allopurinol and uricosuric drugs can be given.

Dose: 100–300 mg OD.

Febuxostat is another xanthine oxidase inhibitor but it is not purine. It reduces the formation of xanthine and uric acid. Like allopurinol, treatment with febuxostat can cause gout flares. It can also cause nausea, diarrhea, headache and altered liver function.

Febuxostat is well absorbed and extensively metabolized in the liver. It is used in the dose of 80–120 mg for the treatment of chronic gout.

Uricase Analogs

Rasburicase: Uricase (Urate Oxidase) is an enzyme present in mammals but absent in human beings. It converts uric acid to allantoin which is a highly soluble product and easily excreted by the kidneys. Rasburicase is recombinant uricase and **pegloticase** is recombinant uricase attached to methoxypolythylene glycol (mPEG). Given IV (4–12 mg) it rapidly reduces uric acid levels in 1–3 days, maintaining it up to 21 days.

$$\text{Uric Acid} \xrightarrow[\text{Rasburicase}]{} \text{Allantoin} \longrightarrow \text{Excreted}$$

Adverse effects include **allergic reactions**, gout flare, nausea, anemia and methemoglobinemia. They are to be avoided in G6PD deficiency. Rasburicase and pegloticase are used in tumor lysis syndrome and refractory chronic gout.

Uricosuric Drugs

Probenecid is an organic acid developed to inhibit the renal tubular secretion of penicillin in order to prolong its action. Probenecid blocks tubular reabsorption of uric acid and thereby promotes its excretion. Plasma urate pool decreases and tophaceous deposits are gradually reabsorbed. It is ineffective in presence of renal insufficiency as it acts through the kidney. It is well-absorbed and well-tolerated. Adverse effects include GI irritation and skin rashes.

Large amounts of water should be given to prevent the formation of renal stones. Probenecid is indicated in chronic gout and secondary hyperuricemia. It is started with 500 mg once a day and gradually increased to 1 g/day. Probenecid may also precipitate acute attacks of gout due to fluctuating urate levels.

Sulphinpyrazone, a pyrazolone derivative, is another uricosuric drug which has actions and adverse effects similar to probenecid. Duration of action is similar to probenecid—given once or twice daily. It is used in chronic gout in an initial dose of 200 mg/day and gradually increased to 400–800 mg/day.

Benzbromarone is a uricosuric drug which acts by inhibiting renal tubular reabsorption of uric acid. It is a potent uricosuric given 40–80 mg, once daily. It is used as an alternative in patients allergic to other drugs.

Benzbromarone can also be used in combination with allopurinol.

IMMUNOSUPPRESSANTS AND IMMUNOSTIMULANTS

Immunosuppressants are drugs which inhibit immunity. They may suppress cell mediated or humural immunity or both. They are:

- **T-cell inhibitors:** Cyclosporine, tacrolimus, sirolimus, mycophenolate mofetil.
- **Cytotoxic drugs:** Azathioprine, methotrexate, cyclophosphamide, chlorambucil, leflunomide.
- **Glucocorticoids**
- **Immunosuppressant antibodies:** Muromonab CD3, antithymocyte globulin.

T-Cell Inhibitors

Cyclosporine is a cyclic peptide produced by a fungus *Beauveria nivea.*

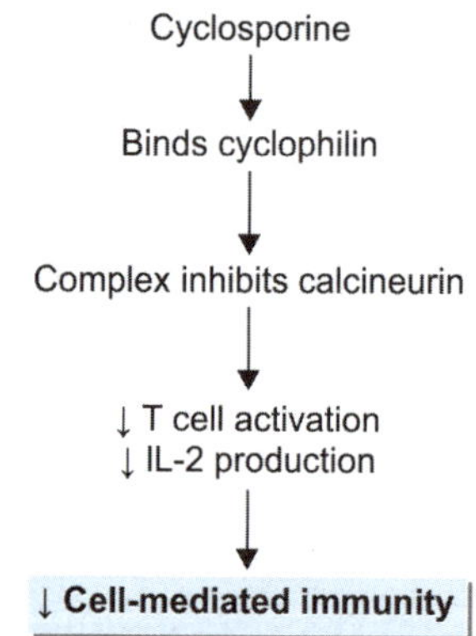

Actions: Cyclosporine acts at an early stage and selectively inhibits T cell-proliferation. It also inhibits interleukin-2 production. Thus cyclosporine selectively suppresses cell mediated immunity but not humoral immunity.

Mechanism of action: Cyclosporin binds to cycliphilin and this complex binds to and inhibits the enzyme calcineurin phosphatase.

This results in inhibition of T-cell activation and IL 2 production. T cells do not respond to specific antigenic stimulation. Cyclosporin also suppresses the proliferation of cytotoxic T cells.

Adverse effects include nephrotoxicity, hepatotoxicity, anorexia, gum hypertrophy and increased susceptibility to infections, hypertension, hyperglycemia, hyperlipidemia and hirsutism.

Uses

- **In organ transplantation:** Cyclosporine is very effective for the prophylaxis and treatment of graft rejection in organ transplantation surgeries—like kidney, liver, bone marrow and other transplants.
- **Autoimmune disorders:** Cyclosporine is also useful in some autoimmune disorders like rheumatoid arthritis, severe psoriasis, atopic dermatitis, inflammatory bowel disease and nephrotic syndrome.

Tacrolimus is a macrolide antibiotic obtained from *Streptomyces tsukubaensis*. Its mechanism of action is similar to cyclosporine. Tacrolimus can be given both orally and parenterally but absorption from the gut is incomplete. It is extensively bound to plasma proteins.

Adverse effects include nephrotoxicity, gastrointestinal disturbances, hypertension, hyperglycemia, tremors and seizures.

Sirolimus obtained from *Streptomyces hygroscopicus* acts by inhibiting the activation of T-cells. Sirolimus may be used in combination with other drugs for immunosuppression.

Toxicity includes hyperlipidemia, gastrointestinal disturbances and an increased risk of infections and lymphomas.

Everolimus is similar to tacrolimus with minor differences.

Uses:

1. Tacrolimus, sirolimus and everolimus are used for the prevention of **graft rejection in organ transplantation.**
2. **Psoriasis:** Topical sirolimus is used
3. **Coronary stents:** Sirolimus or everolimus are incorporated into cardiac stents to inhibit local cell proliferation and to reduce restenosis - these are called drug elluting stents.
4. **Uveoretinitis:** Sirolimus is used to suppress inflammation.

Mycophenolate mofetil a prodrug is converted to mycophenolic acid, which inhibits guanine nucleotide synthesis and inhibits the proliferation and functions of lymphocytes.

Mycophenolate mofetil is indicated as an adjunct to other immunosuppressive drugs in the prophylaxis of transplant rejection.

Cytotoxic drugs like azathioprine, cyclophosphamide and methotrexate inhibit cell mediated immunity (while cyclophosphamide predominantly suppresses humoral immunity). They are used in the prevention of graft rejection and in autoimmune disorders.

Leflunomide is a prodrug. The active metabolite inhibits autoimmune T cell proliferation and production of antibodies by T cells. Leflunomide is orally effective, undergoes enterohepatic circulation and has a long $t\frac{1}{2}$ of 5–40 days.

Leflunomide is used with methotrexate in rheumatoid arthritis patients not responding to methotrexate alone.

Glucocorticoids have potent immunosuppressant activity and are used in the prevention of organ transplant rejection and in autoimmune disorders.

Antibodies as Immunosuppressants

Muromonab CD3 is a monoclonal antibody to CD3 antigens on T lymphocytes. On intravenous administration, T cells disappear from the circulation within minutes. It is used with other immunosuppressants in organ transplantation. Fever, chills and pulmonary edema may occur.

Antithymocyte globulin (ATG) binds to T lymphocytes and deplete them thereby suppressing immune response. It is used in the management of organ transplantation.

Infliximab is a monoclonal antibody and **etanercept** is a protein that blocks TNFα. They are useful in rheumatoid arthritis and Crohn's disease and psoriatic arthritis.

Hydroxycholoquine, an antimalarial drug like chloroquine also has immunosuppressant properties for which it is used in rheumatoid arthritis and systemic lupus erythematosus (SLE).

Interferons

Interferons are cytokines with antiviral and immunomodulatory properties. Recombinant interferons α, β and γ are available for clinical use. They bind to specific receptors and bring about immune activation and increase host defenses. There is an increase in the number and activity of cytotoxic and helper T cells and killer cells.

Interferons α, and β are mainly used for antiviral effects while interferon γ is used for its immunomodulating actions.

Interferons are indicated in several tumors including malignant melanoma, hairy cell leukemia, lymphomas, Kaposi's sarcoma, condylomata acuminata and in viral infections.

Immunostimulants

Immunostimulating or immunomodulating agents are drugs that modulate the immune response and can be used to increase the immune responsiveness of patients with immunodeficiency as in AIDS, chronic illness and cancers. This is still a developing field of pharmacology. The drugs currently used for this purpose are **BCG, levamisole** and interferons. BCG has been tried in cancers. Levamisole used in helminthiasis is also found to enhance cell-mediated immunity in humans. It has been tried in some cancers.

Immunization vaccines are used for active immunization and antisera are used for passive immunization. Both of them impart immunity.

Immunoglobulins are human gamma globulins that carry the antibodies, e.g., normal human gammaglobulin, tetanus Ig, rabies Ig, anti-diphtheria Ig and hepatitis B Ig. Allergic reactions including serum sickness and anaphylaxis can occur with antisera, while it is uncommon with immunoglobulins.

5

CHAPTER

Drugs Acting on the Kidney

CHAPTER HIGHLIGHTS

- Physiology of Urine Formation
- Diuretics
- Antidiuretics

DIURETICS AND ANTIDIURETIC DRUGS

Kidney, the excretory organ of our body serves the important functions of excretion of waste products, regulation of fluid volume and electrolyte content of the extracellular fluid.

PHYSIOLOGY OF URINE FORMATION

Normally about 180 liters of fluid is filtered everyday, of which 99% gets reabsorbed and about 1.5 liters of urine is formed. For simplification, the nephron can be divided into four sites (Fig. 5.1).

Proximal tubule: Sodium bicarbonate, sodium chloride, amino acids and glucose are reabsorbed in the proximal tubule along with water by specific transport mechanisms. Osmotic diuretics act here.

Henle's loop: In the thin descending limb of the loop of Henle, water is reabsorbed by osmotic forces. Hence osmotic diuretics are acting here too. The thick ascending limb actively reabsorbs sodium chloride from the lumen (but is impermeable to water) by $Na^+/K^+/2Cl^-$ co-transporter. 'Loop diuretics' selectively block this transporter.

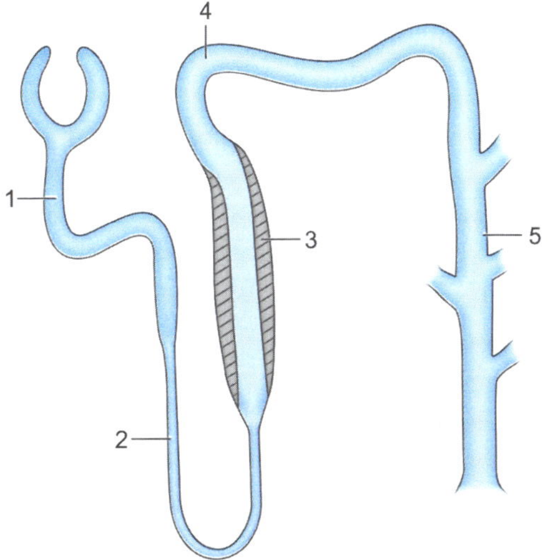

Fig. 5.1: Simplified diagram of a nephron showing sites of action of diuretics: (1) Proximal tubule—acetazolamide, (2) Descending limb of Henle's loop—osmotic diuretics, mannitol, (3) Ascending limb of Henle's loop—loop diuretics, (4) Early distal tubule—thiazides, (5) Distal tubule and collecting duct—K^+ sparing diuretics.

Distal convoluted tubule: In the early distal tubule, sodium chloride is reabsorbed by an electrically neutral Na^+ and Cl^- transporter. This transporter is blocked by thiazide diuretics.

Collecting tubule: In the late distal tubule and collecting duct, $NaCl^-$ is actively reabsorbed, in exchange for K^+ and H^+ to maintain the ionic balance-regulated by aldosterone. Absorption of water is under the control of antidiuretic hormone (ADH).

DIURETICS

Diuretic is an agent which increases urine and solute excretion.

Classification

1. **High efficacy diuretics (loop diuretics)**
   - Furosemide, bumetanide, piretanide, ethacrynic acid, torsemide, azosemide
2. **Moderate efficacy diuretics**
   - **Thiazides:** Benzothiadiazines like chlorothiazide, hydrochlorothiazide, polythiazide, bendroflumethiazide
   - **Thiazide - like diuretics:** Chlorthalidone, clopamide, indapamide, metolazone, xipamide
3. **Low efficacy diuretics**
   - **Potassium sparing diuretics:** Triamterene, amiloride, spironolactone, eplerenone
   - **Carbonic anhydrase inhibitors:** Acetazolamide
   - **Osmotic diuretics:** Mannitol, urea, glycerol
   - **Methylxanthines:** Theophylline

High Efficacy or Loop Diuretics

Loop diuretics act on the ascending limb of the loop of Henle. They are **highly efficacious** as diuretics.

Frusemide (furosemide) is a sulfonamide derivative. It is the most popular loop diuretic.

Mechanism of action: Frusemide acts by inhibiting $NaCl^-$ reabsorption in the thick ascending limb of the Henle's loop (Fig. 5.2). It blocks the Na^+ K^+ $2Cl^-$ symporter in the thick ascending limb of the Henle's loop because of which it is called a loop diuretic. It greatly increases the excretion of Na^+ and Cl^- in the urine. As a large amount of $NaCl^-$ is absorbed in this segment, loop diuretics are highly efficacious. Diuretic response increases with dose (high ceiling of effect) and over-enthusiastic treatment and can cause dehydration (Table 5.1).

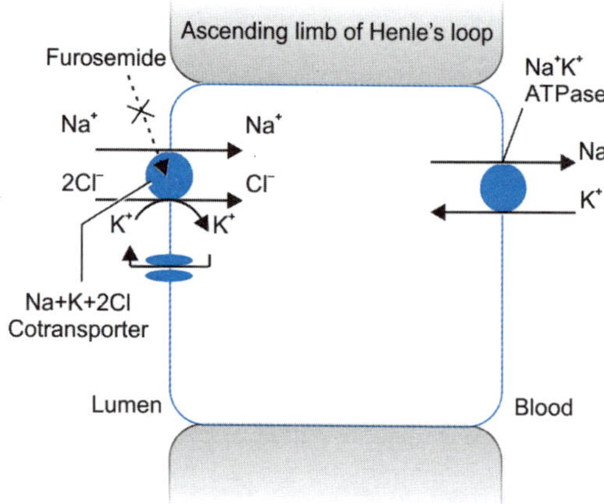

Fig. 5.2: Mechanism of action of loop diuretics.

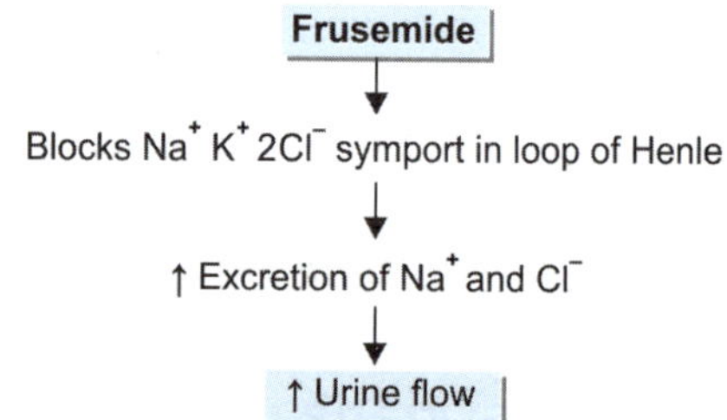

Other actions

- Loop diuretics also increase the excretion of K^+, Ca^{++} and Mg^{++} (but Ca^{++} is reabsorbed in the distal tubule—hence no hypocalcemia).
- They increase reabsorption of uric acid in the proximal tubule.
- They also alter renal hemodynamics to reduce fluid and electrolyte reabsorption in the proximal tubule.
- IV furosemide relieves pulmonary congestion and reduces left ventricular filling pressure by causing venodilation in congestive heart failure and pulmonary edema.

Pharmacokinetics: Furosemide is rapidly absorbed orally, highly bound to plasma proteins and excreted by kidneys. Given intravenously it acts in 2–5 minutes, while following oral use, it takes 20–40 minutes; duration of action is 3–6 hours.

Table 5.1: Compare and contrast hydrochlorothiazide and frusemide.

Features	*Hydrochlorothiazide*	*Frusemide*
Efficacy	Low	High
Site of action	Early distal tubule	Ascending limb of loop of Henle
Mechanism of action	Inhibits Na^+Cl^- symport	Inhibits $Na^+K^+2Cl^-$ cotransport
Onset of action	After 1 hour	In minutes (20–40)
Duration of action	Long (8–12 hours)	Short (3–6 hours)
Response to increasing dose	No significant increase	Increases (Dose dependent)
Hyperuricemia	Higher incidence	Low
Blood glucose	May increase Contraindicated in diabetics	No significant effect Not contraindicated
Ototoxicity	Not known to cause	Can cause
Primary use	Hypertension	Edema

Bumetanide is a sulfonamide like frusemide but is 40 times more potent. Bioavailability is 80% and is better tolerated.

Adverse Effects of Loop Diuretics

1. **Hypokalemia and metabolic alkalosis** (due to loss of H^+) are dose dependent and can be corrected by K^+ replacement and correction of hypovolemia.
2. **Hyponatremia, dehydration, hypovolemia and hypotension** should be treated with saline infusion.
3. **Hyperuricemia** may precipitate acute attacks of gout.
4. **Hypocalcemia and hypomagnesemia:** After prolonged use this may result in osteoporosis.
5. **Ototoxicity:** Loop diuretics cause hearing loss by a toxic effect on the hair cells in the internal ear—more common with ethacrynic acid. It is dose-related and generally reversible. Concurrent use of other ototoxic drugs should be avoided.
6. **Hyperglycemia and hyperlipidemia** are mild in therapeutic doses.
7. **GIT disturbances** like nausea, vomiting and diarrhea are common with ethacrynic acid.
8. **Allergic reactions** like skin rashes are more common with sulfonamide derivatives.
9. Weakness, fatigue, hypotension, dizziness and muscle cramps are mostly due to hypokalemia.

Uses

1. **Edema:** Frusemide is highly effective for the relief of edema of all origins like cardiac, hepatic and renal edema. In chronic congestive cardiac failure, loop diuretics reduce venous and pulmonary congestion.
2. **Acute renal failure:** Loop diuretics increase the urine output and K^+ excretion and therefore useful in acute renal failure.
3. **Acute pulmonary edema** is relieved by IV frusemide due to its immediate vasodilator effect and then by diuretic action.
4. **Cerebral edema:** Frusemide is used as an alternative to osmotic diuretics.
5. **Forced diuresis:** In poisoning due to drugs like barbiturates and salicylates, frusemide is used with IV fluids to induce diuresis and promote the excretion of toxic drugs.
6. **Hypertension** with renal impairment may be treated with loop diuretics.
7. **Acute hypercalcemia and hyperkalemia:** Loop diuretics increase the excretion of Ca^{++} and K^+. But Na^+ and Cl^- should be replaced to avoid hyponatremia and hypochloremia.

Thiazides and Thiazide-like Diuretics

Chlorothiazide was the first thiazide to be synthesized. All thiazides have a sulfonamide group.

Actions and Mechanism of Action

Thiazides act on the early distal tubule. Thiazides have a moderate efficacy because 90% of the filtered sodium is already reabsorbed before reaching the distal tubule. This group of drugs block Na^+/Cl^- co-transport (Fig. 5.3) in the early distal tubule (site 3). They also inhibit carbonic anhydrase activity. Thiazides also increase the excretion of Mg^+ and K^+ (in the distal segments, Na^+ in the lumen is exchanged for K^+ which is then excreted). But they inhibit urinary excretion of Ca^{++} and uric acid resulting in hypercalcemia and hyperuricemia.

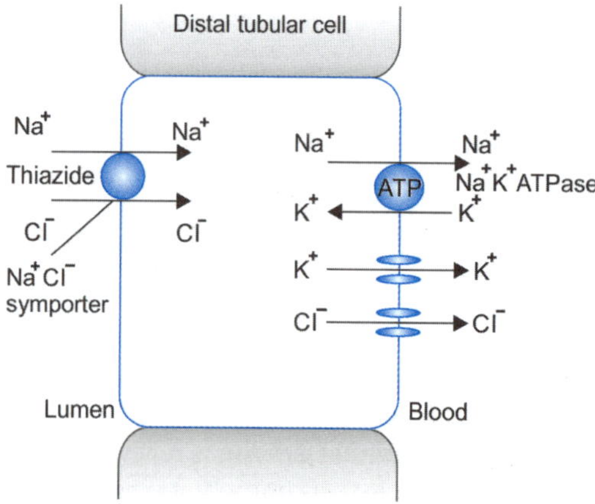

Fig. 5.3: Mechanism of action of thiazide diuretics.

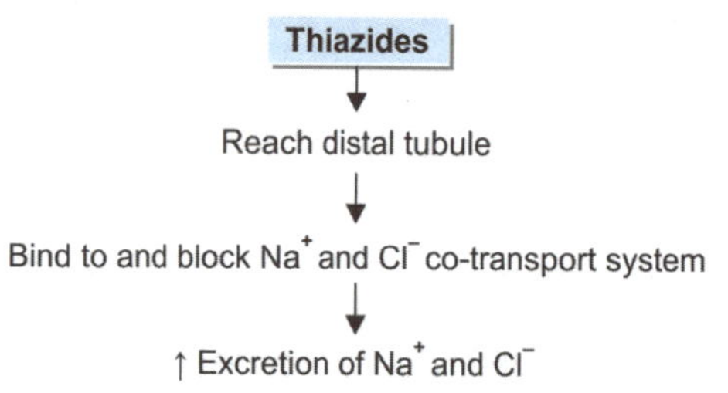

Pharmacokinetics

Thiazides are well-absorbed orally and are rapid acting. Duration varies from 6–48 hours. They are excreted by the kidney.

Adverse Effects

1. **Hypokalemia** is the most important side effect of thiazide use
2. **Metabolic alkalosis, hyperuricemia,** hypovolemia, hypotension, dehydration, hyponatremia, hypomagnesemia, hypochloremia, hypercalcemia, and hyperlipidemia are similar to that seen with loop diuretics
3. **Hyperglycemia** induced by thiazides may precipitate diabetes mellitus probably by inhibition of insulin secretion. It is more common when long-acting thiazides are used for a long time
4. Thiazides can cause **impotence** in men
5. **Weakness**, fatigue, anorexia, gastrointestinal disturbances and **allergic reactions** like rashes and photosensitivity can be seen.

Uses

1. **Hypertension:** Thiazides are the first line drugs.
2. **Congestive heart failure:** Thiazides are the first line drugs in the management of edema due to mild to moderate CHF.
3. **Edema:** Thiazides may be tried in hepatic or renal edema.
4. **Renal stones:** Hypercalciuria with renal stones can be treated with thiazides which reduce calcium excretion.
5. **Diabetes insipidus:** Thiazides reduce plasma volume and GFR and benefit such patients.

Indapamide is particularly suitable in hypertension because it is claimed to lower blood pressure in subdiuretic doses and in such doses adverse effects are milder. It is well absorbed orally and has a long duration of action to permit once a day dosing.

Potassium Sparing Diuretics

Potassium sparing diuretics may act by two ways. They may be aldosterone antagonists or directly inhibit ion channels in distal tubule and collecting duct.

Spironolactone: Aldosterone increases the Na^+ reabsorption through Na^+ channels in the collecting tubule and increases K^+ secretion. It binds aldosterone receptors on distal tubule and collecting duct and competitively inhibits the action of aldosterone.

Spironolactone is an aldosterone antagonist. It binds aldosterone receptors on distal tubule and collecting duct and competitively inhibits the action of aldosterone (aldosterone promotes Na^+ reabsorption and K^+ secretion). As major amount of Na^+ is already reabsorbed in the proximal parts, spironolactone has low efficacy. Spironolactone also reduces K^+ loss due to other diuretics.

It increases the excretion of calcium by a direct action on the renal tubules.

Spironolactone

↓

Binds aldosterone receptors and inhibits its action

↓

↑ Na^+ and water excretion, ↓ K^+ excretion

Adverse effects include gynecomastia, sexual dysfunction in men, drowsiness, hyperkalemia especially in renal insufficiency; metabolic acidosis and skin rashes.

Eplerenone an analog of spironolactone has greater selectivity for mineralocorticoid receptors and milder activity on androgen and progesterone receptors. Thus the hormonal adverse effects are very much milder.

Amiloride and triamterene are directly acting agents which enhance Na^+ excretion and reduce K^+ loss by acting on ion channels in the distal tubule and collecting duct. They block the Na^+ transport through ion-channels in the luminal membrane. Since K^+ secretion is dependent on Na^+ entry, these drugs reduce K^+ excretion.

Adverse effects are gastrointestinal disturbances, hyperkalemia and metabolic acidosis.

Uses of Potassium Sparing Diuretics

1. **With thiazides and loop diuretics** to prevent potassium loss.
2. **Edema:** In cirrhosis and renal edema where aldosterone levels may be high.
3. **Hypertension:** Along with thiazides to avoid hypokalemia and for additive effect.
4. **CCF:** Moderate of severe heart failure along with frusemide.
5. **Primary or secondary aldosteronism:** Spironolactone is used.

Carbonic Anhydrase Inhibitors

Carbonic anhydrase is an enzyme that catalyses the formation of carbonic acid which spontaneously ionizes to H^+ and HCO_3^-. This HCO_3^- combines with Na^+ and is reabsorbed.

$$H_2O + CO_2 \rightleftharpoons H_2CO_3$$

$$H_2CO_3 \rightleftharpoons H^+ + HCO_3^-$$

Carbonic anhydrase is present in the nephron, eyes, gastric mucosa, pancreas and other sites.

Acetazolamide, is a carbonic anhydrase inhibitor. It increases the excretion of sodium, potassium, bicarbonate and water. The loss of bicarbonate leads to metabolic acidosis.

Other Actions

- **Eye:** Bicarbonate and sodium ions are required for the production of aqueous humor. Carbonic anhydrase inhibition results in decreased formation of aqueous humor and thereby reduces intraocular pressure.
- **Brain:** Bicarbonate is secreted into CSF and carbonic anhydrase inhibition reduces the formation of CSF.

Adverse Effects

- **Metabolic acidosis:** Due to HCO_3^- loss
- **Renal stones:** Calcium is lost with HCO_3^- resulting in hypercalciuria. This excess Ca^{++} may precipitate resulting in the formation of renal stones
- Hypokalemia, drowsiness and allergic reactions can occur.

Uses

1. **Glaucoma:** (*See* page 58) Intraocular pressure is decreased by acetazolamide;

it is given orally. Newer ones—*methazolamide, brinzolamide* and *dorzolamide* are better tolerated and are available as eye drops.
2. **To alkalinize the urine:** As required in overdosage of acidic drugs.
3. **Metabolic alkalosis:** Acetazolamide increases HCO_3^- excretion.
4. **Mountain sickness:** In mountain climbers who rapidly ascend great heights, severe pulmonary edema or cerebral edema may occur. Acetazolamide may help by reducing CSF formation.
5. **Epilepsy:** Acetazolamide is used as an adjuvant as it increases the seizure threshold.
6. **Hyperphosphatemia:** When hyperphosphatemia is severe, it can be treated with acetazolamide to increase the urinary phosphate excretion.

Osmotic Diuretics

Mannitol is a pharmacologically inert substance. When given IV (orally not absorbed), mannitol gets filtered by the glomerulus but not reabsorbed. It causes water to be retained in the kidney by osmotic effect resulting in water diuresis. There is also some loss of Na^+.

Adverse effects are dehydration, ECF volume expansion, headache and allergic reactions.

Uses

- To maintain urine volume in conditions like shock.
- To reduce intracranial and intraocular pressure—following head injury and glaucoma respectively.

Glycerol is effective orally—reduces intraocular and intracranial pressure.

Methylxanthines like theophylline have mild diuretic effect.

Newer Drugs

Vasopressin antagonists—conivaptan, tolvaptan and lixivaptan (vaptans) inhibit the effects of ADH in the collecting tubule to cause diuresis. They are useful in hyponatremia and in patients with inappropriate secretion of ADH.

Sodium-glucose cotransporter-2 (SGLT-2) inhibitors: 90% of glucose is reabsorbed through SGLT-2 and inhibition of this transporter increases the excretion of glucose and sodium and causes diuresis.

Dapagliflozin and canagliflozin are SGLT-2 inhibitors used in diabetes mellitus.

Drug Interactions with Diuretics

- Frusemide is highly protein bound and may compete with drugs like warfarin and clofibrate for protein binding sites.
- Other ototoxic drugs like aminoglycosides should not be used with loop diuretics to avoid increased toxicity.
- Hypokalemia induced by diuretics increase digitalis toxicity.
- NSAIDs blunt the effect of diuretics as they cause salt and water retention.
- Diuretics increase lithium toxicity by reducing renal excretion of lithium.
- Other drugs that cause hyperkalemia (ACE inhibitors) and oral K^+ supplements should be avoided with K^+ sparing diuretics because, together they can cause severe hyperkalemia.

ANTIDIURETICS

Antidiuretics are drugs that reduce urine volume. These include:

- Antidiuretic hormone (vasopressin)
- Thiazide diuretics
- Miscellaneous
  - Chlorpropamide
  - Carbamazepine.

Antidiuretic hormone (ADH) is secreted by the posterior pituitary along with oxytocin. It is synthesized in the supraoptic and paraventricular nuclei of the hypothalamus, transported along the hypothalamo-hypophyseal tract to the posterior pituitary and it is stored there. ADH is released in response to two stimuli—dehydration and rise in plasma osmolarity.

Actions

ADH acts on vasopressin receptors and increases water reabsorption, causes vasoconstriction and raises BP. It also acts on other smooth muscles to increase peristalsis in the gut and contracts the uterus.

It is given parenterally as injection or as intranasal spray.

Adverse Effects

When used intranasally ADH can cause nasal irritation, allergy, rhinitis and atrophy of the nasal mucosa. Other effects include nausea, abdominal cramps and backache (due to contractions of the uterus).

Uses

- Diabetes insipidus of pituitary origin—desmopressin is used.
- Bleeding esophageal varices—ADH constricts mesenteric blood vessels and may help.
- Before abdominal radiography—expels gases from the bowel.
- Hemophilia—may release factor VIII.

Vasopressin analogs: Desmopressin is a selective V2 agonist used as nasal spray. terlipressin is longer acting. Felypressin is used with local anesthetics to prolong their duration of action because of its vasoconstrictor properties.

Vasopressin antagonists: Conivaptan, tolvaptan and lixivaptan are used in the treatment of inappropriate secretion of ADH.

Thiazides Paradoxically thiazides reduce urine volume in diabetes insipidus of both pituitary and renal origin by an unknown mechanism.

Chlorpropamide an oral antidiabetic drug, sensitizes the kidney to ADH action.

Carbamazepine an antiepileptic, stimulates ADH secretion.

6

CHAPTER

Cardiovascular Pharmacology

CHAPTER HIGHLIGHTS

- Cardiac Glycosides and Treatment of Cardiac Failure
- Antiarrhythmic Drugs
- Antihypertensive Drugs
- Drugs Used in the Treatment of Ischemic Heart Disease
- Pharmacotherapy of Shock
- Plasma Expanders
- Vasoactive Drugs
- Cerebral Ischemia
- Drugs Used in Treatment of Peripheral Vascular Diseases
- Hypolipidemic Drugs
- Drugs Used in the Disorders of Coagulation
- Thrombolytics (Fibrinolytics)
- Hematinics

CARDIAC GLYCOSIDES AND TREATMENT OF CARDIAC FAILURE

The Heart

The cardiac muscle is a specialized tissue with unique properties like excitability, contractility and automaticity. The myocardium has two types of cells—the contracting cells and the conducting cells. The contracting cells participate in the pumping action of the heart. SA node, AV node and His-Purkinje system comprise the conducting tissue of the heart. Parts of the conducting tissue have the characteristic property of automaticity. **Automaticity** is the ability of the cell to generate electrical impulses spontaneously. Normally the SA node acts as the pace maker. **Excitability** is the ability of the cell to undergo depolarization in response to a stimulus. **Contractility** is the ability of the myocardium to adequately contract and pump the blood out of the heart.

Cardiac action potential When a stimulus reaches the cardiac cell, specific ions move into and out of the cell eliciting an action potential. Such movement of ions across the cardiac cell may be divided into phases (Fig. 6.1).

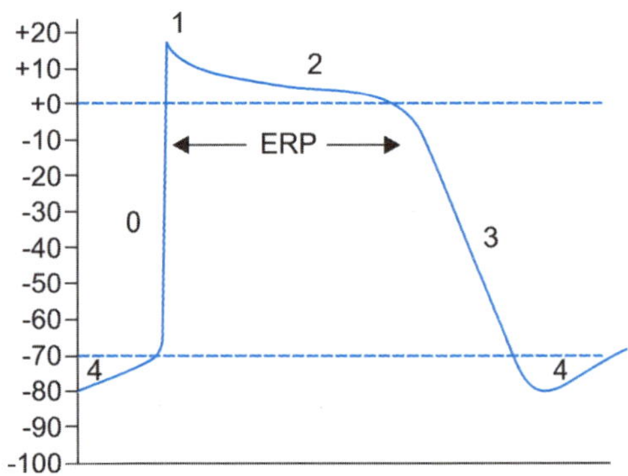

Fig. 6.1: Cardiac action potential phases 0–4: Phase 0—indicates rapid depolarization, Phases 1–3—indicate repolarization, Phase 4—gradual depolarization during diastole.

(ERP: effective refractory period)

Phase 0 is rapid depolarization of the cell membrane during which there is fast entry of sodium ions into the cell through the sodium channels. This is followed by repolarization.

Phase 1 is a short, initial, rapid repolarization due to efflux of potassium ions.

Phase 2 is a prolonged plateau phase due to slow entry of calcium ions into the cell through the calcium channels. Cardiac cell differs from other cells in having this phase of action potential.

Phase 3 is a second period of rapid repolarization with potassium ions moving out of the cell.

Phase 4 is the resting phase during which potassium ions return into the cell while sodium and calcium ions move out of it and the resting membrane potential is restored.

During phases 1 and 2, the cell does not depolarize in response to another impulse, i.e., it is in absolute refractory period. But during phases 3 and 4, the cell is in relative refractory period and may depolarize in response to a powerful impulse.

The cardiac output is determined by heart rate and stroke volume. The stroke volume in turn depends on the preload, afterload and contractility. **Preload** is the load on the heart due to the volume of blood reaching the left ventricle. It depends on the venous return. **Afterload** is the resistance to the left ventricular ejection, i.e., the total peripheral resistance.

Congestive cardiac failure (CCF) is one of the common causes of morbidity and mortality. In congestive cardiac failure, the heart is unable to provide adequate blood supply to meet the body's oxygen demand. The pumping ability of the heart is reduced and the cardiac output decreases. The ventricles are not completely emptied resulting in increased venous pressure in the pulmonary and systemic circulation. This causes pulmonary edema, dyspnea, liver enlargement and peripheral edema. As a compensatory mechanism, there is stimulation of the sympathetic system and renin angiotensin system which help in maintaining the cardiac output. The myocardium also undergoes structural alterations like ventricular hypertrophy and remodelling to adapt itself to the stressful situation. These compensatory changes maintain the cardiac output for sometime.

Depending on the cardiac output, cardiac failure may be of two types—low output failure and high output failure.

Low output failure could result from ischemic heart disease, hypertension, valvular and congenital heart diseases. High output failure results from anemia, thyrotoxicosis, beriberi and certain congenital heart diseases.

The drugs used in CCF include **diuretics, vasodilators** and **cardiac glycosides**. The pharmacology of cardiac glycosides has been discussed first, followed by the role of other drugs in CCF.

Drugs Used in Congestive Cardiac Failure

In congestive cardiac failure, the heart is unable to provide adequate blood supply to meet the demand. The aim of treatment is to reduce morbidity and mortality by restoring cardiac output and relieving congestion.

The drugs used in CCF are:

1. **Diuretics:** Frusemide, bumetanide spironolactone.
2. **Vasodilators:** Hydralazine, nitrates, angiotensin converting enzyme inhibitors, angiotensin receptor blockers, sodium nitroprusside, prazosin, calcium channel blockers.
3. **Inotropes:**
   - **Cardiac glycosides:** Digoxin (Table 6.1)
   - **Beta adrenergic agonists:** Dobutamine, dopamine, dopexamine
   - **Phosphodiesterase (PDE) inhibitors:** Amrinone, milrinone
   - **Newer agents:** Sildenafil, Istaroxime, levosimendan.

1. *Diuretics*

High ceiling diuretics like frusemide are used. They increase salt and water excretion and reduce blood volume. By this they *reduce preload* and venous pressure, improve cardiac performance and relieve edema. Diuretics provide symptomatic relief and may be used for short periods.

Loop diuretics → ↑Salt and water excretion → ↓Plasma volume → ↓Preload < Improve cardiac performance / ↓Edema → Rapid relief in CCF

2. *Vasodilators*

Vasodilators reduce the mortality in patients with cardiac failure. They may be arteriolar or venular dilators or both.

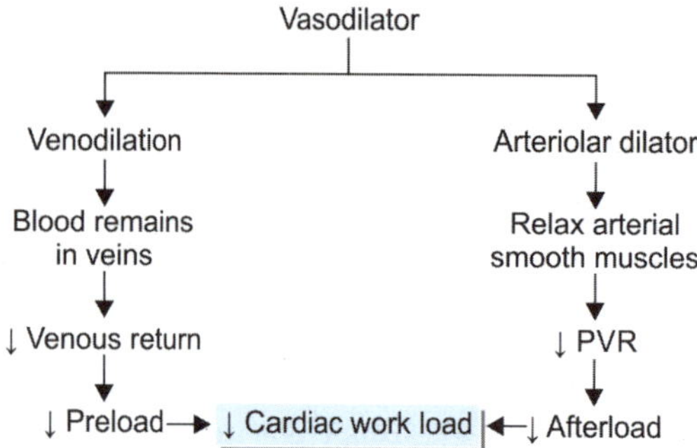

a. **Arteriolar dilators** (↓afterload)—hydralazine relaxes arterial smooth muscles, thus reducing peripheral vascular resistance (↓afterload). As a result, the work load on the heart is reduced.

b. **Venodilators** (↓preload)—nitrates-reduce the venous return to the heart (↓preload) thus reducing the stretching of the ventricular walls and myocardial oxygen requirements.

   Organic nitrates: Nitroglycerine and isosorbide dinitrate are good vasodilators with a rapid and short action. They can be used for short periods to decrease the ventricular filling pressure in acute heart failure. Nitroglycerine can be used IV in acute CCF. Nitrates may be given in combination with hydralazine.

c. **Both arteriolar and venular dilators**: ACE inhibitors, sodium nitroprusside, prazosin, calcium channel blockers—these reduce both preload and afterload.

Angiotensin converting enzyme inhibitors (ACE-I) (*See* page 122) like captopril, enalapril, lisinopril and ramipril act by:

- **Reduction of afterload:** Angiotensin II is a powerful vasoconstrictor present in the plasma in high concentrations in cardiac failure. ACE-inhibitors prevent the conversion of angiotensin I to angiotensin II and thereby reduce the afterload.
- **Reduction of preload:** Aldosterone causes salt and water retention and increases plasma volume. ACE-I prevent the formation of aldosterone (by reducing Ang-II) and thereby reduce the preload.
- **Reversing compensatory changes:** Angiotensin II formed locally in the myocardium is responsible for various undesirable compensatory changes like ventricular hypertrophy and ventricular remodelling seen in CCF. ACE-I reverse these changes.

ACE inhibitors are the **most preferred drugs** in chronic congestive cardiac failure.

3. *Inotropes*

Digoxin: Mild to moderate cases of low output failure are treated with diuretics and vasodilators (ACE-inhibitors preferred). When patients with low output failure are not adequately benefited by diuretics and vasodilators, they may be started on digoxin. Digoxin improves cardiac performance in the dilated, failing heart. If there is associated atrial fibrillation, digoxin is the preferred drug in such patients.

Other inotropic agents like **dobutamine, dopamine** and **dopexamine** increase the force of contraction of the heart and increase cardiac output. They are beta adrenergic agonists and are useful in acute heart failure.

Levosimendan is a phosphodiesterase inhibitor which has inotropic effects as well as vasodilator properties including coronary vasodilation. It is therefore useful in heart failure.

Istaroxime is another inotropic agent being studied for use in heart failure.

Cardiac Glycosides

Cardiac glycosides are obtained from the plants of the foxglove family. William Withering, an English physician first described the clinical effects of digitalis in CCF in 1785.

Source: Digoxin is derived from the leaves of *Digitalis lanata*. The word digitalis is used to mean cardiac glycosides.

Chemistry: The glycosides consist of an aglycon attached to sugars. The aglycon has pharmacodynamic activity while sugars influence pharmacokinetic properties.

Pharmacological Actions

1. **Cardiac actions - Inotropic effects:** Digoxin is a cardiotonic drug. Cardiac glycosides increase the force of contraction of the heart—the stroke volume increases and thereby the cardiac output. The systole is shortened and the diastole is prolonged which allows more rest to the heart. The ventricles are more completely emptied because of more forceful contractions. Thus digoxin is a positive **inotropic drug**.

The **heart rate is reduced** due to:
- Increased vagal tone
- Decreased sympathetic overactivity due to improved circulation
- By a direct action on SA and AV nodes.

Digitalis also produces the characteristic ECG changes.

Blood pressure: No significant effects in CCF patients.

Coronary circulation: Improves due to increased cardiac output and prolonged diastole during which the coronaries get filled better.

2. **Extracardiac actions**
- **Kidney:** Diuresis occurs which relieves edema in CCF patients.
- **Central nervous system (CNS):** High doses stimulate chemoreceptor trigger zone (CTZ) resulting in nausea and vomiting.

Table 6.1: Precautions and contraindications to digitalis therapy.

- Hypokalemia—enhances toxicity
- MI, thyrotoxicosis patients—more prone to arrhythmias
- Acid base imbalance—prone to toxicity

Mechanism of action: Cardiac glycosides inhibit the enzyme Na^+/K^+ ATPase—also called 'sodium pump' present on the cardiac myocytes. This results in an increase in the intracellular Na^+ and Ca^{++}. Thus more calcium is available for contraction, resulting in increased force and velocity of contraction (Flowchart 6.1).

Pharmacokinetics: Digoxin is well-absorbed. Presence of food in the stomach delays absorption. Bioavailability varies with different manufacturers and because the safety margin is low, in any given patient, the preparations from the same manufacturer should be used. Glycosides are cumulative drugs.

Adverse effects: Cardiac glycosides have a low safety margin and adverse effects are common.

Extracardiac: Anorexia, nausea, vomiting and diarrhea are the first symptoms to appear.

Flowchart 6.1: Mechanism of action of cardiac glycosides.

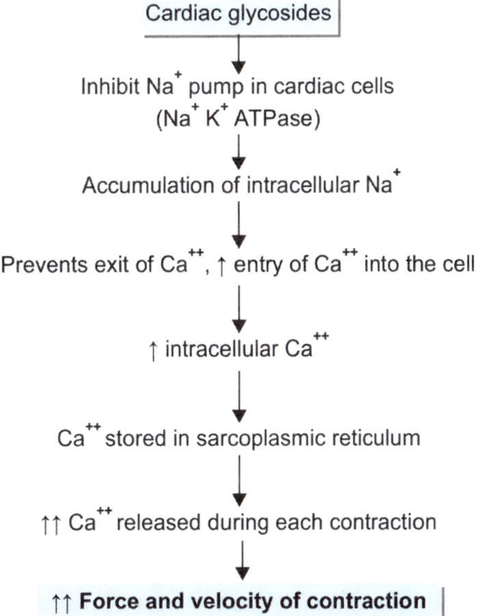

Weakness, confusion, hallucinations, blurred vision and gynecomastia can occur.

Cardiac toxicity: Arrhythmias of any type including extrasystoles, bradycardia, pulses bigeminy and AV block, ventricular tachycardia and fibrillation can be caused by cardiac glycosides. Hypokalemia enhances digitalis toxicity.

Treatment of Toxicity

- Stop digoxin
- Oral or parenteral K^+ supplements are given
- Ventricular arrhythmias are treated with IV lignocaine or phenytoin
- Bradycardia is treated with atropine and supraventricular arrhythmias with propranolol
- Antidigoxin immunotherapy that is antidigoxin antibodies are now available (Table 6.2).

Table 6.2: Drug interactions.

Drugs that enhance digoxin toxicity
• Diuretics (due to hypokalemia), calcium • Quinidine, verapamil, methyldopa—↑digoxin levels
Drugs that reduce digoxin levels
• Antacids, neomycin, metoclopramide—reduce absorption • Rifampicin, phenobarbitone—hasten metabolism due to enzyme induction

Uses

- Congestive cardiac failure - in chronic heart failure, digoxin is used as an alternative or add-on drug when diuretics and vasodilators are not effective.
- Cardiac arrhythmias
  - Atrial fibrillation and atrial flutter—digoxin reduces the ventricular rate
  - Paroxysmal supraventricular tachycardia (PSVT)—digoxin is an alternative to verapamil.

ANTIARRHYTHMIC DRUGS

Arrhythmia is an abnormality of the rate, rhythm or site of origin of the cardiac impulse or an abnormality in the impulse conduction. Cardiac arrhythmias may be due to abnormal generation or conduction of impulses. Factors like hypoxia, electrolyte disturbances, trauma, drugs and autonomic influences can cause arrhythmias (Table 6.3).

Classification

Vaughan Williams classified antiarrhythmics (Flowchart 6.2):

Sodium Channel Blockers

Class IA drugs

All drugs in this class block the sodium channels and prevent the inward movement of sodium ions by blocking Na^+ channels, they depress phase-0 depolarization. They also prolong repolarization by blocking K^+ channels (Fig. 6.2).

Quinidine is the D-isomer of quinine obtained from the cinchona bark.

Flowchart 6.2: Classification of antiarrhythmics.

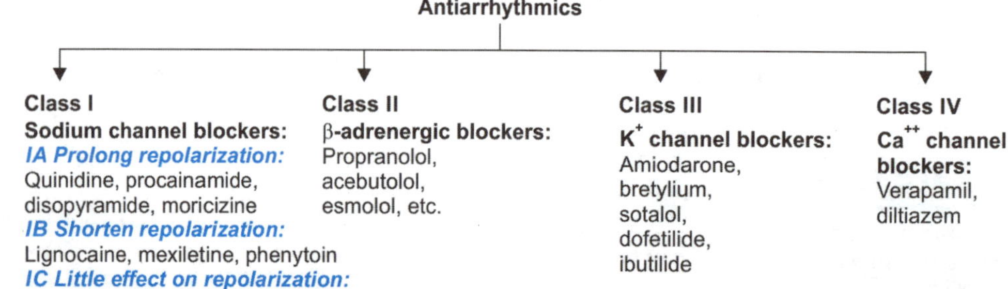

Table 6.3: Choice of drugs in cardiac arrhythmias.

Arrhythmia	*Cause*	*Treatment*
Sinus tachycardia	↑ sympathetic tone, fever, thyrotoxicosis	• Treat the cause • If severe—propranolol
Atrial extrasystoles	Excess caffeine, nicotine, alcohol	• Treat the cause • Reassurance • If severe—propranolol/disopyramide
Atrial flutter/ fibrillation	Rheumatic heart disease, cardiomyopathy, hypertension	• Cardioversion • Propranolol/quinidine/disopyramide/digitalis
PSVT		• Vagal maneuvers like carotid massage • Verapamil/adenosine • β-blockers
Ventricular ectopics	Normal heart—benign; also in cardiomyopathy, ischemic, digitalis induced	• β-blockers • Lignocaine
Ventricular tachycardia	Organic heart disease and ventricular dysfunction, drug-induced	• Cardioversion • Lignocaine
Ventricular fibrillation	Acute MI, organic heart disease, surgical trauma, drug-induced	• Cardioversion • Lignocaine • Class I A drugs for prevention
Digitalis induced tachyarrhythmias	Digitalis toxicity	• Phenytoin • Potassium • Lignocaine
Sinus bradycardia		• Atropine

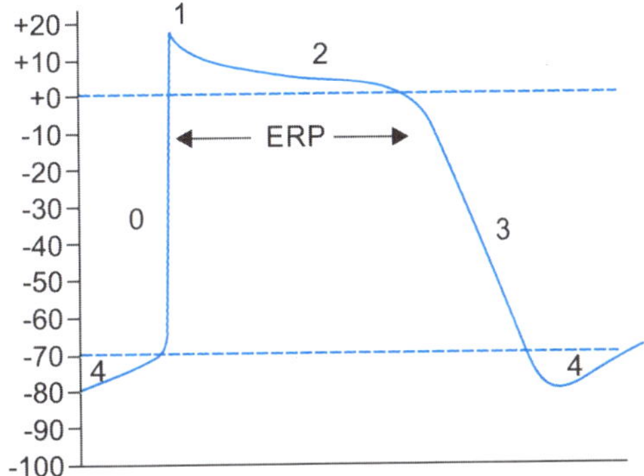

Fig. 6.2: Cardiac action potential: Phase 0—rapid depolarization, Phase 1—initial rapid repolarization, Phase 2—prolonged plateau phase, Phase 3—second rapid repolarization, Phase 4—resting phase.

Mechanism of action: By blocking Na^+ channels, it depresses all cardiac properties—automaticity, excitability, conduction velocity and prolongs repolarization: quinidine thus has membrane-stabilizing activity, i.e., it inhibits the propagation of the action potential.

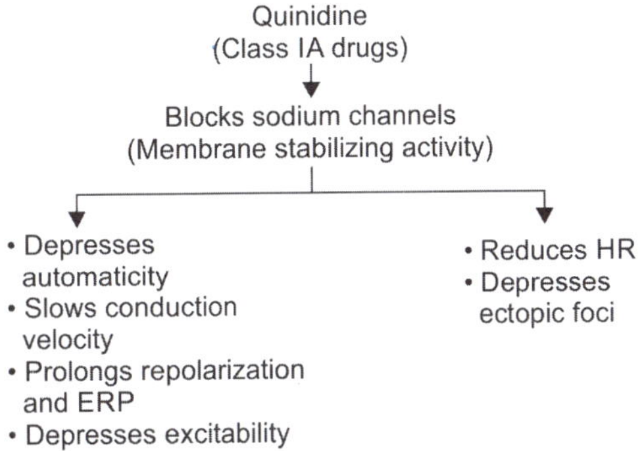

Quinidine also has vagolytic and α-blocking properties. It is also a skeletal muscle relaxant.

Pharmacokinetics: Given orally quinidine is rapidly absorbed, 90% bound to plasma proteins, metabolized in the liver and excreted in the urine.

Adverse effects: Quinidine is not well-tolerated due to adverse effects and may need to be stopped. Adverse effects are:

Cardiac: Quinidine itself can cause arrhythmias, heart block and hypotension. Hence treatment should be monitored.

Non-cardiac: Nausea, vomiting, diarrhea, hypersensitivity and idiosyncratic reactions can occur. Higher doses can cause cinchonism like quinine.

Procainamide: A derivative of the local anesthetic procaine has the advantages over quinidine that it has weak anticholinergic properties and is not an α-blocker. It is better tolerated than quinidine.

Disopyramide: It has significant anticholinergic properties.

Uses of Class IA drugs: Class IA drugs are useful in almost all types of arrhythmias. They are used in atrial fibrillation and atrial flutter and in ventricular arrhythmias. Because of the adverse effects, quinidine and procainamide are not preferred in arrhythmias but quinidine can be used in malaria in place of quinine.

Class IB Drugs

Class IB drugs block the sodium channels and also shorten repolarization.

Lignocaine suppresses the electrical activity of the arrhythmogenic tissues while the normal tissues are not much affected. It is a local anesthetic. Given orally lignocaine undergoes high first pass metabolism and has a short t½—hence used parenterally. It may cause drowsiness, hypotension, blurred vision, confusion and convulsions. Lignocaine is used in the treatment of ventricular arrhythmias, especially that caused by acute myocardial infarction or open heart surgery.

Phenytoin is an antiepileptic also useful in ventricular arrhythmias and digitalis induced arrhythmias.

Mexiletine can be used orally; causes dose related neurologic adverse effects including tremors and blurred vision. Nausea is common. It is used as an alternative to lignocaine in ventricular arrhythmias.

Class IC Drugs

Class IC drugs like encainide and flecainide are the most potent sodium channel blockers. Because of the risk of cardiac arrest, sudden death and other adverse effects, they are not commonly used. They may be used only in severe ventricular arrhythmias.

Class II Drugs

β-blockers like propranolol exert antiarrhythmic effects due to blockade of cardiac β receptors (in high doses has membrane stabilizing activity). They depress myocardial contractility, automaticity and conduction velocity.

Propranolol and cardioselective β-blockers like **atenolol** and **metoprolol** are used in the treatment of supraventricular arrhythmias especially those associated with exercise, emotion or hyperthyroidism.

Esmolol given intravenously is rapid and short-acting and can be used to treat arrhythmias during surgeries, following myocardial infarction and other emergencies.

Sotalol a β-blocker also prolongs the action potential duration and is often preferred when a β-blocker is needed.

Class III Drugs

These drugs prolong the action potential duration and refractory period by blocking the potassium channels.

Amiodarone, an analog of thyroid hormone, is a powerful antiarrhythmic which contains iodine in its structure. It acts by multiple mechanisms. It blocks the K^+ channels and prolongs the action potential duration, it also blocks β adrenergic receptors and sodium as well as Ca^{++} channels.

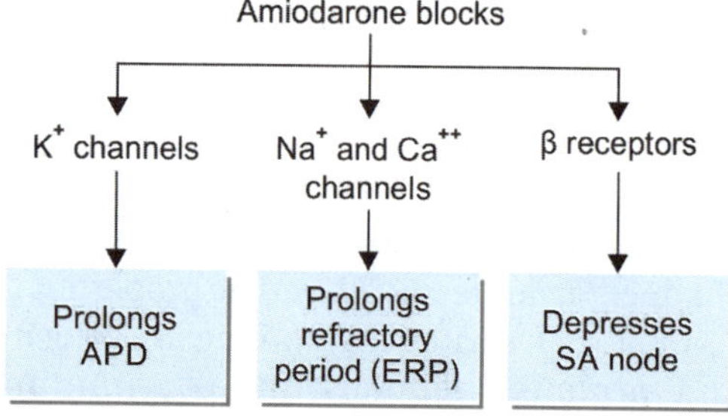

Vasculature: Amiodarone relaxes vascular smooth muscles including coronaries and improves blood flow to the myocardium.

Vasodilation in peripheral vasculature results in a decrease in the preload, myocardial workload and thereby oxygen consumption. IV amiodarone can cause hypotension.

Adverse effects: Amiodarone can cause many adverse effects like heart block, cardiac failure, hypotension, hypothyroidism or hyperthyroidism (analog of thyroid hormone), pulmonary fibrosis and hepatotoxicity.

Uses

Amiodarone is a broad spectrum antiarrhythmic and is the most efficacious antiarrhythmic drug.

However, it is a toxic drug and requires constant monitoring.

- Amiodarone is useful in atrial arrhythmias.
- IV amiodarone is used for the treatment and prophylaxis of life - threatening, resistant ventricular fibrillation and ventricular tachycardia.

Dronedarone: An analog of amiodarone does not contain iodine atoms and therefore does not cause the thyroid related side effects. It is longer acting and is used in atrial fibrillation.

Bretylium is an adrenergic neurone blocker used in resistant ventricular arrhythmias.

Class IV Drugs

Calcium channel blockers inhibit the inward movement of calcium resulting in reduced contractility, automaticity and AV nodal conduction. Verapamil and diltiazem have prominent cardiac effects.

Verapamil is used to terminate paroxysmal supraventricular tachycardia (PSVT). It is also used to control ventricular rate in atrial flutter or fibrillation.

Miscellaneous

Adenosine is a purine nucleotide having rapid and short antiarrhythmic action. Given IV it suppresses automaticity, AV conduction and dilates the coronaries. Adenosine is the drug of choice for acute termination of paroxysmal supraventricular tachycardias (PSVT).

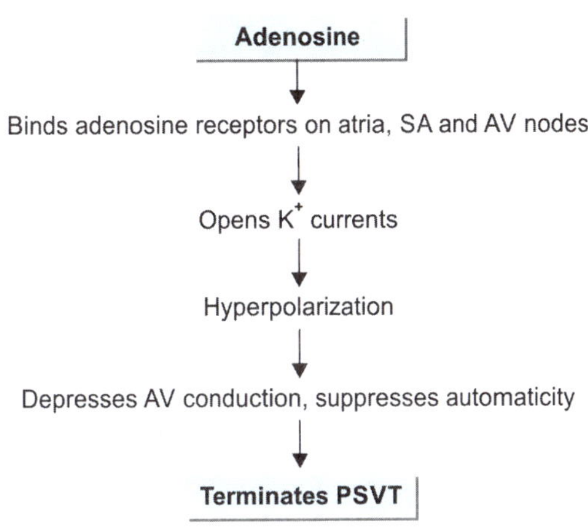

Adverse effects are nausea, dyspnea, flushing and headache but are of short duration.

ANTIHYPERTENSIVE DRUGS

Hypertension is an elevation of systolic and/ or diastolic BP above 140/90 mm of Hg. It is a common cardiovascular condition. Hypertension may be

- *Primary* (essential) hypertension—where the cause is not known or
- *Secondary*—it is secondary to other conditions like renal, endocrine or vascular disorders.

Based on the degree of severity, hypertension can be graded as in Table 6.4:

Table 6.4: Grading of blood pressure.

Category	*SBP mm Hg*		*DBP mm Hg*
Normal	<120	and	<80
Prehypertension	120–139	or	80–89
Hypertension Stage 1	140–159	or	90–99
Hypertension Stage 2	≥160	or	≥100

(SBP: systolic blood pressure; DBP: diastolic blood pressure)

Blood pressure is determined by cardiac output (CO) and total peripheral vascular resistance (PVR). Blood pressure is controlled by baroreceptor reflexes acting through autonomic nervous system along with the renin-angiotensin-aldosterone system.

Prolonged hypertension damages the blood vessels of the heart, brain and the kidneys and may result in several complications like stroke, coronary artery disease or renal failure. Hence hypertension needs to be treated even though as such it does not generally produce obvious troublesome symptoms.

Antihypertensives act by influencing the BP regulatory systems *viz* the autonomic system, renin-angiotensin system, calcium channels or sodium and water balance (plasma volume).

Classification

See below.

Diuretics

The antihypertensive effect of diuretics is mild—BP falls by 15-20 mm Hg over 2-4 weeks. Mode of action of diuretics act as antihypertensives (Flowchart 6.3).

Diuretics increase the excretion of sodium and water resulting in:

- ↓ Plasma volume → ↓ cardiac output → ↓ BP
- ↓ Body sodium → relaxation of vascular smooth muscles (due to Na^+ depletion) → ↓ PVR → ↓ BP.

Flowchart 6.3: Mode of action of diuretics in hypertension.

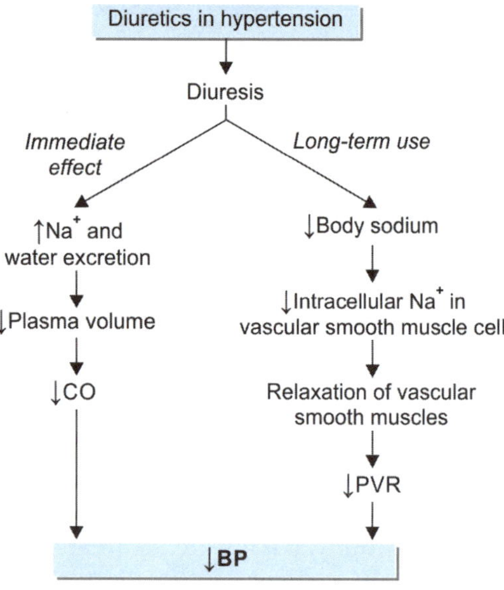

Restriction of dietary salt intake will reduce the dose of the diuretic needed. Thiazides are the first-line antihypertensives. They may be combined with a K^+ sparing diuretic to avoid hypokalemia. Thiazides may also be used in combination with other antihypertensives .

Classification of antihypertensives

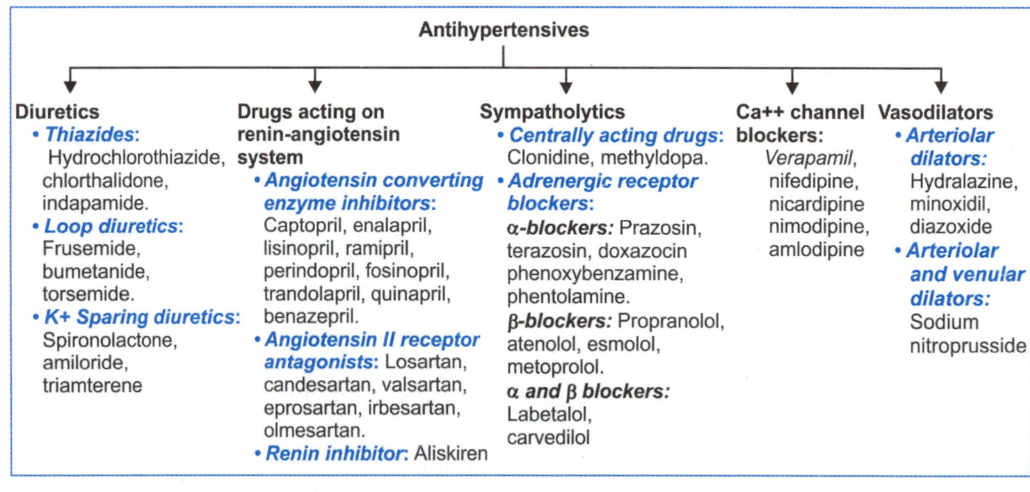

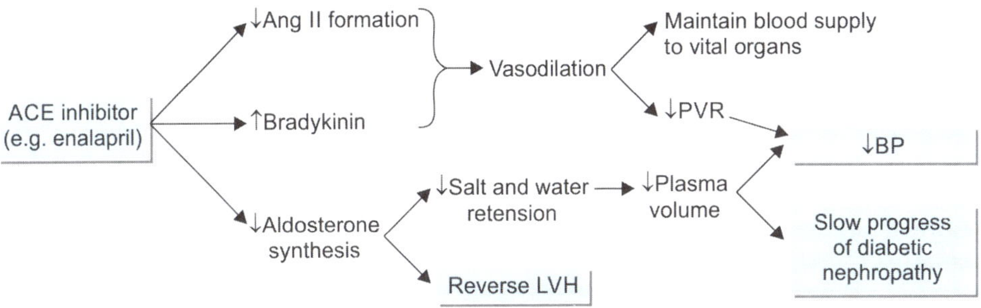

Fig. 6.3: ACE inhibitors in hypertension.

Loop diuretics: Though loop diuretics like frusemide are powerful diuretics, their antihypertensive efficacy is low. They are used only in hypertension with chronic renal failure or congestive heart failure and in hypertensive emergencies to rapidly lower the BP.

Drugs Acting on Renin Angiotensin System

1. Angiotensin Converting Enzyme (ACE) Inhibitors

Angiotensin II is a powerful vasoconstrictor. Aldosterone also raises the BP by increasing the plasma volume (Fig. 6.3). ACE inhibitors prevent the formation of angiotensin II and (indirectly) aldosterone. As a result, there is vasodilation and decrease in PVR leading to a fall in BP. As ACE also degrades bradykinin, ACE inhibitors raise the bradykinin levels which is a potent vasodilator. This also adds to the fall in BP.

The blood flow to the kidneys, brain and heart increases due to selective vasodilation and thus maintains adequate blood supply to these vital organs.

Pharmacokinetics: ACE inhibitors are generally well-absorbed. Except captopril and lisinopril, all others are prodrugs. Duration of action varies (Table 6.5).

Adverse effects: ACE inhibitors are well-tolerated. Adverse effects include persistent **dry cough** (due to raised bradykinin levels), hyperkalemia, alteration of taste sensation, skin rashes, hypotension, headache, nausea, abdominal pain and blood disorders.

Table 6.5: Dose and duration of action of some commonly used ACE inhibitors.

Drug	*Duration of action (in hrs)*	*Daily dose in hypertension (mg)*
Captopril	6–12	12.5–50 mg BD
Enalapril	24	2.5–20 mg OD
Lisinopril	>24	5–40 mg OD
Ramipril	8–48	1.25–10 mg OD

Angioedema though rare can be severe. At the first sign of angioedema ACE inhibitors should be stopped.

Uses

1. **Hypertension:** ACE inhibitors are useful in the treatment of hypertension of all grades due to all causes. Addition of a diuretic like thiazides potentiates their efficacy. They are presently the **first line antihypertensives** (Table 6.6). They are specially indicated as antihypertensives in:
   - Patients with diabetes as ACE-I slow the development of nephropathy.
   - Renal diseases—ACE inhibitors slow the progression.
   - Left ventricular hypertrophy—is gradually reversed by ACE inhibitors.
   - Patients who also have ischemic heart disease.
2. **CCF:** ACE inhibitors are the first line drugs.
3. **Myocardial infarction:** ACE inhibitors started within 24 hours and given for

Table 6.6: Dose and route of administration of some commonly used antihypertensives.

Antihypertensives	*Daily doses*	*Routes*
Hydrochlorothiazide + Amiloride	12.5–25 mg + 1.25–2.5 mg daily	Oral
Clonidine	100–300 μg	Oral
Methyldopa	250–500 mg q 6–12 hr	Oral
Atenolol	25–100 mg OD	Oral
Prazosin	2–20 mg daily	Oral
Hydralazine	25–50 mg q 8–24 hr	Oral
Diazoxide	50–100 mg every 5–10 min	IV
Sodium nitroprusside	0.2–0.3 mg/min	IV
Nifedipine	10 mg 5–20 mg q 8–12 hr	SL Oral
Losartan	50 mg OD	Oral
For ACE inhibitors *See* Table 6.5		

several weeks prevent the development of CCF and reduce mortality.

4. **Coronary artery disease:** In patients who are at a high-risk of ischemic cardiovascular conditions like MI and stroke, ACE inhibitors provide significant benefit by reducing the risk of MI, stroke and sudden death.
5. **Chronic renal failure:** In patients with diabetic nephropathy and chronic renal failure, ACE inhibitors delay the progression of renal disease.
6. **Scleroderma renal crisis:** ACE inhibitors may be life-saving in these patients.

Angiotensin II Receptor Antagonists or Angiotensin II Receptor Blockers (ARBs)

Losartan is an angiotensin II receptor antagonist. AT_1 receptors present in vascular and myocardial tissue, brain, kidney and adrenal glomerular cells are blocked by losartan. Losartan relaxes vascular smooth muscles, promotes salt and water excretion and reduces plasma volume. The advantage of ARBs over ACE inhibitors is that there is no increase in bradykinin levels and its associated adverse effects like dry cough and angioedema.

Adverse effects: Include hypotension and hyperkalemia. Angioedema is rare. It is contraindicated in pregnancy and lactation.

Uses

Hypertension: ARBs are used as first line drugs in the treatment of hypertension in similar indications as that of ACE inhibitors.

CCF: ARBs are alternatives to ACE inhibitors.

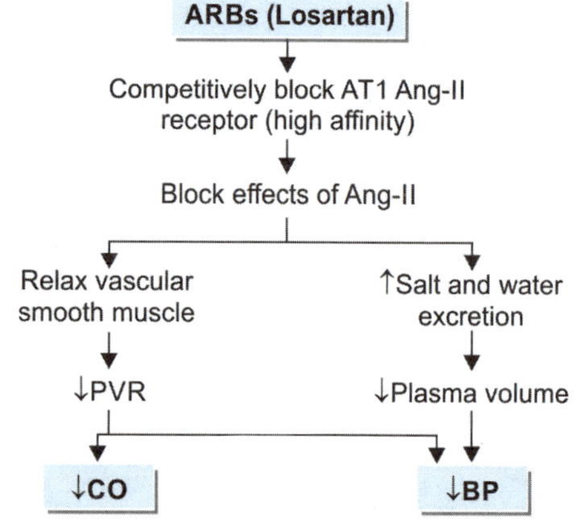

Renin Inhibitor

Aliskiren is a direct renin inhibitor that was recently introduced. Aliskiren blocks the effects of renin thereby reducing the blood pressure. Use of some drugs like ACE inhibitors, ARBs and diuretics tend to bring about a compensatory rise in the plasma renin levels. The antihypertensive action of Aliskiren is synergistic with these drugs. It can also be used as monotherapy and is orally effective. Dose: 150–300 mg once daily. Aliskiren is contraindicated in pregnancy.

Sympatholytics

Sympatholytic drugs may be used to supress sympathetic overactivity at different levels including centrally, at the ganglia, neurons and receptors.

Drugs Acting Centrally

Clonidine is a selective α_2 agonist. Stimulation of α_2 receptors in the CNS (in the vasomotor center and hypothalamus), decreases central sympathetic outflow, blocks the release of noradrenaline from the nerve terminals leading to a fall in BP and bradycardia.

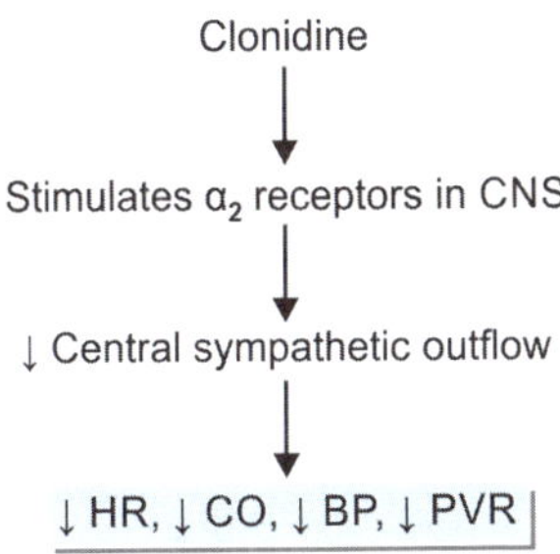

Adverse effects include drowsiness, dryness of mouth, nose and eyes; parotid gland swelling and pain, fluid retention, constipation and impotence. Sudden withdrawal of clonidine will lead to rebound hypertension, headache, tremors, sweating and tachycardia. Hence the dose should be tapered.

Uses: Mild to moderate hypertension.

Other Uses

- **In opioid withdrawal:** Most withdrawal symptoms in opioid addicts are due to sympathetic overactivity and can be benefited by treatment with clonidine.
- **Diabetic neuropathy:** Clonidine controls diarrhea by improving absorption of NaCl and water in the gut by stimulation of α_2 receptors in the intestines.
- **With anesthetics:** Clonidine given preoperatively reduces the dose of the general anesthetic needed due to its analgesic effects.

α-methyl dopa: An analog of dopa, is a prodrug. It is metabolized in the body to α-methyl norepinephrine which is an α_2 agonist and acts like clonidine. Renin levels also fall. Left ventricular hypertrophy is reversed in about 12 weeks of treatment.

Adverse effects are sedation, dryness of mouth and nose, headache, postural hypotension, fluid retention and impotence.

Uses: It is used in mild to moderate hypertension along with a diuretic. **It is safe in hypertension during pregnancy and is preferred in them.**

Ganglion Blockers

These drugs block both sympathetic and parasympathetic ganglia resulting in decreased sympathetic tone and a fall in BP. However, they produce several side effects as they block both ganglia and are not used now. **Trimethaphan** is the only ganglion blocker used intravenously to produce controlled hypotension during certain surgeries for its rapid and short action (15 minutes).

Adrenergic Neuron Blockers

Guanethidine depletes the stores of noradrenaline in the adrenergic neurons and also blocks its release. Because of the adverse effects like postural hypotension, diarrhea and sexual dysfunction, it is **not used**.

Reserpine is an alkaloid obtained from *Rauwolfia serpentina* (Sarpagandhi) that grows in India. In the neurons, it destroys the vesicles that store monoamines like noradrenaline, dopamine and 5-HT and thus depletes the stores of these monoamines. Reserpine also causes various side effects like drowsiness, depression, parkinsonism, postural hypotension, edema and sexual dysfunction. Hence it is **generally not preferred**.

Adrenergic Receptor Blockers

α-blockers: Prazosin is a selective α_1-blocker; it dilates both arterioles and venules. Peripheral vascular resistance is decreased leading to a fall in BP with only mild tachycardia.

'First dose phenomenon' can be avoided by starting with a low dose (0.5 mg) given at bed time. Dose is gradually increased. Prazosin is used in mild to moderate hypertension; it may be combined with diuretics and β-blockers.

β-blockers are mild antihypertensives. Blockade of β1 receptors in the heart results in decreased myocardial contractility and cardiac output. They reduce the BP due to a fall in the cardiac output. They also lower plasma renin activity and have an additional central antihypertensive action.

- They are well-tolerated and are of special value in patients who also have arrhythmias or angina.
- They are also suitable for combination with other antihypertensives.
- They are thus the first line antihypertensive drugs in mild to moderate hypertension.
- **Atenolol** is the preferred β-blocker because of the advantages like
  - once a day dosing
  - absence of CNS side effects
  - β1 selectivity.
- β-blockers should always be tapered while withdrawing.
- **Metoprolol** may be used as a sustained release tablet.
- **Esmolol**, the short acting β-blocker is used in intraoperative and postoperative hypertension and in hypertensive emergencies.

α and β-blockers: Labetalol blocks α_1 and β receptors. It is used intravenously in the treatment of hypertension in pheochromocytoma and in hypertensive emergencies.

Vasodilators

Vasodilators relax the vascular smooth muscles thus reducing BP due to decreased peripheral vascular resistance. Salt and water retention and reflex tachycardia are common with vasodilators.

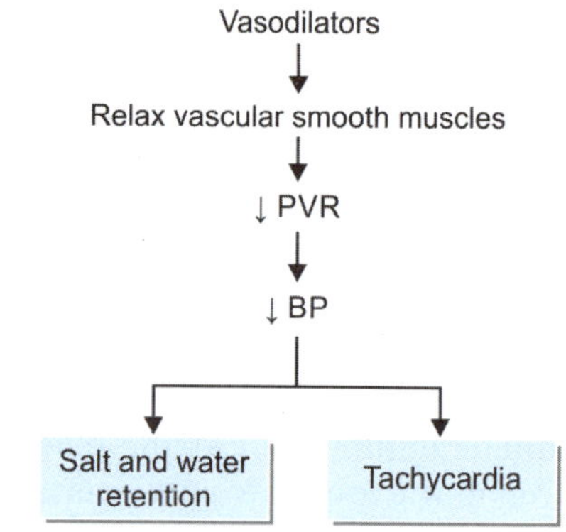

Vasodilators may be:

- **Arteriolar dilators:** Hyralazine, minoxidil, diazoxide, calcium channel blockers.
- **Arteriolar and venular dilators:** Sodium nitroprusside.

Hydralazine is a directly acting arteriolar dilator. The fall in BP is associated with tachycardia, renin release and fluid retention. Coronary, cerebral and renal blood flow are increased.

Adverse effects are headache, flushing, palpitation, salt and water retention. It may precipitate angina in some patients. Hypersensitivity reactions like serum sickness and lupus erythematosus may occur.

Uses: Hydralazine is used with a β-blocker and/or a diuretic in moderate to severe hypertension not controlled by the first line drugs. It can be given in **hypertension during pregnancy**.

Minoxidil is a directly acting arteriolar dilator used in severe hypertension not responding to other drugs. It acts by opening K^+ channels in smooth muscles.

Minoxidil stimulates the growth of hair on prolonged use. Hence it is used topically (2% solution) in *alopecia*. Young men with relative alopecia are more likely to respond.

Minoxidil can cause fluid retention, tachycardia and growth of hair on the face, arms, legs and the back.

Diazoxide is related to thiazide diuretics and is a potent arteriolar dilator. Its mechanism of action is like minoxidil. It is used in hypertensive emergencies where monitoring of infusion is not possible. Diazoxide has a long duration of action (24 hours) and is suitable in such situations.

Sodium nitroprusside is a rapidly acting vasodilator and it relaxes both arterioles and venules. Both peripheral resistance and cardiac output are reduced resulting in lower myocardial oxygen consumption. Nitroprusside acts through the release of nitric oxide which relaxes the vascular smooth muscles. On IV administration, it is rapid (acts within 30 seconds) and short-acting (duration 3 minutes) allowing titration of the dose. This makes it suitable for use in **hypertensive emergencies with close monitoring. It decomposes on exposure to light; the infusion bottle and tubing should be covered with opaque foil.**

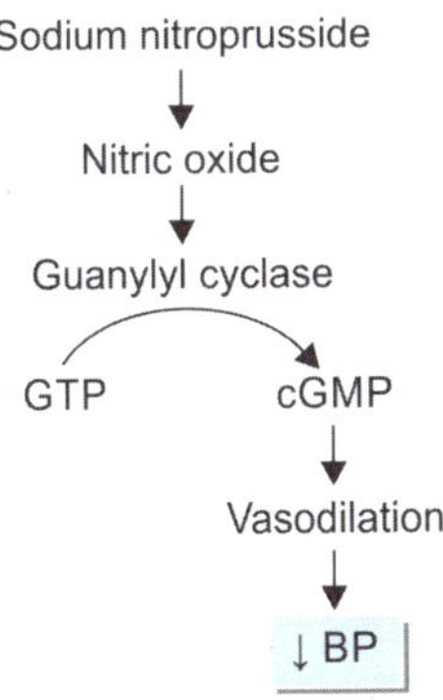

Adverse reactions are palpitation, sweating, weakness, nausea, vomiting and in high doses, accumulation of thiocyanide can result in thiocyanate toxicity including psychosis, muscle spasm and convulsions.

Uses

- Nitroprusside was used in hypertensive emergencies but now not preferred.
- It is used in situations where short-term reduction of myocardial workload is required as in myocardial infarction.

Calcium Channel Blockers

Calcium channel blockers (CCBs) are another important group of antihypertensives. They dilate the arterioles resulting in reduced peripheral vascular resistance. Nifedipine produces some reflex tachycardia while this is not seen with verapamil and diltiazem as they are cardiac depressants. Fluid retention is negligible unlike other arteriolar dilators.

Use in hypertension

- CCBs are well-tolerated, and effective.
- CCBs are particularly effective in elderly patients - in hypertensive emergencies, nifedipine effectively lowers BP in 10 minutes - may be used sublingually or parenterally.
- CCBs are of special value in patients who also have angina.
- Sustained release preparations or long acting CCBs may be used for smoother control of BP.
- CCBs may be used in combination with other antihypertensives in moderate to severe hypertension (stage 2).

Drug Interactions of Antihypertensives

- Sympathomimetics and tricyclic anti-depressants can antagonize the effects of sympatholytics.
- Antihistamines add to sedation produced by clonidine and methyldopa.
- NSAIDs tend to cause salt and water retention and may blunt the effect of antihypertensives.

Treatment of Hypertension

The aim of treatment in hypertension is to prevent complications by maintaining the blood pressure at near normal levels. Since treatment is generally prolonged (may be life-long) and all antihypertensives can cause side effects, initially nonpharmacological measures should be used. If drugs are required, minimum possible dose should be used.

Stage 1 hypertension is treated with a thiazide diuretic or an ACE inhibitor/ARB/CCB. If uncontrolled by adequate doses of one drug, a second drug may be added.

Stage 2 hypertension would require a combination of 2 drugs—a thiazide with ARB/ACEI/CCB. In patients with chronic kidney disease, treatment should be initiated with an ACE inhibitor/ARB with or without other antihypertensives.

Hypertensive emergencies: Conditions like hypertensive encephalopathy and acute cardiac failure due to hypertension require immediate treatment in an ICU. Parenteral drugs are preferred. BP should be lowered gradually to avoid ischemia to vital organs. Directly acting vasodilators and some adrenergic blockers are commonly used. IV **nicardipine** produces rapid and reliable antihypertensive effects and is the preferred drug. **IV labetalol and esmolol** are alternatives. Because of the toxicity, sodium nitroprusside is generally not preferred. As soon as possible switch over to oral drugs like amlodipine or labetalol.

Hypertension in pregnancy: The drugs found safe are—**methyldopa** orally for maintenance and **hydralazine** (parenteral) for reduction of BP in emergency. However they should be used only after the first trimester. Cardio-selective β-blockers (atenolol) α-blocker prazosin and α_2 agonist clonidine can also be used.

Combination of antihypertensives: When it is not possible to achieve adequate control of BP with a single drug, a combination may be used. Antihypertensives may also be combined to overcome the side effects of one another. This also allows use of lower doses of each drug.

Sympatholytics and vasodilators cause fluid retention which can be overcome by adding a diuretic.

Vasodilators like nifedipine and hydralazine can lead to reflex tachycardia. This can be countered by β-blockers, while propranolol may cause initial rise in PVR which is countered by vasodilators.

Combination of ACE inhibitors and diuretics is synergistic.

Non-pharmacological measures: Low salt diet, weight reduction, transidental meditation, all go a long way in controlling the blood pressure. Smoking and alcohol should be given up. These measures also help in reducing the dose of the antihypertensive needed.

DRUGS USED IN ISCHEMIC HEART DISEASE

Ischemic heart disease is a common cause in death across the world. It may manifest as:

- Angina pectoris
- Unstable angina
- Myocardial infaction (MI).

Drugs Used in the Treatment of Angina Pectoris

Angina pectoris is the symptom of ischemic heart disease (IHD) characterized by sudden, severe, substernal discomfort or pain which may radiate to the left shoulder and along the flexor surface of the left arm. Myocardial oxygen consumption is mainly determined by preload (venous return and stretching of the heart), afterload (peripheral arterial resistance) and heart rate. When the oxygen supply to the myocardium is insufficient for its needs, myocardial ischemia develops. Pain is due to accumulation of metabolites in the cardiac muscle. Two forms of angina are:

1. **Classical angina (stable angina, angina of effort):** Pain is induced by exercise or emotion, both of which increase myocardial oxygen demand. As there is

narrowing of the coronary arteries due to atherosclerosis, they cannot dilate to increase the blood supply during exercise. Hence there is imbalance between oxygen supply and demand.

2. **Variant or Prinzmetal's angina** occurs at rest and is caused by spasm of the coronary artery.

Acute coronary syndrome is anginal pain occuring at rest due to rupture of the atherosclerotic plaque leading to coronary thrombosis and includes unstable angina and myocardial infarction.

Antianginal Drugs

Drugs are used to improve the balance between oxygen supply and demand either by increasing oxygen supply to the myocardium (coronary dilation) or by reducing the oxygen demand (reducing preload/afterload/heart rate or all of these).

1. **Nitrates:** Nitroglycerine, isosorbide dinitrate, isosorbide mononitrate, pentaerythritol tetranitrate.
2. **Calcium channel blockers:** Verapamil, diltiazem, amlodipine, nifedipine.
3. **β-blockers:** Propranolol, atenolol, etc.
4. **Potassium channel openers:** Nicorandil pinacidil, cromakalim.
5. **Miscellaneous:** Aspirin, dipyridamol, clopidogrel, trimetazidine, ranolazine, ivabradine.

Nitrates

Mechanism of action: Nitrates are vasodilators (mainly venodilators) (Fig. 6.4). They are converted to nitric oxide which leads to relaxation of the vascular smooth muscles. Venodilation reduces venous return to the heart thereby reducing preload. Arteriolar dilation reduces vascular resistance thus decreasing afterload. As both preload and afterload are reduced, work load of the heart is decreased thereby reducing oxygen requirement of the heart.

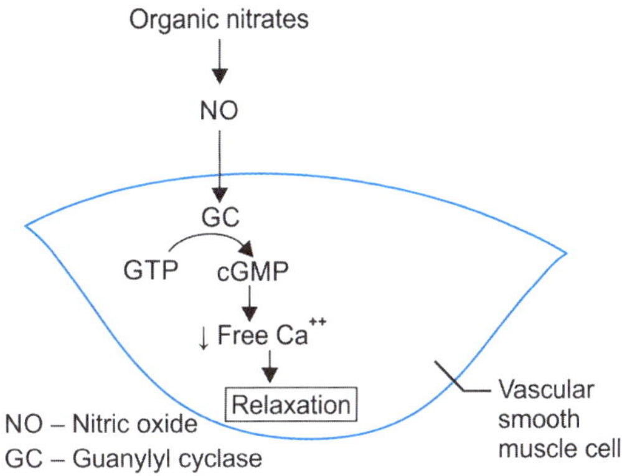

Fig. 6.4: Mechanism of action of nitrates.

In variant angina, nitrates relieve vasospasm due to coronary vasodilation.

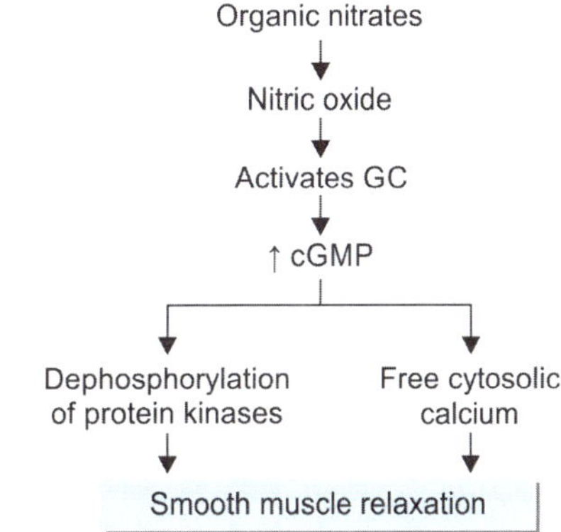

Nitrates also cause dilation of blood vessels in the skin—resulting in **flushing**; dilatation of the meningeal vessels result in **headache**.

Bronchial smooth muscles are also **relaxed**.

Adverse effects: Headache is common; **flushing, sweating, palpitation,** weakness, postural hypotension and rashes can occur. Tolerance to vascular effects develops on repeated long-term use. Nitrates should be gradually withdrawn after long-term use.

Uses

1. **Exertional angina:**
   - **Acute episode:** Sublingual nitroglycerine is the drug of choice for acute anginal attacks (Table 6.7). It

Table 6.7: Some nitrates used in angina pectoris.

Drug	Dose and route	Duration of action
Nitroglycerine glyceryl trinitrate (GTN) (Angised)	0.5 mg SL 5 mg oral 2% Skin ointment applied 1–2 inches on the precardial region	15–40 min 4–8 hr 4–6 hr
Isosorbide dinitrate (Sorbitrate)	5–10 mg SL 10–20 mg oral	20–40 min 2–3 hr
Isosorbide mononitrate (ISMO)	10–20 mg oral	6–8 hr

(SL: sublingual)

relieves pain in 3 minutes. If the pain is not relieved, the dose may be repeated (up to 3 tablets in 15 minutes).

The patient should be advised to take the tablet in a sitting position, since the sudden reduction in BP can result in fall due to syncope.

– **Prophylaxis:** NTG can be used for acute as well as chronic prophylaxis. When patient is expected to have a known exertion like walking uphill, a tablet of sublingual NTG can be used for (acute prophylaxis) prevention of angina.

  Isosorbide dinitrate may be used orally for prevention of nocturnal angina. Nitroglycerine **ointment** may be applied over the chest. **Transdermal** nitroglycerine patch delivers nitroglycerin constantly for 24 hours.

2. **Vasospastic angina:** Nitroglycerin relieves pain by relieving coronary vasospasm.
3. **Unstable angina:** Intravenous nitroglycerin helps to relieve pain. The benefit could be both due to reduction in cardiac work load and coronary vasodilation.
4. **Cardiac failure:** Nitrates are useful due to their vasodilator property.
5. **Myocardial infarction:** IV nitroglycerine is used by many physicians.
6. **Cyanide poisoning:** Cyanide rapidly binds to cytochrome oxidase and other vital enzymes resulting in inhibition of cellular respiration and blocks the utilization of oxygen. It requires immediate treatment. Amylnitrite is given by inhalation and sodium nitrite by IV injection (10 mL of 3% solution). Sodium thiosulfate is given IV (50 mL of 25% solution). It reacts with cyanmethemoglobin to form thiocyanate which is easily excreted by the kidneys. Nitrates convert hemoglobin to methemoglobin which has a high affinity for cyanide and binds to cyanide forming cyanmethemoglobin. It thus protects the important enzymes from binding to cyanide. Amyl nitrite is preferred. Early treatment is very important.

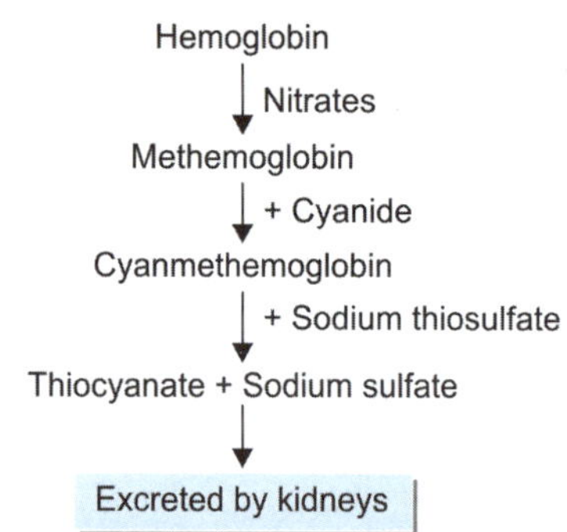

7. **Antispasmodic:** Nitrates relieve esophageal spasm when taken sublingually before meals. Nitrates also relieve biliary colic.

Calcium Channel Blockers

The depolarization of cardiac and vascular smooth muscle cells depend on the entry of extracellular calcium into the cell through calcium channels. This calcium triggers the release of intracellular calcium from the sarcoplasmic reticulum. All these calcium ions cause contraction. Calcium channel blockers (CCBs) inhibit the entry of Ca^{++} by blocking the Ca^{++} channels. This results in the following actions:

- **Smooth muscle relaxation:** Arteriolar dilatation reducing peripheral vascular resistance, leading to a fall in BP. Reflex tachycardia may occur with some.
- **Heart:** CCBs depress myocardial contractility, reduce heart rate, cardiac work and myocardial O_2 consumption.
- **Coronary circulation:** Coronary vasodilation occurs, increasing coronary blood flow. Hence CCBs are useful in variant angina.

CCBs include

1. **Dihydropyridines:** Nifedipine, nimodipine, nicardipine, amlodipine, felodipine, isradipine, nitrendipine, nisoldipine.
2. **Others:** Verapamil, diltiazem.

Verapamil has prominent myocardiac depressant actions. AV conduction is depressed and usually bradycardia is seen. Hence, it should not be combined with β-blockers. Fall in BP is mild as the vasodilator effect of verapamil is less potent.

Adverse effects include constipation, bradycardia, heart block and hypotension. It may precipitate CCF in patients with diseased heart. Diltiazem has mild vasodilator effects but is a myocardiac depressant like verapamil.

Nifedipine a dihydropyridine, is a potent vasodilator and causes a significant fall in BP and evokes reflex tachycardia. Myocardiac depressant effect is weak. It can be given sublingually.

Adverse effects are headache, flushing, palpitation, dizziness, fatigue, hypotension, leg cramps and ankle edema.

Other CCBs like amlodipine, felodipine, nitrendipine and nicardipine are similar to nifedipine with some pharmacokinetic variations. They have higher vascular selectivity. **Nimodipine** selectively relaxes cerebral vasculature.

Pharmacokinetics: CCBs are well-absorbed but undergo extensive first pass metabolism. They are all highly plasma protein bound and are metabolized in the liver.

Uses of CCBs

1. **Ischemic heart diseases:** CCBs—verapamil and diltiazem are used in the treatment of **stable angina**. They are very effective in relieving the pain, as CCBs are coronary vasodilators they relieve spasm in **vasospastic angina**. Verapamil is also useful in **unstable angina**.
2. **Hypertension:** Verapamil, nifedipine, amlodipine and diltiazem can be used. Nifedipine is used sublingually in hypertensive crisis.
3. **Arrhythmias:** Verapamil is the drug of choice in PSVT.
4. **Peripheral vascular disease:** Nifedipine is useful in Raynaud's disease due to its vasodilator effects.
5. **Hypertrophic cardiomyopathy:** Verapamil is used.
6. **Migraine:** Verapamil can be used in the prophylaxis of migraine.
7. **Subarachnoid hemorrhage:** Vasospasm that follows subarachnoid hemorrhage is believed to be responsible for neurological defects. As nimodipine brings about cerebral vasodilation, it is used to treat neurological deficits in patients with cerebral vasospasm.
8. **Atherosclerosis:** Dihydropyridines may slow the progress of atherosclerosis.
9. **Diabetic nephropathy:** Verapamil is an alternative to ACE inhibitors to slow the development of diabetic nephropathy.
10. **Preterm labor:** Nifedipine inhibits uterine contractions and is useful in delaying labor in premature contraction.
11. **Smooth muscle hypertrophy:** As seen in achalasia may respond to CCBs.

Mnemonic for uses

verapamil's HIP HAD SPASM
H—**Hypertrophic cardiomyopathy**
I— **Ischemic heart diseases**
P—**Peripheral vascular disease**
H—Hypertension
A—**Arrhythmias**
D—Diabetic nephropathy
S—**Subarachnoid hemorrhage**
P—Pre-term labor
A—Atherosclerosis
S—Smooth muscle hypertrophy
M—**Migraine**

β-blockers

β-blockers reduce the frequency and severity of attacks of exertional angina and are useful in the prevention of angina. Exercise, emotion and similar situations increase sympathetic activity leading to increased heart-rate, force of contraction and BP, thereby increasing O_2 consumption by the heart. β-blockers prevent angina by blocking all these actions. They are used for the long-term prophylaxis of classical angina and may be combined with nitrates. β-blockers should always be tapered after prolonged use. They are *not* useful in variant angina.

Potassium Channel Openers

Nicorandil is an arterial and venous dilator. Opening of the K^+ channels results in hyperpolarization and therefore relaxation of the vascular smooth muscles. In addition nicorandil also acts through nitric oxide to cause vasodilatation. Adverse effects are headache, flushing, dizziness and hypotension. Nicorandil is used as an alternative to nitrates in the treatment of angina. It is used in the dose of 10–20 mg twice daily. Pinacidil is similar to nicorandil and is also useful in hypertension. Minoxidil and diazoxide are K^+ channel openers used in hypertension.

Miscellaneous

1. **Aspirin:** Low dose aspirin is given for a long period for its **antiplatelet aggregatory property**. It has been shown to prevent myocardial infarction in patients with angina.
   Clopidogrel, an antiplatelet drug, is also used either alone or along with aspirin.
2. **Dipyridamole:** Dipyridamole is a coronary vasodilator but it diverts the blood from ischemic zone and is therefore not beneficial. It inhibits platelet aggregation for which it is used in post-MI and post-stroke patients for prevention of coronary and cerebral thrombosis.
3. **Trimetazidine** is a calcium channel blocker claimed to have a protective effect on the ischemic myocardium and to maintain left ventricular function. Trimetazidine belongs to a new class of drugs that modulate the metabolism in the myocardium. Trimetazidine inhibits the enzyme involved in fatty acid oxidation pathway in the myocardium. It also inhibits the cytotoxicity to the myocardial cells. Trimetazidine thus protects the myocardium from ischemic damage. It is orally effective and is well tolerated with occasional gastric irritation, fatigue and muscle cramps. Trimetazidine is used as an add on drug along with other antianginal drugs in the treatment of angina pectoris.
4. **Ranolazine** is a recently introduced trimetazidine derivative with a unique mechanism of action. Ranolazine inhibits the late sodium current in the myocardium and prevents calcium overload in the myocardium during ischemia. It thus reduces myocardial oxygen demand. Due to this **cardioprotective properties**, ranolazine is used for the prevention of angina in patients who do not respond to first line drugs. Ranolazine in orally effective. It can cause weakness, postural hypotension, QT prolongation, dizziness, headache and constipation. Dose 500 mg sustained release tablets twice daily.

5. **Ivabradine** decreases the heart rate by a direct effect (direct-bradycardiac agent) and may be used as an alternative to β-blockers.

Pharmacotherapy of Angina

Coronary angioplasty with the insertion of a stent is the preferred treatment in the presence of significant narrowing of the coronary arteries. Coronary artery bypass surgery is done when there is severe narrowing. Pharmacotherapy may be an alternative in some patients.

Acute attack: Sublingual nitroglycerine is the drug of choice. If the pain does not subside in 5 minutes, repeat the dose. After the relief of pain, the tablet should be discarded.

Acute prophylaxis: Sublingual nitroglycerine given 15 minutes before an exertion (e.g. walking uphill) can prevent the attack. The prophylactic effect lasts for 30 minutes.

Chronic prophylaxis: Long-acting nitrates or β-blockers (preferred) or calcium channel blockers can be used. All are given orally.

If one drug is not effective, a combination of drugs may be used.

Combination of Drugs in Angina

1. Nitrates + β-blockers—very effective in exertional angina.
   Reflex tachycardia due to nitrates is countered by β-blockers. Ventricular dilatation due to β-blockers is opposed by nitrates.
2. Nifedipine + β-blockers. The antianginal effects are additive. Reflex tachycardia due to nifedipine is countered by β-blockers.
3. Nitrates + CCBs—nitrates decrease preload, CCBs reduce afterload and the combination reduces cardiac workload.
4. CCBs + β-blockers + Nitrates—if the angina is not controlled by 2 drug combinations, 3 drugs can be used. Nitrates reduce preload, CCBs reduce afterload while β-blockers decrease heart rate. This combination is useful in severe angina.

Unstable angina includes:
- Patients with exertional angina developing angina at rest
- Severe, prolonged anginal attacks without ECG evidence of MI
- Angina developing after myocardial infarction.

Such patients with unstable angina are at a high risk of developing MI or sudden death and need hospitalization and rigorous treatment for its prevention.

Drugs used in unstable angina: Aspirin, heparin and IV nitroglycerine may be used in unstable angina. Long-term administration of β-blockers like atenolol or a CCB like verapamil is beneficial.

Drugs used in myocardial infarction: Rupture of an atheromatus plaque in the coronary artery results in the formation of a thrombus which blocks the artery leading to loss of blood supply to the concerned part of the heart. This results in acute myocardial infarction.

Drugs used are:
- IV opioid analgesics like morphine/pethidine to relieve pain and anxiety
- Thrombolytics like streptokinase to dissolve the thrombus
- Aspirin for its antiplatelet aggregatory effect.
- Atenolol and ACE inhibitors are employed both for acute episode and long-term use.

PHARMACOTHERAPY OF SHOCK

Shock is acute circulatory failure with underperfusion of tissues. Symptoms of sympathetic overactivity are generally seen—like pallor, sweating, cold extremities and tachycardia. Shock may be:

1. **Hypovolemic shock:** Decreased fluid volume due to sudden loss of plasma or blood as in hemorrhage, burns or dehydration—results in hypovolemic

shock. Treatment is by replacement of fluids and electrolytes.

2. **Septic shock** is precipitated by severe bacterial infection. It may be due to release of bacterial toxins. Immediate treatment of shock and appropriate IV antibiotics should be started.
3. **Cardiogenic shock** is due to failure of heart as a pump as in myocardial infarction.
4. **Anaphylactic shock:** Type I hypersensitivity reaction causing release of massive amounts of histamine which is triggered by antigen-antibody reaction.
5. **Neurogenic shock** is due to venous pooling as following spinal anesthesia, spinal cord injury, abdominal or testicular trauma.

Treatment

Shock of any type needs immediate treatment:

- The cause should be identified and treated
- Maintain BP and plasma volume
- Correct the acid base and electrolyte disturbances
- Ensure adequate urine output.

In shock due to myocardial infarction, **IV morphine** is the drug of choice to relieve pain and anxiety. Thrombolytic therapy and oxygen inhalation should be started immediately. Absolute bed rest, prevention of arrhythmias and maintenance of cardiac output are all important.

Septic shock should be treated with appropriate antibiotics.

Anaphylactic shock—treatment—*See* page 49.

PLASMA EXPANDERS

When there is a sudden loss of blood or plasma as in road traffic accidents, the plasma volume falls, resulting in reduced blood supply to the tissues and can be rapidly fatal.

To restore the intravascular volume, the component lost should ideally be replaced like—plasma in burns and blood after hemorrhage. However, in emergency, immediate volume replacement is important. In such situations plasma expanders are used. Plasma expanders are high molecular weight substances which when infused IV exert oncotic pressure and remain in the body for a long time to increase the volume of circulating fluid.

An ideal plasma expander should exert oncotic pressure comparable to plasma, be long-acting, non-antigenic and pharmacologically inert.

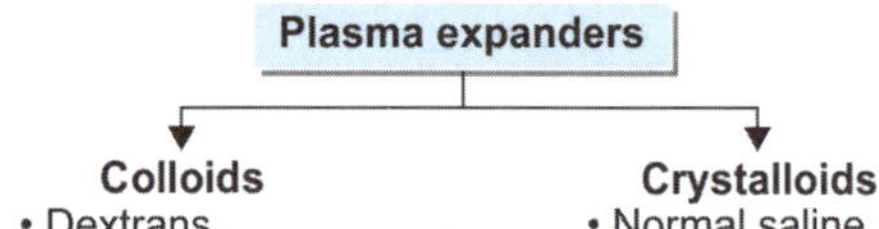

Colloids

Dextrans (Dextran 70 mol. wt. 70,000 and dextran 40 mol. wt. 40,000) are commonly used. Allergic reactions are common. It interferes with coagulation, blood grouping and cross-matching.

Gelatin products have a mol. wt. of 30,000 and a duration of action of 12 hours. Allergic reactions are rare.

Hydroxyethyl starch maintains blood volume for a long period and allergic reactions are rare.

Polyvinyl pyrrolidone (PVP) is a synthetic polymer. It is not preferred due to various disadvantages like—it provokes histamine release and interferes with blood grouping.

Crystalloids

Crystalloids include normal saline, Ringer lactate and dextrose solution.

Normal saline solution (0.9% sodium chloride) remains in the ECF because the electrolytes make up its osmolality. It is used in hyponatremia. It should be avoided in

Compare and contrast colloids and crystalloids		
	Colloids	**Crystalloids**
Molecular size	Large molecules	Small crystals or salts dissolved in solution
On infusion	Remain in vascular system for long periods	Easily filtered by glomerulus and excreted
Duration of action	Long (12–36 hrs)	Short (1–2 hrs)
Plasma volume expansion	Potent plasma expanders	Less effective
Oncotic pressure	Exerted	Only by hypertonic solution
Movement across semipermeable membrane	Not possible	Possible
Cost	More expensive	Less expensive
Disadvantages	• Some of them interfere with coagulation, blood grouping and cross matching • Allergic reactions can occur	• Short acting • Volume expansion not effective
Use	To restore intravascular volume as in burns and bleeding	Replacement of fluid, electrolytes, nutrition and to dilute drugs
Examples	Dextrans, gelatin polymer, hetastarches, polyvinylpyrrolidone, **Natural colloids**-whole blood, plasma, human albumin	Normal saline, dextrose, ringer lactate solution

heart failure, pulmonary edema and renal impairment.

Lactated Ringer's solution contains potassium, calcium and sodium chloride. The lactate provides bicarbonate and helps to correct acidosis. It is used to correct dehydration, hyponatremia and replace gastrointestinal fluids. Many other similar solutions including diarrhea treatment solutions (DTS) are available with minor changes in the electrolyte content.

5% Dextrose in normal saline or lactated Ringer's solution is a hypertonic solution. They should be infused slowly to avoid volume overload. 50% dextrose is used in hypoglycemia or to supplement calories.

Uses of plasma expanders These are used as plasma substitutes in hypovolemic shock, burns and extensive fluid loss—as an emergency measure to restore plasma volume.

VASOACTIVE DRUGS

Drugs that affect the vascular smooth muscles are vasoactive drugs and include vasoconstrictors and vasodilators.

Some prostaglandins, angiotensin and antidiuretic hormone are natural vasoconstrictors released in the body (endogenous). They are released in hypotension and hypovolemia.

Vasoconstrictors

1. **Endogenous:** Noradrenaline, prostaglandins (TXA_2), angiotensin, ADH, 5-HT
2. **Drugs**
   - **α-agonists:** Dopamine, adrenaline, ephedrine, phenylephrine, mephentermine, metaraminol, methoxamine
   - **5-HT agonist:** Sumatriptan, ergot alkaloids.

In general vasoconstrictors bring about a rise in blood pressure with bradycardia. α_1 agonists are used in hypotension and topically as nasal decongestants.

Vasodilators

1. **Endogenous:** Prostaglandins, acetylcholine, nitric oxide
2. **Drugs**
   - **ACE inhibitors:** Captopril, enalapril, ramipril, etc.

- **Angiotensin II receptor antagonists:** Losartan, candesartan, etc.
- **Ca^{++} channel blockers:** Nifedipine, nimodipine, etc.
- α **blockers:** Prazosin, phentolamine, phenoxybenzamine
- **Nitrates:** Nitroglycerine, sodium nitroprusside
- **K^+ channel openers:** Minoxidil, cromakalim, nicorandil
- **Others:** Hydralazine, theophylline.

In general the effects of vasodilators include hypotension and reduced cardiac workload. However, they may cause reflex tachycardia. Adverse effects to vasodilators generally include palpitation, flushing, dizziness, headache, hypotension and edema.

Vasodilators are used in the treatment of hypertension, angina pectoris, cardiac failure, myocardial infarction and peripheral vascular diseases.

CEREBRAL ISCHEMIA

Stroke is due to sudden reduction of blood flow for a brief period (few seconds to few minutes) in the brain which if continues for more than a few minutes results in infarction of the brain tissue. Stroke results from focal ischemia of a part of the brain, or intracranial hemorrhage. Ischemia could be due to a thrombus or embolus occluding a blood vessel in the brain. Stroke is the most common cause of severe physical disability and about 50% of patients who survive acute stroke suffer from physical disability.

Risk factors include prolonged hypertension, diabetes mellitus, old age, heredity, hyperlipidemia, atherosclerosis and smoking.

Manifestations of stroke include hemiplegia which may be associated with signs of focal cerebral dysfunction like aphasia, sensory loss and visual field defects. Transient ischemic attack is stroke which resolves in 24 hours. The cause should be detected and efforts should be made to prevent its recurrence.

Treatment of Ischemic Stroke

1. **Thrombolytics:** Though thrombolytics seem to be helpful in dissolving the clot and restoring the blood supply, it carries the risk of hemorrhagic transformation of the infarct which could be fatal. However, thrombolysis carried out within 3 hours of onset of stroke in selected patients after ruling out hemorrhage results in improvement. Intravenous infusion of recombinant tissue plasmogen activator is started. Blood supply may also be restored by alternative methods like intra-arterial thrombolysis, mechanical dissolution or removal of the clot.
2. **Antiplatelet drugs:** Low dose aspirin (300 mg) should be started immediately if tPA is not given. If thrombolytics are given, aspirin may be started on the second day and should be continued - alternatively, clopidogrel or ticlopidine can be used.
3. **Anticoagulants:** After ruling out hemorrhage by MRI, heparin is started intravenously to prevent recurrence. Heparin is given for a week and then anticoagulation is continued with oral anticoagulants. However it carries the risk of hemorrhage and the benefits have not been proved. Therefore routine heparin use is not recommended.
4. Maintenance of airway, circulation and blood pressure are important in acute stroke, risk factors if any like hypertension, uncontrolled diabetes mellitus, hyperlipidemia should be taken care of.
5. **Rehabilitation** includes physiotherapy, speech therapy and if needed occupational therapy.
6. To reduce the risk of recurrence antiplatelet drugs should be continued for long-term. Carotid angioplasty and stenting also prevent restenosis.

DRUGS USED IN TREATMENT OF PERIPHERAL VASCULAR DISEASES

Peripheral vascular diseases (PVD) result from reduced blood supply to the lower limbs. Reduction in blood supply may be due to:

1. Organic occlusion or obstruction (e.g. thrombus)
2. Vasospasm.

Obstruction to the blood flow in the peripheral circulation due to any cause can result in ischemia of the area distal to it with its related consequences. Drugs are not of much help in vascular disease due to organic obstruction. Vasospastic peripheral vascular diseases include thromboangitis obliterans (TAO, Buerger's disease), Raynaud's phenomenon, frost bite, vascular complications of diabetes mellitus like gangrene, leg and foot ulcers.

Drugs used in peripheral vascular diseases include:

1. **Vasodilators**
   - CCBs - nifedipine
   - Adrenergic blockers - prazosin, tolazoline
   - β adrenergic agonists - isosxuprine
2. **Anticoagulants and antiplatelet drugs:** Heparin, warfarin, aspirin, clopidogrel.
3. **Other drugs:** Hypolipidemics (Statins), pentoxiphylline, naftidofuryl oxalate, cilostazol, cyclandelate, xanthinol nicotinate.

Vasodilators are of no significant value in obstructive peripheral vascular diseases because they do not enhance the blood flow to the ischemic areas. In fact they may even harm such an area because general vasodilation may shift the blood to other nonischemic areas described as 'steal' syndrome. However, vasodilators may be used in vasospastic diseases like Raynaud's phenomenon. The strategy is to bring about dilation of the arterioles to allow better blood flow to the limbs with minimum hypotension.

- **Calcium channel blockers**—like nifedipine are good vasodilators and are beneficial in patients with peripheral vascular diseases. Nifedipine is given in the dose 5-20 mg thrice daily.
- **Alpha adrenergic blockers**—like prazosin may be used in the dose of 0.5 mg twice daily.
- **Beta adrenergic agonists**—like isoxsuprine also help to relieve symptoms.

Anticoagulants and antiplatelet drugs like heparin and warfarin prevent the formation of clot. They are of value particularly in obstructive peripheral vascular disease. Aspirin 75-150 mg once a day or clopidogrel 10 mg twice daily may be used for this purpose.

Pentoxiphylline an analog of xanthine is a phosphodiesterase inhibitor. It reduces the viscosity of the blood and enhances blood flow to the ischemic areas. It is also claimed to improve the flexibility of the RBCs - (called hemorrheological action) resulting in an improvement of microcirculation and is devoid of steal phenomenon. It potentiates the action of anticoagulants.

Uses: Pentoxiphylline is used in transient ischemic attacks, nonhemorrhagic stroke, chronic cerebrovascular insufficiency, trophic leg ulcers, gangrene, intermittent claudication (which could be due to diabetes, atherosclerosis or inflammatory vascular disease). Pentoxiphylline is also used in AIDS patients with increased TNF (because pentoxiphylline can inhibit the production of TNF-α) and to improve sperm motility.

Dose: 400 mg 2-3 times a day with food.

Naftidofuryl oxalate is found to be useful in peripheral vascular diseases like TAO and in cerebrovascular disorders. Though not a vasodilator, it is said to improve the supply of ATP to the skeletal muscles and reduce their lactate levels—it is called a 'metabolic enhancer'—thus it improves performance in patients with TAO or intermittent claudication where it increases the walking distance.

Naftidofuryl oxalate also blocks $5HT_2$ receptors and inhibits 5HT induced vasoconstriction and platelet aggregation.

However, it is found to increase the blood flow to the skin rather than the muscles. It has beneficial effects in the treatment of venous leg ulcers.

Dose: 100 mg BD - TDS oral.

Xanthinol nicotinate: Both xanthine and nicotinic acid are vasodilators and xanthinol nicotinate increases blood flow in several vascular beds. Therefore it has been tried in cerebrovascular insufficiency and peripheral vascular diseases. However clinically it is not proved to be useful.

Dose: 300-600 mg TDS oral/300 mg IM/ slow IV.

Cilostazol is a phosphodiesterase III inhibitor. It has vasodilator and antiplatelet effects - improves pain free walking and maximum walking distance. It is used in the dose of 100 mg BD to be taken 30 minutes before breakfast and dinner. It can cause headache, diarrhea, dizziness and tachycardia and is contraindicated in heart failure.

Thromboangitis obliterans: Atheroma of the peripheral arteries results in reduced blood supply to the concerned part—usually lower limbs. Historically, localized inflammatory changes can be seen in the walls of the arteries and veins leading to thrombosis. Initially there is pain in the legs on walking (intermittent claudication) but later pain even at rest while in severe cases there could be gangrene of the feet and legs.

The goal is to prevent pain, arrest progression of the disease and decrease the risk of cardiovascular and cerebrovascular events. Patients should first stop smoking. Hyperlipidemia if any should be corrected. Vasodilators may be tried.

Night cramps - quinine has been tried in a low dose of 200 mg at night to relieve night cramps.

Surgical treatment is the preferred option. Angioplasty of iliac or superficial femoral arteries (with stent placement) is often effective. Other options include arterial bypass grafting or endarterectomy and lastly amputation of the leg in severe cases.

Raynaud's phenomenon is a vasospastic disorder. A vasodilator like nifedipine, topical nitroglycerine, indoramin, prazosin or slow infusion of prostacyclin (epoprostenol) help to relieve symptoms. Regular exercises to improve blood supply to the muscles may help. Because β blockers can worsen PVD including Raynaud's phenomenon (due to reduced cardiac output), they should be avoided in these patients. Exposure to cold should also be avoided.

HYPOLIPIDEMIC DRUGS

Lipids and proteins form complexes called lipoproteins and circulate in the blood vessels. There are four types of lipoproteins:

- Low density lipoproteins (LDL)
- High density lipoprotein (HDL)
- Very low density lipoproteins (VLDL)
- Chylomicrons

Hyperlipoproteinemias (HPL) are conditions in which the concentration of cholesterol or triglyceride (TG) carrying lipoproteins in the plasma is elevated above normal (Table 6.8). When the lipoproteins increase, the development of atherosclerosis is faster and is a risk factor for myocardial infarction. Low density lipoprotein (LDL) is the primary carrier of cholesterol while very low density lipoprotein (VLDL) is the carrier of triglycerides. Along with reduction of body weight and low cholesterol diet, hypolipidemic drugs may be given in patients with hyperlipoproteinemias.

Table 6.8: Plasma lipid levels (mg/dL).

Grade	*Total cholesterol*	*Triglycerides*
Normal	< 200	< 150
Borderline	200–239	150–199
High	> 240	> 200

Hypolipidemics

1. **HMG CoA reductase inhibitors**
   - Lovastatin
   - Simvastatin
   - Pravastatin
   - Atorvastatin
   - Rosuvastatin
   - Fluvastatin
   - Pitavastatin
2. **Fibric acids**
   - Gemfibrozil
   - Clofibrate
   - Fenofibrate
   - Bezafibrate
   - Ciprofibrate
3. **Bile acid binding resins**
   - Cholestyramine
   - Colestipol
   - Colesevalam
4. **Miscellaneous**
   - Ezetimibe
   - Probucol
   - Nicotinic acid.

HMG-CoA Reductase Inhibitors (Statins)

Hydroxymethylglutaryl-CoA (HMG-CoA) is the rate controlling enzyme in the biosynthesis of cholesterol. Lovastatin and its congeners are competitive inhibitors of the enzyme HMG-CoA reductase. They lower plasma LDL cholesterol and triglycerides. The concentration of high density lipoprotein (HDL) cholesterol (the protective lipoprotein) increases by 10%.

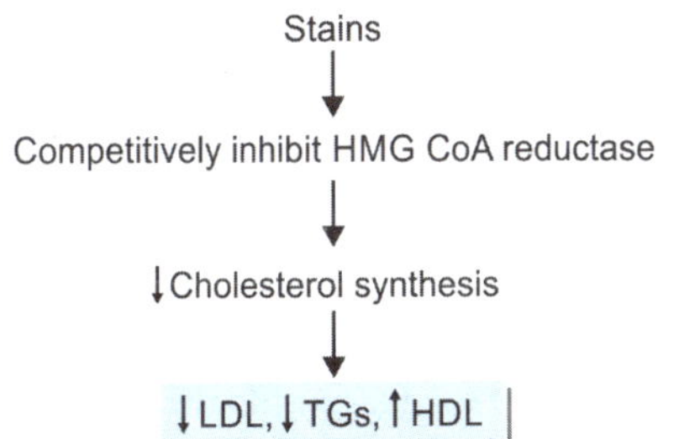

Pleiotropic effects: Statins can produce many beneficial effects in reducing the risk of CV diseases—called pleiotropic effects of statins.

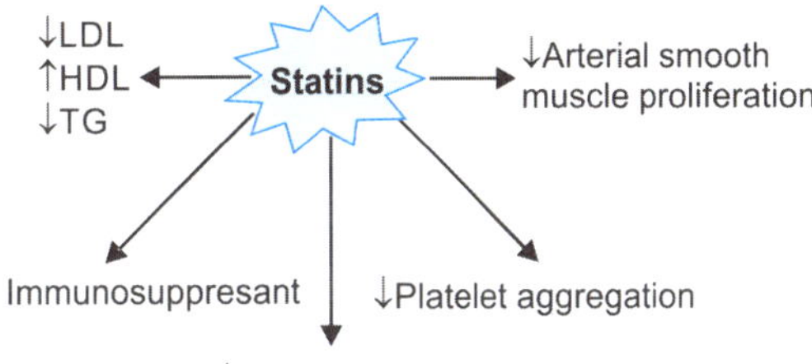

All the above actions contribute to the useful effects of statins

Pharmacokinetics: Statins are well absorbed when given orally but may undergo extensive first pass metabolism in the liver. Simvastatin is a prodrug converted to its active metabolite in the liver.

Adverse effects include gastrointestinal disturbances, headache, insomnia, rashes and angioedema.

Treatment with statins can cause hepatotoxicity though not very common. Serum transaminases may be elevated on prolonged therapy. Patients should be watched for hepatotoxicity while on statins. All statins can cause **muscle tenderness** and **myopathy** (with myalgia and weakness), **rhabdomyolysis** though the incidence is low (<0.1–0.1%). Use with other drugs that also cause myopathy including fibrates and niacin should be avoided.

Statins are contraindicated in pregnancy and lactation as they are not proved to be safe in them.

Mnemonic for ADRs

HMG-CoA Reductase **I**nhibitors
H—Hepatotoxicity
M—Myopathy, myositis
G—Gastrointestinal disturbances
Co—↑ CPK levels
A—Alcoholics—caution
R—Rashes
I—Insomnia

Uses (Table 6.9)

1. Statins are used in patients with MI, angina, stroke and transient ischemic attacks to lower cholesterol levels. Statins reduce morbidity and mortality in such patients.
2. HMG CoA reductase inhibitors are the first line drugs for **hyperlipidemias** both for familial and secondary hyperlipidemias as in diabetes mellitus.

Table 6.9: Choice of hypolipidemics.

Elevated TG levels	Gemfibrozil
Elevated LDL cholesterol	Lovastatin; adjuvants-binding resins/nicotinic acid
Elevated TG + cholesterol	Lovastatin + Gemfibrozil

Fibric Acids

Fibric acids increase the activity of the enzyme lipoprotein lipase which degrades VLDL resulting in lowering of triglycerides. They also increase HDL levels. Gemfibrozil is the drug of choice in patients with increased TG levels.

Fibrates ⟶ ↑ Lipoprotein lipase activity ⟶ VLDL degraded ⟶ ↓ TG

Adverse effects include gastrointestinal (GI) upset, skin rashes, headache, muscle cramps, **rhabdomyolysis and blurred vision.**

Bile Acid Binding Resins

They bind bile acids in the intestine and increase their excretion. Bile acids are required for intestinal absorption of cholesterol. Plasma cholesterol and LDL levels fall. Bile acid binding resins are unpleasant to take; they may cause GI upset, constipation and piles. They also bind many drugs in the intestines thereby reducing their absorption.

Ezetimibe

Ezetimibe selectively inhibits the absorption of cholesterol from the intestines by inhibiting a specific transport protein [Niemann-Pick C1-Like1 (NPC1L1)] which takes up cholesterol from intestinal lumen. The plasma LDL cholesterol decreases by 15–20% with a marginal increase in HDL cholesterol.

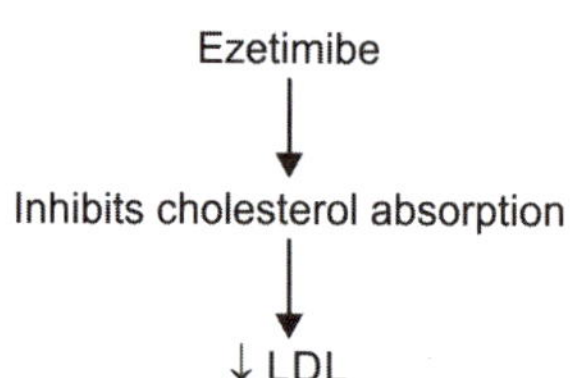

The effects are synergistic with statins and the combination can bring about a significant (up to 60%) decrease in LDL cholesterol level.

Ezetimibe can cause hepatic dysfunction and myositis.

Ezetimibe may be used in patients with mild hypercholesterolemia or in combination with a low dose of statins in patients who have not had adequate response with statins alone.

Probucol is a synthetic antioxidant which lowers plasma cholesterol, LDL and HDL levels. It is used with other hypolipidemics.

Miscellaneous

Nicotinic acid—a B group vitamin, inhibits lipolysis and increases lipoprotein lipase activity resulting in lowering of TGs and LDL levels. It reduces the synthesis of VLDL.

Niacin is used in hypertriglyceridemia with low HDL levels.

Neomycin forms insoluble complexes with bile acids in the intestines and thus lowers cholesterol levels.

DRUGS USED IN THE DISORDERS OF COAGULATION

Hemostasis is the spontaneous arrest of bleeding from the damaged blood vessels. In the process, complex interactions take place between the injured vessel wall, platelets and clotting factors.

Following an injury, there is local vasoconstriction and platelets stick to one another. A clot forms on this with the help of fibrin forming a plug which temporarily stops bleeding. This is reinforced by fibrin for long-term hemostasis.

Classification

Classification of anticoagulants is given in Flowchart 6.4.

Clotting factors are proteins synthesized by the liver. Two systems—the extrinsic and the intrinsic system are involved in the process of coagulation (Fig. 6.5). Several proteins interact in a cascading series to form the clot. Several drugs are used to modify the process of coagulation including procoagulants and anti-coagulants, antiplatelet drugs, fibrinolytics and antifibrinolytics (Flowchart 6.5).

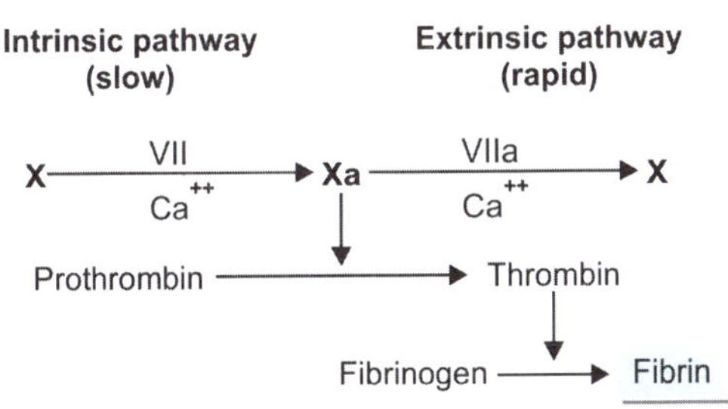

Fig. 6.5: Major reactions of blood coagulation.

ANTICOAGULANTS

Anticoagulants are drugs that reduce the coagulability of the blood.

Heparin

Heparin was discovered by McLean, a medical student in 1916. It was named 'heparin' as it was first extracted from the liver. It is found in the mast cells of the liver, lungs and intestinal mucosa. Heparin is the strongest acid in the body.

Actions: Heparin is a powerful anticoagulant that acts instantaneously both *in vivo* and *in vitro*.

Mechanism of action: Heparin activates plasma antithrombin III (Fig. 6.6) which binds to the clotting factors and inactivates them. Clotting time is prolonged.

Pharmacokinetics: Heparin is not effective orally. It is given IV or SC. Treatment is monitored by the clotting time. Heparin is metabolized by heparinase in the liver.

Adverse Reactions

- **Bleeding** is the most common, major adverse effect of heparin. Careful

Flowchart 6.4: Classification of anticoagulants.

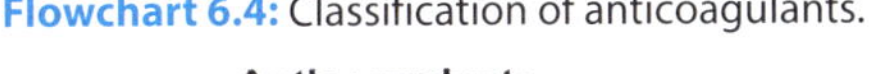

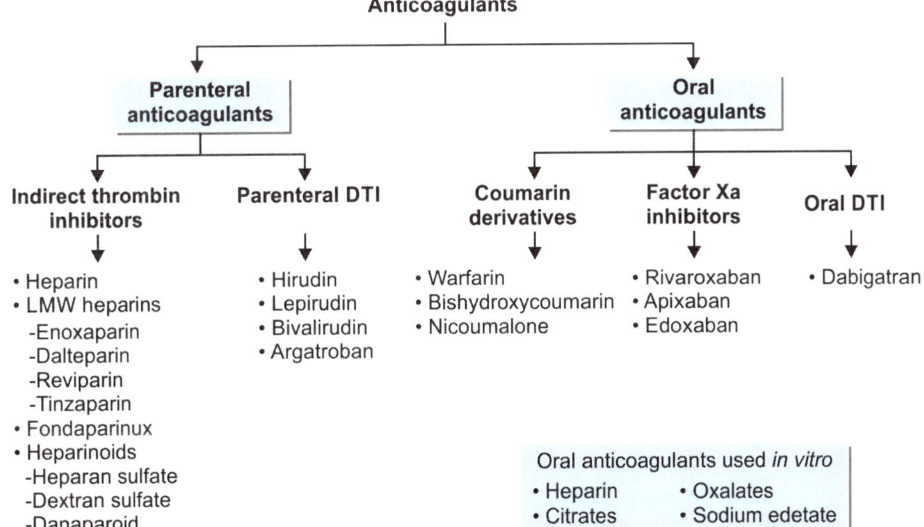

(DTI: direct thrombin inhibitors)

Flowchart 6.5: Drugs used in the disorders of coagulation.

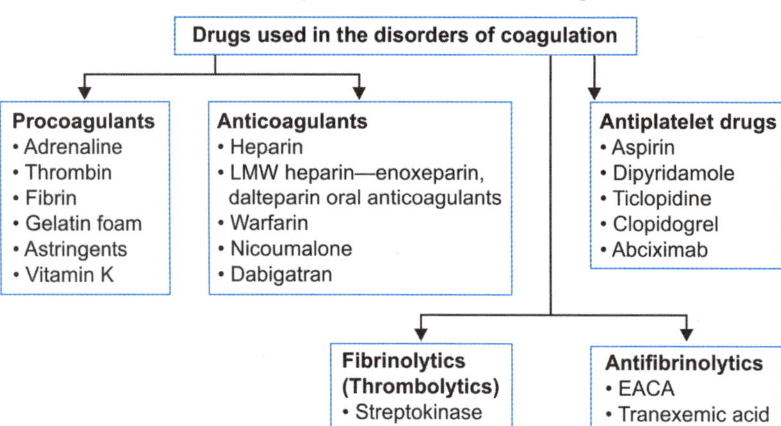

(EACA: epsilon-aminocaproic acid; LMW: low molecular weight)

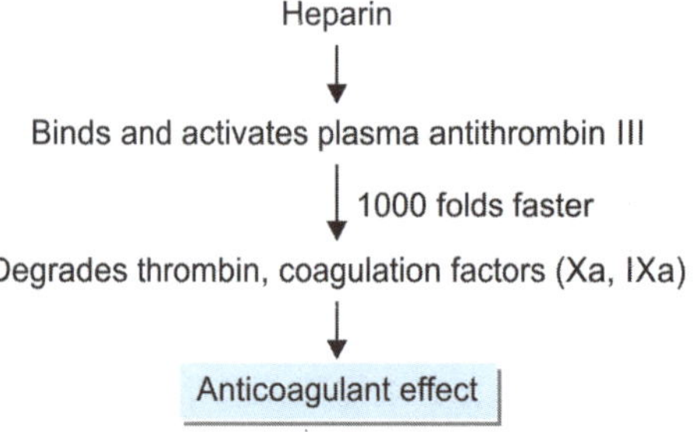

Fig. 6.6: Mechanism of action of heparin.

monitoring and dose control will prevent this to a great extent.

- **Hypersensitivity reactions**—for commercial use heparin is obtained from bovine lung or porcine intestine. Because of its animal origin allergic reactions are quite common.
- **Heparin induced thrombocytopenia (HIT):** Heparin induced platelet aggregation and formation of antiplatelet antibodies can both result in thrombocytopenia. Though rare it can be serious. Heparin should be stopped immediately at the first sign of thrombocytopenia.

'H' for Heparin ADRs
H—Hemorrhage
H—Hypersensitivity reactions
H—Hair loss
H—HIT
H—Hyperkalemia
H—Hypoaldosteronism

- **Hair loss or alopecia** is reversible.
- **Osteoporosis:** On long-term use.
- **Hypoaldosteronism:** Heparin can inhibit the synthesis of aldosterone and may result in hyperkalemia.

Contraindications to Heparin Therapy

Bleeding disorders, thrombocytopenia, hemophilia, severe hypertension, intracranial hemorrhage, cirrhosis, ulcers in the gut, renal failure and neurosurgery.

Low molecular weight (LMW) heparins, e.g., enoxaparin, dalteparin, tinzaparin, ardeparin and reviparin have a mol. wt. of 4000–7000. LMW heparins (unfractionated

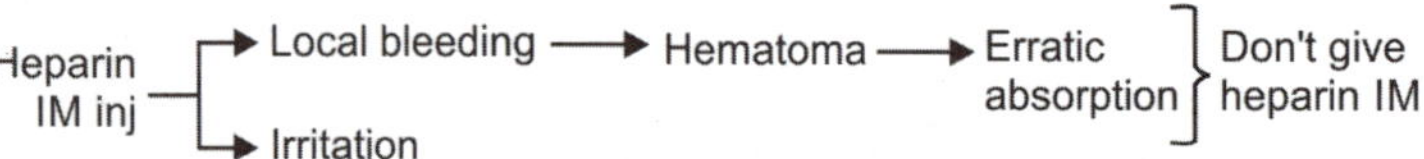

heparin, UFH) are obtained by chemical/enzymatic treatment of standard heparin or unfractionated heparin. LMW heparins inhibit factor Xa like conventional heparin but differ from it in many ways. In therapeutic doses (Table 6.10), LMW heparins do not inhibit thrombin activity (because they are too short). In therapeutic doses, LMW heparins do not have significant effect on the tests of clotting. Therefore laboratory monitoring is not required. Apart from being equally efficacious, LMW heparins have a favorable pharmacokinetic profile and have the following advantages over standard heparins:

- Better bioavailability following SC injection
- Longer action
- Lower risk of bleeding (because of less interaction with platelets)
- Lower risk of osteoporosis
- Lower incidence of thrombocytopenia (because less antigenic) and thrombosis
- Routine lab monitoring not required.

Uses: LMW heparins are used in:

1. The prevention and treatment of venous thrombosis and pulmonary embolism
2. In unstable angina
3. To maintain the patency of tubes in dialysis patients.

Synthetic Heparin Derivative

Fondaparinux is longer acting, risk of thrombocytopenia is less and does not require frequent monitoring. It is being used in place of heparin.

Heparin antagonist - Mild heparin overdosage can be treated by just stopping heparin because heparin is short acting. In severe heparin overdose, an antagonist may be needed to arrest its anticoagulant effects.

Protamine sulfate is a protein obtained from the sperm of certain fish. Given intravenously, it neutralizes heparin and acts as heparin antagonist in heparin overdosage. Whole blood transfusion may be needed.

Heparin antagonist protamine sulfate is a protein obtained from the sperm of certain fish. Given intravenously, it neutralizes heparin and acts as heparin antagonist in heparin overdosage.

Heparinoids

Heparan sulfate present in some tissues is similar to heparin. It is believed to be responsible for antithrombotic activity on the vascular endothelium.

Danaparoid is a mixture of heparinoids and acts by inhibiting factor Xa. It does not prolong aPTT and is longer acting. It is used subcutaneously in the treatment of deep vein

Table 6.10: Compare and contrast standard heparin and LMW heparin.

Features	*Standard Heparin*	*LMW Heparin*
Molecular weight	10,000–20,000	4,000–7,000
Source	Natural	Semisynthetic (chemical treatment of standard heparin)
Thrombin activity in therapeutic doses	Inhibited	Not inhibited
Effect on tests of clotting	Significant	Not significant
Laboratory monitoring	Required	Not required
SC bioavailability	Low (20–30%)	High (70–90%)
Duration of action	Short (2–4 hours)	Long (18–24 hours)
Frequency of administration	Every 4–6 hours	Once a day
Dose dependent clearance	Yes	No
Thrombocytopenia	Can occur (++++)	Lesser chances (++)
Risk of bleeding	Present	Lower

thrombosis and in other conditions as an alternative to heparin.

Direct Thrombin Inhibitors

Direct thrombin inhibitors (DTIs) can be parenteral or oral. Parenteral DTIs include:

Hirudin is the anticoagulant found in the salivary glands of leeches. It is a powerful direct thrombin inhibitor. **Lepirudin** is produced by recombinant DNA technology and can be used in patients allergic to heparin but it has no antagonist yet. Other drugs in this group are **desirudin, bivalirudin and argatroban**.

Oral Anticoagulants

Bishydroxycoumarin was the first oral anticoagulant to be identified in North America. Many related compounds were then developed and are also being used as rat poisons.

Warfarin

Warfarin is a commonly used oral anticoagulant.

Mechanism of Action

Warfarin and other coumarin derivatives prevent the synthesis of vitamin K dependent clotting factors (factors II, VII, IX and X) in the liver.

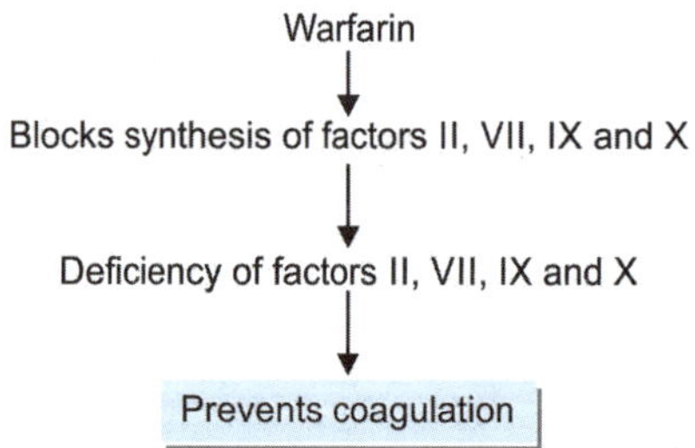

The onset of action is slow; it develops over 1-3 days because oral anticoagulants do not destroy the already circulating clotting factors. Prothrombin time (PT) is measured to monitor the treatment. It takes 5-7 days for PT to return to normal after stopping oral anticoagulants.

Pharmacokinetics

Warfarin is completely absorbed orally and is 99% bound to plasma proteins (Table 6.11).

Adverse Effects

- Hemorrhage is the main adverse effect. Bleeding in the intestines, brain, nose and gums can occur.
  Treatment: Depends on the severity:
  - Stop the anticoagulant.
  - Fresh blood transfusion is given to supply the clotting factors.
  - **Antidote:** The specific antidote is **vitamin K_1 oxide** which allows synthesis of clotting factors. However, the response to vitamin K_1 oxide needs several hours. Hence in emergency, **fresh whole blood** is necessary to counter the effects of oral anticoagulants.
- Other adverse effects include allergic reactions, gastrointestinal disturbances and teratogenicity.

Drug Interactions

Many drugs increase warfarin action

1. **Drugs that inhibit platelet function:** NSAIDs like aspirin increase the risk of bleeding.
   NSAIDs + warfarin →↑ bleeding
2. Drugs that inhibit hepatic drug metabolism like cimetidine, chloramphenicol and metronidazole increase the plasma levels of warfarin.
3. Drugs that displace warfarin from plasma protein binding sites like NSAIDs enhance plasma levels of warfarin.

Table 6.11: Factors influencing oral anticoagulant activity.

Factors enhancing activity	*Factors reducing activity*
Poor diet, bowel disease, liver disease and chronic alcoholism—result in vitamin k deficiency	Pregnancy—there is increased synthesis of clotting factors Hypothyroidism—there is reduced degradation of clotting factors

4. Drugs like broad spectrum antibiotics inhibit gut flora thus decreasing vitamin K synthesis.

Some drugs *reduce* the effect of oral anticoagulants.

1. **Drugs that increase the metabolism of oral anticoagulants:** Microsomal enzyme inducers like barbiturates, rifampicin, griseofulvin increase the metabolism of oral anticoagulants. When these drugs are suddenly withdrawn, excess anticoagulant activity may result in hemorrhages.

   Drugs that inhibit the metabolism of drugs like chloramphenicol, allopurinol, erythromycin, increase the plasma levels of warfarin.
2. **Drugs that increase the synthesis of clotting factors**, e.g., oral contraceptives.

Factor Xa Inhibitor

Rivaroxaban directly binds to factor Xa and inactivates it. Since the binding is direct, its onset of action is faster (3–4 hours). Constant laboratory monitoring is not required and is orally effective. It is useful in the prophylaxis of postoperative deep vein thrombosis and following stroke. Apixaban and edoxaban are similar.

Oral Direct Thrombin Inhibitor

Dabigatran binds directly to thrombin and inactivates it.

Advantages are:

- Orally effective (given as dabigatran etexilate)
- Fast onset of action (<2 hours)
- No need for constant lab monitoring
- Long-acting given once daily
- An antidote **idarucizumab** is recently made available which can quickly reverse its effects.

Though currently dabigatran is being used for the prevention of deep vein thrombosis postoperatively, it could soon be one of the popular anticoagulants.

Uses of anticoagulants: Anticoagulants can prevent extension of the thrombus but cannot destroy the existing clots. Heparin has rapid and short-action which makes it suitable for initiating treatment while warfarin is suitable for long-term maintenance due to its slow and prolonged action and convenience of oral use.

1. **Venous thrombosis and pulmonary embolism:** Anticoagulants prevent extension of thrombus and recurrence of embolism.
2. **Postoperative, post-stroke patients; bedridden patients:** Due to leg fractures and other causes—who cannot be ambulant for several months—anticoagulants prevent venous thrombosis and pulmonary embolism in such patients.
3. **Rheumatic heart disease:** Anticoagulants prevent embolism.
4. **Unstable angina:** heparin reduces the risk of myocardial infarction in patients with unstable angina.
5. **Vascular surgery, artificial heart valves and hemodialysis:** Anticoagulants prevent thromboembolism.

Contraindications to Anticoagulant Therapy

- Bleeding disorders including thrombocytopenia
- Severe hypertension
- Malignancies
- Bacterial endocarditis
- Liver and kidney diseases.
- Recent surgery (in the last 10–15 days)
- History of cerebrovascular accident

THROMBOLYTICS (FIBRINOLYTICS)

Thrombolytics lyse or dissolve the clot or thrombi by activating the natural fibrinolytic system.

Plasminogen circulates in the plasma and also some of it is bound to fibrin. Tissue plasminogen activator (tPA) activates plasminogen which is converted to plasmin. Plasmin degrades fibrin thereby dissolving the clot. Thrombolytic agents are **streptokinase, urokinase, alteplase, duteplase, teneteplase**, and **reteplase anistreplase**.

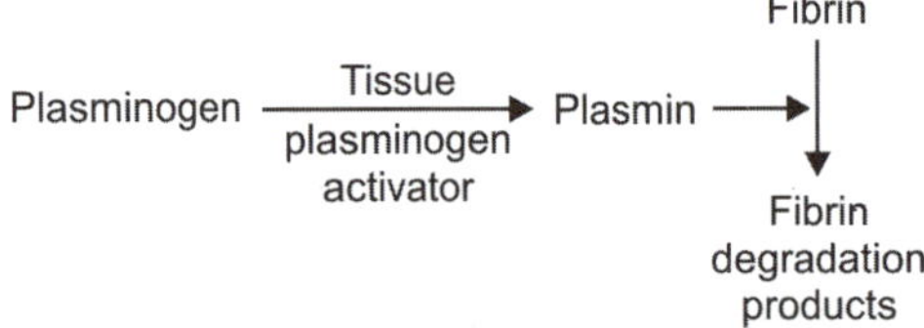

Streptokinase obtained from β-hemolytic streptococci activates plasminogen. Antistreptococcal antibodies present in the blood due to previous streptococcal infections inactivate a large amount of streptokinase. Allergic reactions are common (because of source).

Anistreplase is a form of streptokinase which is long acting and can be given in a single IV bolus dose.

Urokinase is an enzyme prepared from cultures of human kidney cells (it was first isolated from human urine—hence the name). It activates plasminogen.

Tissue plasminogen activator (tPA) selectively activates plasminogen that is bound to clot which means circulating plasminogen is largely spared.

Alteplase and duteplase are tPA produced by recombinant DNA technology.

Reteplase is modified human tPA obtained by genetic engineering. It has less bleeding tendency when compared to other fibrinolytics.

Tenecteplase is longer acting and can be given as an IV bolus injection. Its ability to bind fibrin is very good. Other newer fibrinolytics are similar to alteplase with minor differences.

Adverse effects of thrombolytics: Bleeding is the major toxicity of all thrombolytics. Hypotension and fever can occur. Allergic reactions are common with streptokinase.

Uses

- **Acute myocardial infarction:** Intravenous thrombolytics reduce the morality rate in acute MI.
- **Deep vein thrombosis** and large pulmonary emboli are also treated with fibrinolytics.

Contraindications to Thrombolytic Therapy

- Recent surgery, injury, gastrointestinal bleeding, stroke
- Severe hypertension
- Bleeding disorders.

Antifibrinolytics

Antifibrinolytics inhibit plasminogen activation and thus prevent fibrinolysis.

Epsilon aminocaproic acid (EACA) and its analogue **tranexemic acid** are antifibrinolytics. Tranexemic acid can be given by oral, topical and intravenous routes. Aprotinin is another fibrinolytic drug which acts by inhibiting proteolytic enzymes.

Uses

Tranexemic acid is used in:

- Overdosage of fibrinolytics.
- Menorrhagia, postpartum hemorrhage.
- After cardiac surgeries including cardiopulmonary bypass.
- Bleeding peptic ulcer.
- Following dental procedures to prevent bleeding in patients with hemophilia as a mouth wash.
- After prostate surgery, tonsillectomy.
- Epistaxis, bleeding from eye injury.
- Hereditary angioedema—this rare condition is associated with plasmin induced uncontrolled activation of the complement system.

Antiplatelet Drugs

Platelets form the initial plug at the site of vascular injury and are also involved in the formation of atherosclerosis. By inhibiting the platelet function, thrombosis and atherosclerotic vascular disease can be largely prevented.

Antiplatelet drugs or drugs interfering with platelet function are aspirin, dipyrida-

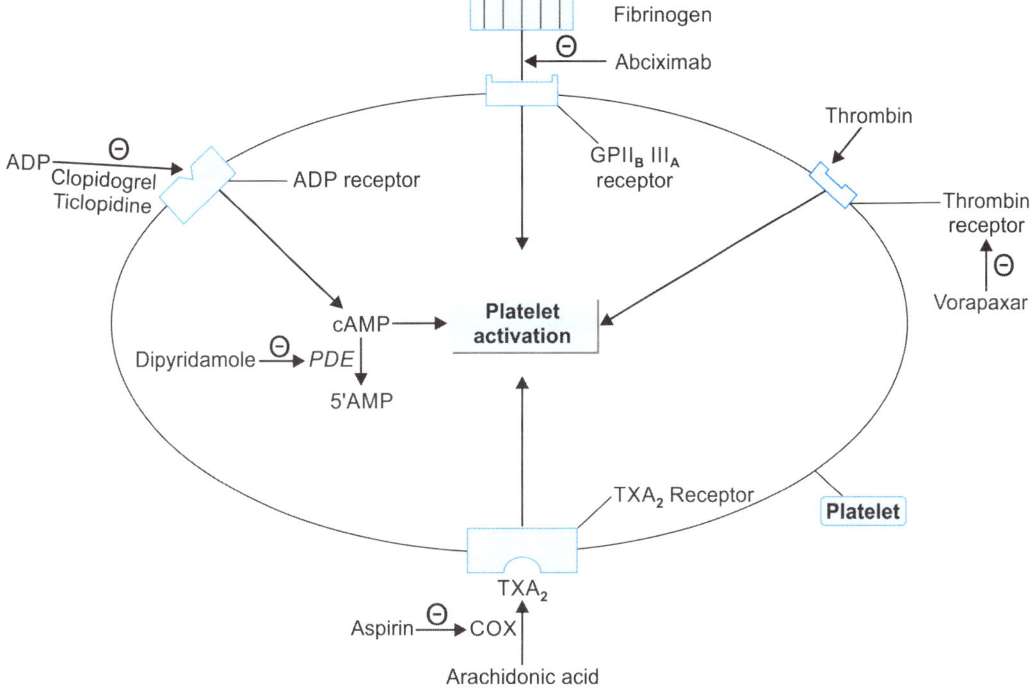

Fig. 6.7: Sites of action of antiplatelet drugs.

mole, sulphinpyrazone and ticlopidine (Fig. 6.7).

Classification:

- **PG synthesis inhibitors:** Aspirin.
- **Phosphodiesterase inhibitor:** Dipyridamole.
- **Adenosine diphosphate (ADP) antagonists:** Ticlopidine, clopidogrel, prasugrel.
- **Glycoprotein IIb/IIIa receptor antagonists:** Abciximab, eptifibatide, tirofiban.
- **Others:** Prostaglandin I_2, cilostazol.

1. *Aspirin*

ThromboxaneA$_2$ promotes platelet aggregation. Aspirin inactivates cyclo-oxygenase (COX) and thereby inhibits the synthesis of thromboxane A$_2$ even in low doses (75 mg/day). The COX inhibition is irreversible and the effect lasts for 7 to 10 days—till fresh platelets are formed. Aspirin is the most commonly used antiplatelet drug. Dose 50–300 mg daily.

2. *Dipyridamole*

Dipyridamole is a phosphodiesterase inhibitor which interferes with platelet function by increasing platelet cyclic AMP levels. It is used along with aspirin for the prophylaxis of thromboemboli in patients with prosthetic heart valves.

3. *ADP Antagonists*

Clopidogrel and ticlopidine: ADP binds to receptors on platelets to bring about platelet aggregation. Clopidogrel and ticlopidine are prodrugs and their active metabolites block ADP receptors and thereby prevent platelet aggregation. Onset of action is slow (7–11 days) and the antiplatelet effect remains for some days even after stopping the drug. Clopidogrel is used as an alternative when aspirin cannot be used. It is also used in combination with aspirin for additive effects. Ticlopidine is not preferred due to its side effects.

Prasugrel has faster and better antiplatelet activity. However, bleeding is a frequent side effect.

4. *Glycoprotein IIb/IIIa Receptor Antagonists*

Fibrinogen and Von Willebrand factor bind to glycoprotein IIb/IIIA receptors on the platelets and mediate the action of platelet agonists like thrombin, collagen and TXA_2. Drugs that block these receptors inhibit platelet aggregation induced by all platelet agonists.

Abciximab is a monoclonal antibody which binds glycoprotein IIb/IIIA receptors and inhibits platelet aggregation. It can cause bleeding and allergic reactions. It is used in patients undergoing coronary angioplasty.

Eptifibatide and **tirofiban** are peptides given as IV infusion. They are short acting and are tried in unstable angina and myocardial infarction.

5. *Others*

Epoprostenol (PGI_2) can be used during hemodialysis to prevent platelet aggregation as an alternative to heparin.

Uses of Antiplatelet Drugs

1. **Myocardial infarction:** Aspirin with thrombolytics improve survival in acute MI. Long-term treatment with aspirin reduces reinfarction in post-MI patients.
2. **Unstable angina and stable angina pectoris:** Aspirin reduces the risk of acute MI. Clopidogrel may be added to aspirin in unstable angina.
3. In patients with prosthetic heart valves, valvular heart disease, coronary artery bypass surgery–long-term use of low dose aspirin is recommended.
4. **Cerebral thrombosis and TIA:** In patients with transient ischemic attacks aspirin reduces the incidence of stroke and mortality. In cerebral thrombosis aspirin prevents recurrence.
5. **Atrial fibrillation:** If oral anticoagulants cannot be given, aspirin is useful.
6. **Cardiac procedures:** After coronary angioplasty, stenting and coronary bypass.
7. **Hemodialysis:** PGI2 is injected into blood entering dialysis unit to prevent clot formation.
8. **Peripheral vascular diseases:** For thromboprophylaxis.
9. **Vascular grafts:** To prevent occlusion and maintain patency of the vascular grafts.

Coagulants

Coagulants are drugs that promote coagulation (procoagulants) and control bleeding. They are also called *hemostatics.* They may be used locally or systemically. Local hemostatics are called *styptics.* Physical methods like application of pressure, tourniquet or ice can control bleeding.

Styptics are local hemostatics that are used on bleeding sites like tooth socket. They are:

1. **Adrenaline:** Sterile cotton soaked in 1:10,000 solution of adrenaline is commonly used in tooth sockets and as nasal packs for epistaxis. Adrenaline arrests bleeding by vasoconstriction.
2. **Thrombin** powder is dusted over the bleeding surface following skin grafting. It is obtained from bovine plasma.
3. **Fibrin** obtained from human plasma is available as sheets. It is used for covering or packing bleeding surfaces.
4. **Gelatin foam** is porous spongy gelatin used with thrombin to control bleeding from wounds. It gets completely absorbed in 4 to 6 weeks and can be left in place after suturing of the wound.
5. **Thromboplastin powder** is used in surgery as a styptic.
6. **Astringents** like tannic acid are used on bleeding gums.

Coagulants used Systemically

Vitamin K

Vitamin K is a fat-soluble vitamin essential for the biosynthesis of clotting factors (factors II, VII, IX and X by the liver).

Vitamin K deficiency results in bleeding tendencies.

Uses

- Vitamin K deficiency.
- **Newborn babies** lack intestinal flora and have low levels of prothrombin and other clotting factors. Routine administration of vitamin K—1 mg IM prevents hemorrhagic disease of the newborn.
- Oral anticoagulant toxicity.

Other Coagulants

Fresh plasma or **whole blood** is useful in most coagulation disorders as it contains all the clotting factors. Other concentrated **plasma fractions** like fibrinogen, factors II, VII, VIII, IX and X are available for the treatment of specific deficiencies.

Snake venoms: Some venoms like Russel's viper venom stimulate thrombokinase and promote coagulation.

Ethamsylate is used orally to arrest bleeding. The exact mode of action is not known but it is thought that it acts by inhibiting the synthesis of prostacycline (PGI2) and correct the abnormal platelet function. It may also stabilize the wall of the capillaries and reduce capillary bleeding. Ethamsylate is given orally to control bleeding in:

- Procedures, such as dental extraction in patients with coagulation disorders
- Menorrhagia
- Postpartum hemorrhage
- Hematemesis and malena.

HEMATINICS

Hematinics are compounds required in the formation of blood and are employed in the treatment of anemias. Iron, vitamin B_{12} and folic acid are essential for normal erythropoiesis (Table 6.12).

Table 6.12: Daily requirement of iron.

Adult male	0.5–1 mg
Adult female	1–2 mg
Pregnancy and lactation	3–5 mg

Iron

Iron is essential for hemoglobin production. It is also present in myoglobin, the cytochromes and other enzymes. Total body iron is about 2.5 to 5 grams.

Dietary sources of iron: Food that is rich in iron are liver, egg yolk, meat, fish, chicken, spinach, dry fruits, wheat and apple.

Absorption: The average Indian diet provides about 10–20 mg of iron. Ten percent of this iron is absorbed. It is mostly absorbed from the upper gut in the ferrous form. During deficiency, absorption is better.

Factors that Influence Iron Absorption

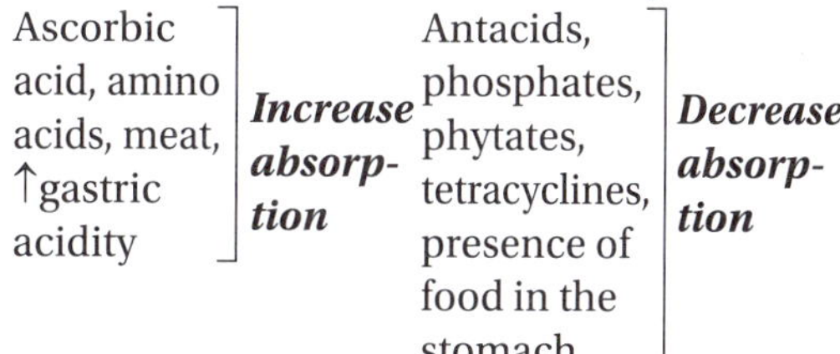

Transport and distribution: Iron is transported with the help of a glycoprotein *transferrin* and stored as *ferritin* and *hemosiderin*, in liver, spleen and bone marrow.

Excretion: Daily 0.5–1 mg of iron is excreted. In females, iron is also lost in menstruation.

Preparations of Iron

Iron is generally given orally and but can be given parenterally when required.

Oral Iron Preparations

- Ferrous sulphate—200 mg tab
- Ferrous fumarate—200 mg tab
- Ferrous gluconate—300 mg tab

- Ferrous succinate—100 mg
- Iron calcium complex—5% iron
- Ferric ammonium citrate—45 mg.
  - Ferrous salts are better absorbed than ferric salts and are cheaper.
  - Expensive preparations of iron with vitamins, liver extract, amino acids, etc. are available but have no clear advantages.

Dose: Ferrous sulphate 200 mg 3 tablets daily.

Adverse effects of oral iron: Epigastric pain, nausea, vomiting, gastritis, metallic taste, constipation (due to astringent effect) or diarrhea (irritant effect) are the usual adverse effects. The stool gets blackened but is harmless. Liquid preparations of iron cause staining of the teeth.

Parenteral iron: Iron is given parenterally only in some situations. Intramuscular injection of iron is given deep IM. Intravenous iron is given slowly over 5–10 minutes or as infusion after a test dose.

Iron dextran can be given IM and IV.

Iron-sorbitol-citric acid complex is given only IM. This preparation should **not** be given IV because it quickly saturates the transferrin stores. As a result, free iron levels in the plasma rises and can cause toxicity. It can cause hypersensitivity reactions and a test dose should be given before the full dose.

Iron sucrose and sodium ferric gluconate can be given IV.

Indications for Parenteral Iron

- When oral iron is not tolerated
- Failure of absorption—as in malabsorption, chronic bowel disease
- When patients do not take regularly
- Severe deficiency with bleeding.

Adverse Effects of Parenteral Iron

Local: Pain at the site of injection and pigmentation of the skin.

Systemic: Fever, headache, joints pain, palpitation, and rarely anaphylaxis.

Acute iron poisoning is common in infants and children in whom about 10 tablets (1–2 g) can be lethal. Manifestations include vomiting, abdominal pain, hematemesis, bloody diarrhea, shock, drowsiness, cyanosis, acidosis, dehydration, cardiovascular collapse and coma. Immediate diagnosis and treatment are important as death may occur in 6–12 hours.

Treatment

- Stomach wash with sodium bicarbonate solution.
- Desferrioxamine is the antidote.
- Correction of acidosis and shock.

Uses of Iron

- **Iron deficiency anemia:** The cause for iron deficiency should be identified. Treatment should be continued depending on the response for 3–6 months to replenish the iron stores.
- **Prophylaxis:** Iron is given in conditions with increased iron requirement as in pregnancy, infancy and professional blood donors.

Vitamin B_{12} and Folic Acid

Vitamin B_{12} and folic acid are water soluble vitamins, belonging to the B-complex group. They are essential coenzymes for many important metabolic reactions and for normal DNA synthesis. Their deficiency leads to impaired DNA synthesis and abnormal maturation of RBCs and other rapidly dividing cells. This results in **megaloblastic anemia**, characterized by the presence of red cell precursors in the blood and bone marrow. Other manifestations of deficiency include glossitis, stomatitis and malabsorption; neurological manifestations can also result.

Vitamin B_{12}

Vitamin B_{12} (cyanocobalamin) is synthesized by microorganisms. Liver, fish, egg yolk, meat, cheese and pulses are the dietary sources of vitamin B_{12}.

Vitamin B_{12} or extrinsic factor is absorbed with the help of intrinsic factor, a protein secreted by the stomach. It is carried in the plasma by B_{12} binding proteins called *transcobalamin* and is stored in the liver. Requirement: Table 6.13.

Table 6.13: Daily requirement of vitamin B_{12} and folic acid.

	Adults	*Pregnancy and lactation*
Vitamin B_{12}	1–3 µg	3–5 µg
Folic acid	50–100 µg	200–400 µg

Deficiency

B_{12} deficiency may be due to:

- **Addisonian pernicious anemia:** Thomas Addison first described cases of anemia not responding to iron. There is deficiency of intrinsic factor resulting in failure of B_{12} absorption.
- **Other causes:** Chronic gastritis, malabsorption and fish tapeworm infestation (consumes B_{12}).

Uses

- **Vitamin B_{12} deficiency:** Prevention and treatment of megaloblastic anemia due to B_{12} deficiency.
- **Vitamin B_{12} neuropathies:** Like subacute combined degeneration respond to vitamin B_{12}.

Folic Acid

Folic acid was first isolated from spinach and therefore named as folic acid (from leaf).

Dietary source: Green vegetables, liver, yeast, egg, milk and some fruits. Prolonged cooking with spices destroys folic acid.

Deficiency

Folate deficiency may be due to dietary folate deficiency, malabsorption and other diseases of the small intestine or drug induced. Phenytoin, phenobarbitone, oral contraceptives, methotrexate and trimethoprim can induce folate deficiency. Increased requirement as in growing children, pregnancy and lactation can also cause deficiency. Manifestations include megaloblastic anemia, glossitis, diarrhea and weakness.

Uses

- **Megaloblastic anemia** due to folate as well as B_{12} deficiency—folic acid is given orally along with vitamin B_{12}.
- In **pregnancy, lactation**, infancy and other situations with increased requirement of folic acid.

Hematopoietic Growth Factors

These are glycoprotein hormones that regulate erythropoiesis. Erythropoietin, and myeloid growth factors like granulocyte colony-stimulating factor (G-CSF), granulocyte macrophage colony-stimulating factor (GM-CSF) are the hematopoietic growth factors available for clinical use. Erythropoietin stimulates red cell production and is used in anemia in AIDS, cancer patients on chemotherapy, chronic renal failure, multiple myeloma and aplastic anemia.

Myeloid growth factors are useful in the prevention and treatment of anemia and neutropenia in AIDS, aplastic anemia, following cancer chemotherapy and bone marrow transplantation.

7 CHAPTER

Central Nervous System

CHAPTER HIGHLIGHTS

- Sedative Hypnotics
- Antiepileptics
- Drugs Used in Parkinsonism
- Opioid Analgesics and Antagonists
- Drugs Used in Psychiatric Disorders: Antipsychotics, Antidepressants and Antianxiety Agents
- CNS Stimulants

Other Drugs Acting on the CNS
- General Anesthetics
- Local Anesthetics
- Alcohols

SEDATIVE HYPNOTICS

Sedative is a drug that produces a calming or quietening effect and reduces excitement. It may cause drowsiness. **Hypnotic** is a drug that produces sleep resembling natural sleep. Both sedation and hypnosis may be considered as different grades of CNS depression. All human beings need sleep. Approximately one-third of our life is spent in sleep.

Sleep can be classified into two types depending on the physiological characteristics.

1. Non-Rapid Eye Movement (NREM) sleep.
2. Rapid Eye Movement(REM) sleep.

Throughout the night, NREM and REM sleep cycles repeat alternately for brief periods.

Insomnia is sleeplessness. Since centuries man has sought the help of drugs and other remedies for insomnia.

Classification of Sedative Hypnotics

1. **Benzodiazepines**

   Long-acting (24–48 hours)

Diazepam	Flurazepam
Chlordiazepoxide	Chlorazepate
Clonazepam	Clobazam

   Short-acting (12–24 hours)

Temazepam	Nitrazepam
Lorazepam	Alprazolam
Oxazepam	Halazepam

   Ultra short-acting (<6 hours)

Triazolam	Midazolam

2. **Newer agents**

   a. **Melatonin and congeners**

Melatonin	Ramelteon
	Tasimelteon

   b. **'Z' hypnotics**

Zolpidem	Eszopiclone
Zopiclone	Zaleplon

   c. **Orexin receptor antagonists**

Suvorexant	Almorexant

3. **Barbiturates**

Phenobarbitone	Pentobarbitone
Mephobarbitone	Thiopentone
Secobarbitone	Hexobarbitone

Benzodiazepines

Chlordiazepoxide was the first benzodiazepine (BZD) to be introduced into clinical medicine in 1961 and since then thousands of BZDs have been synthesized of which 35 are now in clinical use.

Pharmacological Actions

The most important actions of BZDs are on the CNS and include:

1. Sedation and hypnosis
2. Reduction in anxiety
3. Muscle relaxation
4. Anticonvulsant effects
5. Anesthesia
6. Amnesia

Hypnosis: With BZDs, onset of sleep is faster and they also increase the duration of sleep. The quality of sleep resembles natural sleep more closely when compared to barbiturates. Tolerance develops to this effect gradually.

Anxiolytic/antianxiety/sedative effects: BZDs reduce anxiety and aggression and thus produce a calming effect. Alprazolam has additional antidepressant properties.

Muscle relaxant action: BZDs reduce muscle tone by a central action. Generally anxiety is associated with an increased muscle tone and may be responsible for aches and pains in these patients. The muscle relaxation by BZDs adds to the beneficial effects in such patients.

Anticonvulsant effects: BZDs have anticonvulsant properties. Diazepam is used intravenously in status epilepticus and rectally in febrile convulsions. Clonazepam is used in the treatment of absence seizures and myoclonic seizures in children. Nitrazepam and lorazepam are also used as antiepileptics.

Anesthesia: In higher doses BZDs produce general anesthesia. Diazepam, midazolam and triazolam are used IV.

Amnesia: BZDs produce loss of memory for events happening after their use. This property is an advantage when BZDs are used in surgical procedures as the patient does not remember the unpleasant events.

Other actions:

- In higher doses BZDs decrease BP and increase heart rate
- Diazepam decreases nocturnal gastric acid secretion
- BZDs in higher doses can cause respiratory depression.

Mechanism of Action

Gamma aminobutyric acid (GABA) is the principle inhibitory neurotransmitter in the CNS and it acts on the GABA receptors. BZDs bind to the GABA receptors and increase the effects of GABA. They increase the frequency of chloride channel opening leading to increased flow of chloride ions into the neurons. This results in hyperpolarization.

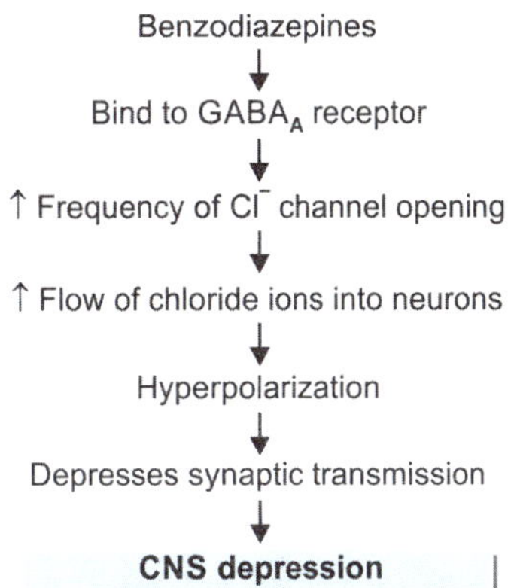

BZDs as hypnotics—when compared to barbiturates:

1. BZDs induce sleep which more closely resembles natural sleep and has less hangover.
2. In hypnotic doses they do not affect respiration or cardiovascular functions.
3. BZDs have a higher safety margin and are safer than barbiturates even in overdoses. The respiratory depression in overdoses is milder.
4. In case of BZD overdosage, a specific BZD antagonist—**flumazenil** can be used to reverse the symptoms.
5. BZDs do not cause microsomal enzyme induction and therefore do not alter the blood levels of other drugs.
6. BZDs have lower abuse liability.

Because of the above reasons, BZDs are the most preferred sedative hypnotics.

Pharmacokinetics

There are significant pharmacokinetic differences among BZDs due to their difference in lipid solubility. They are all completely absorbed on oral use, extensively bound to plasma proteins and metabolised in the liver.

Adverse Effects

BZDs are generally well tolerated. The common side effects include drowsiness, confusion, amnesia, lethargy, ataxia, day time sedation and impaired motor coordination such as driving skills—therefore, while on BZDs driving should be avoided.

In some patients it may cause irritability and anxiety.

Tolerance and dependence: Both tolerance and risk of dependence are less with BZDs as compared to barbiturates. Patients develop tolerance to the sedative effects. On long-term use, dependance develops. If BZDs are suddenly stopped after long-term administration, withdrawal symptoms like anxiety, sleeplessness, irritability and sweating can occur but are milder and slower in onset because most BZDs have a long t 1/2.

Uses of BZDs

1. **Insomnia:** BZDs are used in the treatment of insomnia.
2. **In anxiety states:** BZDs are the most commonly used anxiolytics for the treatment of anxiety states and anxiety neuroses.
3. **As anticonvulsants:** IV diazepam is the drug of choice in the treatment of status epilepticus. Clonazepam is used with other antiepileptic drugs.
4. **Muscle relaxant:** BZDs are centrally acting muscle relaxants used in chronic muscle spasm and spasticity.
5. **As preaneshetic medication** BZDs are useful for their sedation, amnesia and anxiolytic effects.
6. **As an anesthetic** intravenous diazepam or midazolam may be used for short surgical procedures and to supplement general anesthetics.
7. **During alcohol withdrawal:** BZDs are useful in patients during withdrawal of alcohol or other sedative-hypnotics.

Benzodazepine overdose: Overdose induces sleep but respiratory depression is mild. Hence BZDs are safe and availability of a specific antidote flumazenil makes it safer to use BZDs as poisoning can be reversed.

Flumazenil is a BZD receptor antagonist which competes with BZDs for the receptor and reverses all the actions of BZDs.

Uses

- To reverse BZD sedation/anesthesia
- In BZD overdosage.

NEWER HYPNOTICS

1. Melatonin and Congeners

Melatonin: The hormone secreted by the pineal gland is known to regulate sleep. It is secreted at night and plays an important role in the circadian rhythm. There are two types of melatonin receptors—melatonin 1 (MT1) and melatonin 2 (MT2) and melatonin acts on these receptors; it does not depress the CNS; it improves the quality of sleep and helps in withdrawing benzodiazepines after long-term use. However, its role in the maintenance of sleep is not proved.

Uses

- *Insomnia:* Administered orally at bed time in the dose of 2–10 mg, melatonin is considered a natural remedy for insomnia and is free from the disadvantages of BZDs
- *Jet lag:* Melatonin may be used to overcome jet lag and other conditions of disturbed biorhythm
- *To help withdraw hypnotics in elderly dependents:* The secretion of melatonin decreases with age and therefore it is supplemented with the hope that it retards aging.

Ramelteon an agonist at the melatonin receptors (both MT1 and MT2) is a novel hypnotic drug. Ramelteon reduces the latency of persistent sleep. Advantages are that it does not modify the sleep architecture, there is no rebound insomnia or other major withdrawal symptoms.

Adverse effects include dizziness and fatigue. There could be an increase in prolactin levels and decrease in testosterone.

2. 'Z' Hypnotics

Include zolpidem, zopiclone, eszopiclone and zaleplon.

- They are not BZDs but produce their effects by binding to benzodiazepine site on the $GABA_A$ receptors and facilitate the inhibitory actions of GABA
- They are specific hypnotics and do not have antianxiety, anticonvulasant and muscle relaxant properties unlike BZDs.
- They are all rapid and short-acting agents and produce minimum hangover.
- The sleep produced is more closer to natural sleep
- The risk of tolerance and dependence is lower than BZDs
- They are well tolerated with minor side effects
- They are well-absorbed from the gut and metabolized in the liver
- Their actions are blocked by flumazenil
- They are used for short periods when short-acting hypnotics are needed.

Zolpidem is a good hypnotic. It is short-acting (t½–2 hours) but the effects on sleep continue for a long time even after stopping zolpidem.

Dose should be reduced in hepatic dysfunction.

Zaleplon has rapid onset and short duration of action. It has the advantages that no withdrawal symptoms are reported after stopping it and no tolerance develops.

Zopiclone actions resemble those of BZDs.

Eszopiclone is the S enantiomer of zopiclone; it prolongs the total sleep time. It has a half-life of 6 hrs.

Adverse effects include dryness of mouth, metallic taste; higher doses can cause impaired psychomotor performance.

Uses of 'Z' hypnotics: 'Z' hypnotics have similar efficacy as BZDs in the treatment of insomnia with the advantages of rapid action and minimum day—after drowsiness and less amnesia. They are recommended for short periods for the treatment of insomnia.

Orexin Receptor Antagonists

Orexins are neurotransmitters in the CNS which control wakefulness. Orexin levels are high in the day and low at night. Orexins act on the receptors OX1 and OX2. Orexin receptor antagonists **suvorexant**, **almorexant** and **filorexant** are new class of drugs useful in insomnia. They block the binding of wake-promoting orexin A and orexin B to the orexin receptors.

BARBITURATES

Barbiturates are derivatives of barbituric acid and were the largest group of hypnotics in clinical use until the 1960s.

Classification

Barbiturates can be classified based on their duration of action as:

- **Long-acting:** Phenobarbitone, mephobarbitone
- **Short-acting:** Pentobarbitone, butobarbitone
- **Ultrashort-acting:** Thiopentone, hexobarbitone, methohexitone

Mechanism of Action

Barbiturates bind to GABA receptors and increase the inhibitory activity of GABA.

Pharmacological Actions

CNS

1. **Sedation and hypnosis:** Barbiturates cause sedation and induce sleep. They reduce anxiety and impair memory.
   They can produce **euphoria** and are drugs of addiction while some people may experience dysphoria. Barbiturates produce **hyperalgesia** (increased sensitivity to pain). Therefore barbiturates, when given as hypnotics for a patient

in pain may be more troublesome than being of any benefit.

Anesthesia: In higher doses barbiturates produce general anesthesia. The ultra short-acting barbiturates like thiopentone sodium are used intravenously for this effect.

Anticonvulsant effects: All barbiturates have anticonvulsant effects. Phenobarbitone is used in the treatment of epilepsy.

2. **Respiratory system:** Barbiturates depress the respiration. High doses paralyze the respiratory center and can be fatal.
3. **Cardiovascular system:** Barbiturates cause mild hypotension.
4. **Skeletal muscles:** Higher doses of barbiturates depress the excitability of the neuromuscular junction.

Pharmacokinetics

Barbiturates are well-absorbed and widely distributed in the body and metabolized in the liver. They are hepatic microsomal **enzyme inducers**. The metabolites are excreted in the urine.

Adverse Reactions

Drowsiness, prolonged sleep, amnesia and confusion are common. Barbiturates produce respiratory depression which can be dangerous in patients with respiratory disorders.

Hangover may be accompanied by nausea, vomiting, vertigo and diarrhea. Changes of mood, impaired judgement and fine motor skills may be seen. Hence driving should be avoided while on barbiturates. Hypersensitivity reactions are common with skin rashes, swelling of lips and eyelids and rarely exfoliative dermatitis.

Tolerance and dependence: On repeated administration, tolerance develops to the effects of barbiturates.

Development of dependence to barbiturates makes them one of the drugs of abuse. Withdrawal symptoms include anxiety, restlessness, abdominal cramps, hallucinations, delirium and convulsions.

Acute barbiturate poisoning: In acute barbiturate poisoning, there is severe respiratory depression, hypotension and shock. It can be fatal. There is no specific antidote for treatment. Stomach wash, forced alkaline diuresis and hemodialysis should be done.

Uses: Because of respiratory depression and risk of abuse, barbiturates are generally not preferred.

1. **Neonatal jaundice:** Phenobarbitone is a microsomal enzyme inducer. It increases the production of the enzyme required for metabolism and excretion of bilirubin. It therefore helps in the clearance of jaundice in the neonates.
2. **Antiepileptic:** Phenobarbitone is used as an antiepileptic.
3. **Anesthesia:** Thiopentone sodium is used IV for the induction of general anesthesia.
4. **Sedation and hypnosis:** Barbiturates are not preferred as sedative hypnotics.

ANTIEPILEPTICS

Epilepsy is a common neurological abnormality that affects about 0.5–1 percent of the population. **Epilepsy** is a chronic disorder characterized by recurrent seizures often accompanied by episodes of unconsciousness and/or amnesia. It is a disorder of brain function. **Convulsions** are involuntary, violent spasms series of jerking or prolonged contractions of the skeletal muscles.

Seizure is an alteration in behavior because of abnormal firing of some brain neurons. In most of the cases, the cause is not known. It may be due to various reasons including trauma during birth process, head injury, childhood fevers, brain tumors, meningitis or drug induced (e.g. chlorpromazine, methylxanthines).

Types of Seizures

Seizures were classified into partial and generalized seizures. New classification

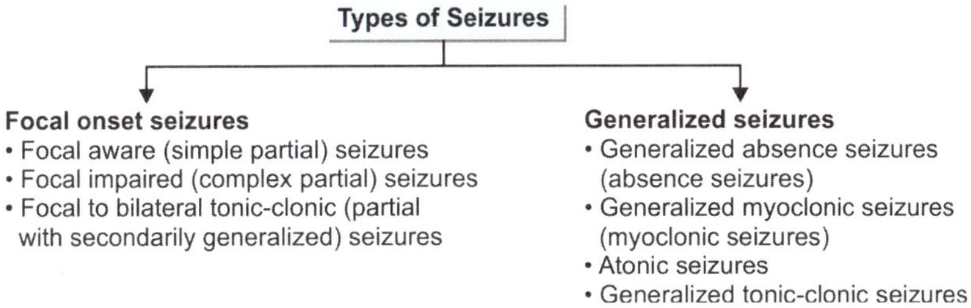

Types of Seizures

Focal onset seizures
- Focal aware (simple partial) seizures
- Focal impaired (complex partial) seizures
- Focal to bilateral tonic-clonic (partial with secondarily generalized) seizures

Generalized seizures
- Generalized absence seizures (absence seizures)
- Generalized myoclonic seizures (myoclonic seizures)
- Atonic seizures
- Generalized tonic-clonic seizures

of seizures has been introduced. Older terminology is given in brackets.

1. **Focal onset seizures (partial seizures)** account for about 60% of all epilepsies and they involve focal brain regions. They are classified as simple partial in which there is no impairment of consciousness and complex partial seizures with impairment of consciousness. When reticular formation is affected unconsciousness results.
   - **Focal aware seizures:** There is no impairment of consciousness. The manifestation depends on the site in the cortex that is activated by the seizure, e.g., if the motor cortex representing the right thumb is involved, there is recurrent contractions of the right thumb. If the sensory area representing the left palm is involved, there is numbness or paresthesia of the left palm. This type of seizures lasts for 20-60 seconds.
   - **Focal with impaired awareness seizures (complex partial)** are the most common types of epilepsy. They are characterized by purposeless movements, such as lipsmaking, hand wringing or swallowing that lasts for 30 seconds to 2 minutes. Consciousness is impaired and may be preceded by an aura.
   - **Focal to bilateral tonic-clonic seizures:** Simple or complex partial seizure may evolve into a generalized seizure.
2. **Generalized seizures:** Account for 40% of all epilepsies and is usually of genetic etiology. Generalized seizures affect the whole brain. They may be:
   - **Generalized absence seizures (petit mal):** In this, there is a sudden onset of impaired consciousness associated with staring. The person stops all ongoing activities and the episode lasts for a brief period usually less than 30 seconds.
   - **Generalized myoclonic seizures** involve a sudden, brief, shock, such as contraction of muscles. It may be limited to a part of the body or may affect the whole body.
   - **Generalized atonic seizures** (drop attacks) are characterized by sudden loss of postural tone and the head may drop for a few seconds or the person may drop to the ground for no obvious reasons.
   - **Generalized tonic-clonic seizures (grand mal epilepsy)** is characterized by sudden loss of consciousness followed by sustained contraction of muscles throughout the body (known

Mnemonic for groups

this Happy BirthDay Is Surely Going To Be Naughty, Memorable One

H—Hydantoins
B—Barbiturates
D—Deoxybarbiturate
I—Iminostilbene
S—Succinimide
G—GABA transaminase inhibitors
B—Benzodiazepines
N—Newer ones
M—Most commonly used
O—Others

as tonic phase), lasting for 1 minute and then, a series of jerks, i.e., periods of muscle contraction alternating with periods of relaxation (clonic phase) lasting for 2–4 minutes follow. Central nervous system (CNS) depression then occurs and the person goes into sleep. Injury may occur during the convulsive episode.

3. **Status epilepticus** is continuous or recurrent seizures of any variety without recovery of consciousness between the attacks.

Classification

1. **Hydantoins:** Phenytoin, mephenytoin
2. **Barbiturates:** Phenobarbitone, mephobarbitone
3. **Deoxybarbiturate:** Primidone
4. **Iminostilbene:** Carbamazepine, oxcarbazepine, eslicarbazine
5. **Succinimide:** Ethosuximide
6. **GABA transaminase inhibitors:** Valproic acid, vigabatrin
7. **Benzodiazepines:** Diazepam, clonazepam, lorazepam, clorazepate
8. **Newer agents:**
   a. **Most commonly used:** Levetiracetam, lamotrigine, topiramate, lacosamide
   b. **Others:** Gabapentin, tiagabine, vigabatrin, zonisamide, felbamate, perampanel.

Phenytoin (Diphenylhydantoin)

Pharmacological Actions

CNS: Phenytoin has good antiseizure activity. It is one of the most effective drugs against generalized tonic-clonic seizures and partial seizures.

Mechanism of Action

Phenytoin causes blockade of the sodium channels and stabilizes the neuronal membrane. It inhibits the generation of repetitive action potentials.

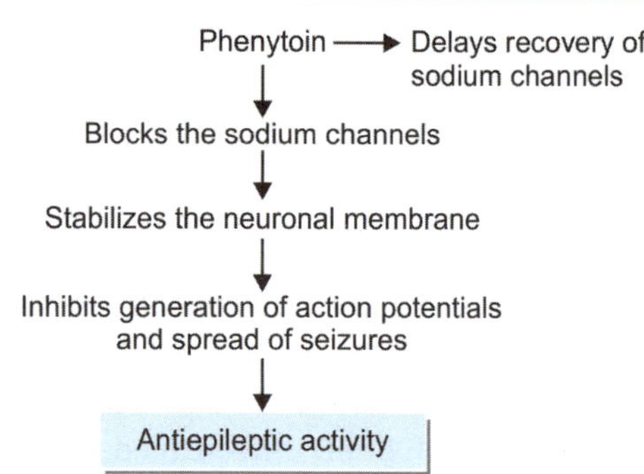

Pharmacokinetics

Phenytoin is poorly water-soluble—hence absorption is slow. Phenytoin is 90% bound to plasma proteins. It is metabolized in the liver initially by first order and later by zero order kinetics as the dose increases. Therefore, monitoring of plasma concentration is useful. Phenytoin is an enzyme inducer.

Adverse Effects

Adverse effects depend on the dose, duration and route of administration.

1. **Nausea**, vomiting, epigastric pain, anorexia.
2. **Nystagmus**, diplopia, ataxia are common.
3. **Gingival hyperplasia** is more common in children on prolonged use.
4. **Peripheral neuropathy.**
5. **Endocrine**
   - Hirsutism, acne, coarsening of facial features.
   - Hyperglycemia—as phenytoin inhibits insulin release.
   - ↓ release of ADH.
   - Osteomalacia, hypocalcemia due to altered metabolism of vitamin D and inhibition of intestinal absorption of Ca^{++}. Phenytoin also reduces target tissue sensitivity to vitamin D.

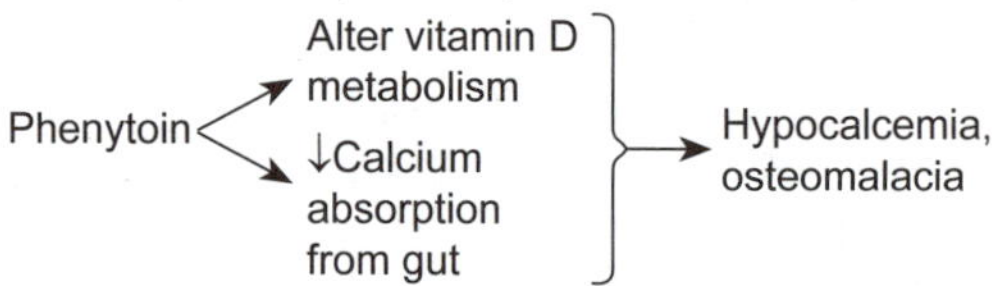

6. **Hypersensitivity**—rashes, systemic lupus erythematosus, hepatic necrosis, lymphadenopathy and neutropenia.
7. **Megaloblastic anemia**—as phenytoin decreases absorption and increases excretion of folates.
8. **Teratogenicity**—when taken by the pregnant lady, phenytoin produces **fetal hydantoin syndrome** characterized by hypoplastic phalanges, cleft palate, harelip and microcephaly in the offspring.

Toxic doses—cerebellar and vestibular effects are prominent; drowsiness, delirium, confusion, hallucinations, altered behavior and coma follow.

Uses

1. Generalized tonic-clonic seizures and partial seizures (not useful in absence seizures).
2. Status epilepticus—phenytoin is used by slow IV injection.
3. Trigeminal neuralgia—as an alternative to carbamazepine.
4. Cardiac arrhythmias—phenytoin is useful in digitalis induced arrhythmias.

Drug Interactions

- Phenytoin is an enzyme inducer. Given with phenobarbitone, both increase each other's metabolism. Also phenobarbitone competitively inhibits phenytoin metabolism.
- Carbamazepine and phenytoin increase each other's metabolism.
- Valproate displaces protein bound phenytoin and may result in phenytoin toxicity.
- Cimetidine and chloramphenicol inhibit the metabolism of phenytoin resulting in toxicity.
- Antacids ↓ absorption of phenytoin.

Fosphenytoin is a prodrug of phenytoin that has certain advantages over phenytoin for parenteral use:

- It is quickly converted to phenytoin in the body
- More potent
- Less cardiotoxic
- Safer on the intestine
- It can be injected into a glucose drip unlike phenytoin
- It can be given IM.

Because of the above advantages, fosphenytoin is preferred over phenytoin in status epilepticus. Dose: 20 mg/kg IV.

Phenobarbitone

Phenobarbitone was the first effective antiepileptic drug to be introduced in 1912. It's use as an antiepileptic is declining.

Antiepileptic actions: Phenobarbitone has specific antiepileptic activity and raises the seizure threshold. Primidone which is rarely used now is metabolized to phenobarbitone.

Mechanism of action: Barbiturates increase the inhibitory activity of GABA in the CNS.

Pharmacokinetics: Oral absorption of phenobarbitone is slow but complete. It is a microsomal enzyme inducer.

Uses: Phenobarbitone is one of the widely used antiepileptics because of its efficacy and low cost. It is used in:

- Generalized tonic-clonic seizures.
- Partial seizures.
- In neonatal jaundice.

Carbamazepine

Carbamazepine is closely related to imipramine.

Antiseizure activity: Carbamazepine has good antiseizure activity. Its mechanism of action is similar to phenytoin, i.e., it blocks sodium channels.

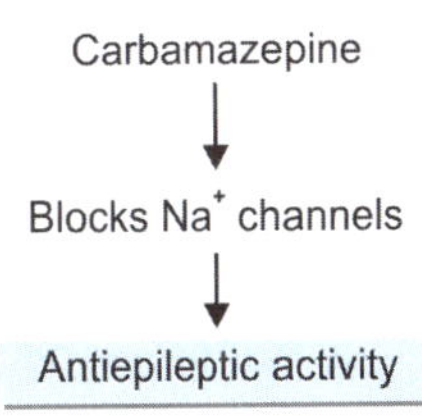

Carbamazepine is also useful in the treatment of trigeminal neuralgia (severe pain along the distribution of the trigeminal nerve) and glossopharyngeal neuralgia.

Carbamazepine is found to be beneficial in mood disorders too.

Pharmacokinetics: Absorption is slow and erratic; has a t½ of 10–20 hours. It is a microsomal enzyme inducer and increases its own metabolism.

Adverse effects: Drowsiness, vertigo, ataxia, diplopia, blurring of vision, nausea, vomiting and dizziness are common. Driving is dangerous for patients on carbamazepine. Hypersensitivity reactions—like skin rashes may occur. Hematological toxicity includes leukopenia, thrombocytopenia and rarely agranulocytosis and aplastic anemia. It is a teratogen.

Mnemonic for uses of Carbamazepine

Carbamzepine Bro's Good Hands Fight To Get rid of Chronic neuropathic and Tabetic Pain
Carbamazepine
Bro's—Bipolar disorder
Good—Generalised tonic clonic seizures
Heart—Hemifacial spasm
Fight—Focal onset seizures
To—Trigeminal neuralgia
Get rid of—Glossophayngeal neuralgia
Chronic neuropathic and Tabetic Pain.

Uses

1. **Generalized tonic clonic seizures** (grand mal epilepsy).
2. **Focal onset seizures**—especially temporal lobe epilepsy.
3. **Trigeminal neuralgia** and glossopharyngeal neuralgia—carbamazepine is the drug of choice for these neuralgias and has to be given for several months.
4. **Chronic neuropathic** pain and **tabetic pain** also respond to carbamazepine
5. **Hemifacial spasm** following facial palsy.
6. **Bipolar mood disorder**—carbamazepine is used as an alternative to other antidepressants.

Ethosuximide

Ethosuximide is the primary agent for absence seizures. It raises the seizure threshold.

Mechanism of action: Ethosuximide reduces the calcium currents (T-currents) in the thalamic neurons. These T-currents are thought to be responsible for absence seizures.

Pharmacokinetics: Absorption is complete on administration of oral dosage forms. It is metabolized in the liver.

Adverse effects: The most common adverse effects are nausea, vomiting, epigastric pain, gastric irritation and anorexia. These can be avoided by starting with a low dose and gradually increasing it. Central nervous system (CNS) effects like drowsiness, fatigue, lethargy, euphoria, dizziness, headache and hiccough are dose-related effects. Hypersensitivity reactions like rashes, urticaria, leukopenia, thrombocytopenia or pancytopenia have been reported.

Uses: Ethosuximide is considered the drug of choice for generalized absence seizures but valproate is preferred now.

Valproic Acid

Valproic acid (salt→sodium valproate) is a very effective antiepileptic drug useful in many types of epilepsies including generalized absence seizures, focal onset and generalized tonic-clonic seizures.

Mechanism of action: Valproic acid acts by multiple mechanisms.

- It increases the level of GABA by:
  - Increasing the synthesis of GABA—by increased activity of GABA synthetase enzyme.
  - Decreasing the metabolism of GABA—by inhibiting GABA transaminase enzyme.
- Like phenytoin, it blocks the sodium channels.
- Like ethosuximide, it suppresses the calcium 'T' currents in the hypothalamus.

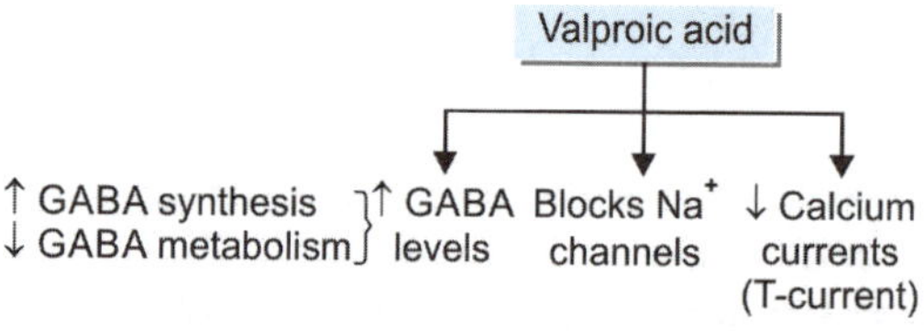

Mechanism of action of valproate

Adverse effects: Gastrointestinal symptoms like nausea, vomiting, epigastric distress occur initially. Tremors, sedation, ataxia, rashes and alopecia are rare. Valproic acid can cause fulminant hepatitis—though rare can be fatal. Hence careful monitoring of liver functions is mandatory. Valproic acid is teratogenic, it can cause neural tube defects including spina bifida.

Uses: Useful in focal onset and generalized seizures. Valproic acid is particularly useful in absence seizures. In patients with both absence seizures and generalized tonic-clonic attacks, valproate is the drug of choice.

Valproate is also useful as a mood stabilizer in bipolar mood disorder.

BENZODIAZEPINES

Benzodiazepines have useful anticonvulsant properties. **Lorazepam** is the drug of choice in status epilepticus and diazepam is used in febrile convulsions. **Clonazepam** is a potent antiepileptic useful in absence and myoclonic seizures. But tolerance develops to its antiepileptic effects. **Clobazam** causes less sedation and is effective in most types of epilepsies.

Newer Antiepileptics

Newer antiepileptics act by -

Blocking Na⁺ channels

Lamotrigine, topiramate lacosamide rufinamide, zonisamide

Increasing GABA activity

Tiagabin, Gabapentin

Vigabatrin

Topiramate

Stiripentol

Decreasing excitatory neurotransmission

Topiramate

Felbamate

Perampanel

Mechanism not understood

Levetiracetam

1. **Levetiracetam** is effective against focal onset and secondarily generalized seizures. Its mechanism of action is not known. Advantage is that it is not an enzyme inducer—hence no related drug interactions. Levetiracetam is used focal seizures, generalized tonic-clonic seizures and myoclonic seizures. It is also being used as an antiepileptic in pregnancy.

2. **Lamotrigine** has a broad spectrum of antiepileptic activity. It inhibits the sodium channels and also inhibits the release of the excitatory amino acids like glutamate. It is completely absorbed from the gut. Lamotrigine may cause skin rashes, nausea, ataxia and dizziness. It is used either alone or with other drugs in partial and generalized seizures.

3. **Lacosamide** has been recently introduced for the treatment of focal onset seizures. It acts on the sodium channels, is completely absorbed when given orally and can cause headache, nausea, dizziness and blurred vision. It can be used in focal onset seizures.

4. **Topiramate** acts by multiple mechanisms. It blocks the sodium channels, increases GABA receptor currents, and blocks AMPA receptors (glutamate receptor). It is effective in focal onset and generalized seizures. Topiramate can be used as add-on therapy in refractory epilepsy. It can also be used for prophylaxis of migraine.

5. **Gabapentin** and **pregabalin** are GABA analogs. They are effective in tonic clonic seizures. Their exact mechanism of action is not known, but they do not act directly on GABA receptors. They are well tolerated and do not change the plasma concentrations of other antiepileptics.

Adverse effects include ataxia, fatigue, drowsiness and dizziness. Tolerance develops to these effects in 1–2 weeks. Gabapentin and pregabalin are used in combination with other antiepileptic drugs in partial seizures. It is also used in migraine, neuropathic pain and in bipolar mood disorder.

6. **Tiagabine:** Tiagabine a GABA analog, inhibits the reuptake of GABA into neurons and thereby increases GABA levels. It may

cause drowsiness and dizziness. Tiagabine can be used as add-on drug for refractory partial seizures.

7. **Vigabatrin** is a GABA analog which acts by irreversibly inhibiting the enzyme GABA transaminase thereby raising brain GABA levels. It can cause depression in some patients. Vigabatrin is useful in patients not responding to other antiepileptics.

8. **Zonisamide** a acts by inhibiting the T type Ca^{++} currents and also by blocking Na^{+} channels. It is well tolerated and is indicated in refractory partial seizures.

9. **Felbamate** an analogue of meprobamate is found to have good antiepileptic action. But felbamate can sometimes cause serious adverse effects like aplastic anemia and hepatitis because of which it is used only in refractory epilepsy.

10. **Other drugs:** Other newer antiepileptics like perampanel, retigabine, rufinamide are available for use in refractory onset seizures.

- Newer antiepileptics include levetiracetam, lamotrigine, topiramate, lacosamide, gabapentin, pregabalin, tiagabine, vigabatrin, zonisamide, felbamate.
- Gabapentin, vigabatrin and lamotrigine act by influencing GABA.
- Lamotrigine, topiramate and zonisamide act on sodium channels.
- The newer antiepileptic levetiracetam is used in focal onset, generalized and myoclonic seizures. It is also used as an antiepileptic in pregnancy. Other newer antiepileptics are being used either alone or as add on drugs in epilepsies. Some of them are preferred over older drugs.

Treatment of Epilepsies (Table 7.1)

Most patients with epilepsy require prolonged treatment, and adverse effects from antiepileptics are expected because of the long duration of treatment needed.

Febrile convulsions: 2–4% of children experience convulsions during fever; of them 2–3% become epileptics. Treatment is controversial. If convulsions occur, diazepam rectally or intravenously can be used. Children < 18 months developing febrile convulsions, those with neurological abnormalities and those with seizures lasting for > 15 minutes, complex seizures—all these have greater risk of recurrence. In recurrent cases, Diazepam (0.5 mg/kg) given orally or rectally at the onset of fever prevents convulsions. Timely use of paracetamol and tepid sponging prevents high fever.

Table 7.1: Choice of antiseizure drugs.

Types of epilepsy	*Preferred drugs*
Generalized tonic-clonic	Valproate, carbamazepine, lamotrigine, levetiracetam, phenytoin
Focal onset seizures	Carbamazepine, valproate, lamotrigine, levetiracetam, phenytoin
Absence seizures	Valproate, Ethosuximide, lamotrigin
Tonic-clonic + absence seizures	Valproate
Myoclonic seizures	Valproate, topiramate, levetiracetam
Focal impaired seizures	Carbamazepine, phenytoin, valproate
Febrile convulsions	Diazepam
Status epilepticus	Lorazepam, diazepam, fosphenytoin, general anesthesia

Status epilepticus: It is a neurological emergency which may be fatal. **Lorazepam** 4 mg IV is the drug of choice. Alternative is diazepam IV (5–10 mg every 10–15 minutes up to 30 mg). Fosphenytoin is preferred to phenytoin as it is faster acting. Phenytoin given intravenously takes 15–20 minutes to act. Some prefer to combine diazepam and phenytoin. If seizures continue—general anesthesia is the last resort. Airway maintenance is important. After the control of seizures, long-term antiepileptic therapy is needed.

In pregnancy: Antiepileptics should be continued in pregnancy because abrupt discontinuation increases the risk of status epilepticus which is hazardous to the fetus. However many of them are teratogenic and the right drugs should be considered.

Lamotrigine and **levetiracetam** are used in the prevention and treatment of epilepsy in pregnancy.

DRUGS USED IN PARKINSONISM

Parkinsonism is a chronic, progressive, motor disorder characterized by rigidity, tremors and bradykinesia. Other symptoms include excessive salivation, abnormalities of posture and gait, seborrhea and mood changes. It was described by James Parkinson in 1817 and is therefore named after him.

The incidence is about 1 percent of population above 65 years of age. It is usually idiopathic in origin but can also be drug induced. In idiopathic parkinsonism, there is degeneration of nigrostriatal neurons in the basal ganglia resulting in dopamine deficiency. The balance between inhibitory dopaminergic neurons and excitatory cholinergic neurons is disturbed.

Antiparkinsonian drugs can only help to reduce the symptoms and improve the quality of life. The two strategies in the treatment are
(i) to increase dopamine activity
(ii) to decrease cholinergic overactivity.

Classification

See Flowchart 7.1.

Drugs that Increase Dopamine Levels

Dopamine Precursor

Levodopa

Though parkinsonism is due to dopamine deficiency, dopamine is of no therapeutic value because it does not cross the blood-brain barrier. Levodopa is a prodrug which is converted to dopamine in the body. It crosses the BBB and is taken up by the surviving nigrostriatal neurons.

$$\text{Levodopa} \xrightarrow{\text{Dopa decarboxylase}} \text{Dopamine}$$

Antiparkinsonian effect: On administration of levodopa, there is an overall improvement in the patient as all the symptoms subside.

Other Actions

Large portion of levodopa is converted to dopamine in the periphery which is responsible for the side effects.

- **Chemoreceptor triggor zone (CTZ):** Dopamine stimulates the CTZ to induce vomiting.
- **Cardiovascular system (CVS):** Large amounts of levodopa converted to dopamine in the periphery causes

Flowchart 7.1: Classification.

Drugs used in parkinsonism

1. **Drugs that increase dopamine levels**
   - **DA precursor**
     Levodopa
   - **Dopaminergic agonists**
     - Bromocryptine, pergolide
     - Lisuride
     - Ropinirole
     - Pramipexole
   - **Inhibit dopamine metabolism**
     - **MAO inhibitors**
       Selegiline, rasagiline
     - **COMT inhibitors**
       Tolcapone, entacapone
   - **Dopamine releaser**
     Amantadine
2. **Drugs that act on cholinergic system**
   - **Central anticholinergics**
     - Benztropine
     - Benzhexol (Trihexyphenidyl)
     - Biperidine
   - **Antihistamines**
     - Diphenhydramine
     - Orphenadrine
     - Promethazine

postural hypotension and tachycardia—dopamine is a catecholamine.

- **Endocrine:** Dopamine (DA) suppresses the prolactin secretion.

Pharmacokinetics: Levodopa is rapidly absorbed. Presence of food delays absorption. It undergoes first pass metabolism in the gut and the liver. Its t½ is 1–2 hours.

Adverse reactions: As 95% of levodopa is converted to dopamine in the periphery, several adverse effects are expected. Nausea, vomiting, postural hypotension, tachycardia and occasionally arrhythmias can occur. Tolerance develops to these effects after sometime. Behavioral effects like anxiety, depression, hallucinations and sometimes psychosis can occur.

Abnormal involuntary movements like facial tics, grimacing, choreoathetoid movements of the limbs may develop after a few months of use and require reduction in the dose of levodopa.

Fluctuation in response to levodopa can occur after 2–5 years of use—known as **'on-off' phenomenon**—where the patient has alternately good response and severe disease.

Uses: Levodopa is the most effective drug in idiopathic parkinsonism but is not useful in drug induced parkinsonism.

Drug Interactions

- Pyridoxine increases the peripheral metabolism (decarboxylation) of levodopa and thus reduces its availability to the CNS.
- Phenothiazines, metoclopramide and reserpine are DA antagonists. They reverse the effects of levodopa.

Carbidopa and benserazide are peripheral dopa decarboxylase inhibitors. When carbidopa or benserazide are given with levodopa, they prevent the formation of dopamine in the periphery. They do not cross the BBB and hence allow levodopa to reach the CNS. The combination is synergistic and therefore levodopa is always given with carbidopa/benserazide.

Advantages of combining carbidopa/benserazide—with levodopa.

1. Dose of L-dopa can be reduced by 75%.
2. Response to L-dopa appears earlier.
3. Side effects like vomiting and tachycardia are largely reduced.
4. Pyridoxine does not interfere with treatment.

Dopamine Receptor Agonists

Bromocriptine and **pergolide** are ergot derivatives having dopamine agonistic activity. The newer agents **ropinirole** and **pramipexole** are:

- selective D2 agonists,
- better tolerated,
- quickly reach therapeutic levels
- adverse effects are milder except some sleep disorders.

Adverse effects include nausea, vomiting, hallucinations and skin eruptions. Ergot derivatives can cause postural hypotension and 'first dose phenomenon'—that is sudden cardiovascular collapse.

DA agonists are used:

- In the treatment of **'on-off' phenomenon**.
- As alternatives in the initial treatment of parkinsonism.

Lisuride and pergolide are similar to bromocriptine.

Drugs that Inhibit DA Metabolism

Monoamine oxidase inhibitors

Selegiline (Deprenyl) is a selective MAO-B inhibitor. MAO-B is present in DA containing regions of the CNS. Selegiline prolongs the action of levodopa by preventing its destruction. Selegiline and **rasagiline** may delay the progression of parkinsonism.

Adverse effects include nausea, postural hypotension, confusion and hallucinations.

Uses: Mild cases of parkinsonism are started on selegiline/rasagiline. It is also used along with levodopa.

COMT inhibitors: Tolcapone and entacapone inhibit the peripheral metabolism of levodopa thereby increasing its bioavailability.

Tolcapone crosses the BBB and enhances the availability of levodopa in the brain.

Adverse effects are nausea, orthostatic hypotension, confusion and hallucinations. Tolcapone can also cause hepatotoxicity.

Amantadine is an antiviral drug. It increases the release of DA in the brain and reduces the re-uptake of DA. The response starts early and its adverse effects are minor. Large doses produce insomnia, dizziness, vomiting, postural hypotension, hallucinations, ankle edema and livido reticularis.

Amantadine is used in mild cases of parkinsonism. It can also be used along with levodopa.

Drugs Acting on Cholinergic System

Anticholinergics

The cholinergic overactivity is overcome by anticholinergics. Tremors, seborrhea and sialorrhea are reduced more than rigidity. Atropine derivatives like **benzhexol, benztropine** (trihexyphenidyl) and biperidine are used. Antihistamines are useful in parkinsonism because of their anticholinergic properties. Atropine-like side effects such as dry mouth, constipation, blurred vision may be encountered.

Uses: Anticholinergics are used as:

i. Adjunct to levodopa
ii. Drugs of choice in drug-induced parkinsonism.

Drug induced parkinsonism:

Drugs like reserpine, metoclopramide and phenothiazines can induce parkinsonism. Reserpine depletes catecholamine stores, while metoclopramide and phenothiazines (like chlorpromazine) are dopamine antagonists.

Treatment: Withdrawal of the parkinsonism inducing drug usually reverses the symptoms. When drugs are needed, one of the anticholinergics are effective.

Levodopa or other dopamine agonists are not effective because DA receptors are already blocked by drugs like metoclopramide and phenothiazines.

OPIOID ANALGESICS AND ANTAGONISTS

Opioid Analgesics

Opioid analgesics are one of the oldest remedies for relief of pain. **Opium** is the dark brown gummy substance obtained from the poppy capsule *(Papaver somniferum)*. On incising the unripe seed capsule, a milky juice comes out which turns brown on drying and this is crude opium. Opium has been in use since 4000 BC both for medicinal and recreational purposes as it causes euphoria. It was Serturner who isolated a pure opium alkaloid in 1806. He named it **Morphine** after Morpheus, the Greek God of dreams. As the research progressed, opium was found to contain 20 alkaloids. Efforts were made to obtain an opioid that is only analgesic and has no euphoric effects. In the process, various agonists, antagonists and partial agonists were synthesized. 'Opioid' is the term used for drugs with morphine-like actions. They were earlier called narcotic analgesics.

Classification

- **Agonists:**
  - **Natural opioids**—Morphine, codeine, noscapine
  - **Synthetic opioids**—Heroin, pethidine, fentanyl, diphenoxylate, loperamide, methadone, dextropropoxyphene tramadol.
- **Antagonists:**
  Naloxone, naltrexone, nalmefene.
- **Mixed agonist-antagonists:**
  Pentazocine, nalbuphine, butorphanol, buprenorphine, nalorphine.

Morphine

Morphine is the most important alkaloid of opium. Though many new opioids with actions similar to morphine have been synthesized. None of them are superior to morphine as an analgesic.

Mechanism of Action

Morphine and other opioids produce their effects by acting on specific opioid receptors *mu* (μ) *kappa* (κ) and *delta* (δ). These receptors are abundant in the CNS and other tissues.

It is found that there are 3 families of opioid peptides released in the body (endogenous) viz *enkephalins, endorphins* and *dynorphins*. This indicates that we have a natural system in the body that releases various opioid peptides in response to pain.

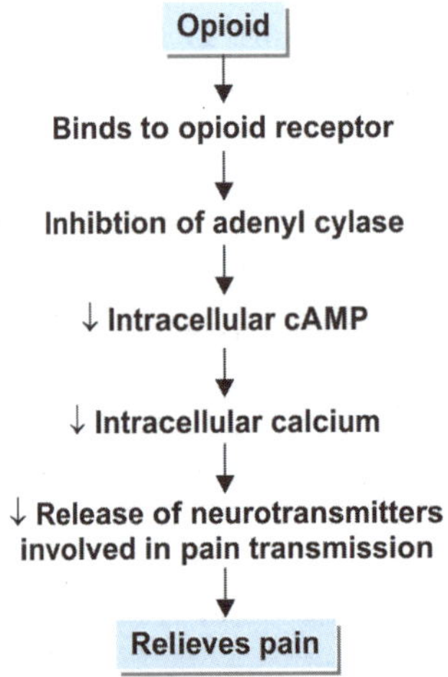

Most pharmacological effects of opioids are due to stimulation of **μ (mu)** opioid receptors.

Pharmacological Actions

1. **Central Nervous System**
   a. **Analgesia:** Morphine is a potent analgesic and relieves pain without loss of consciousness. Dull aching visceral pain is relieved better than sharp pricking pain. In higher doses it relieves even the severe pain as that of biliary colic. Morphine alters both the perception and reaction to pain. It raises the pain threshold and thus increases the capacity to tolerate pain. Further it alters the emotional reaction to pain.
   Euphoria and sedation add to its analgesic effects.
   b. **Euphoria, sedation and hypnosis:** Morphine produces a feeling of well-being termed *euphoria*. It is this effect which makes it an important drug of abuse. Rapid intravenous injection of morphine produces a warm flushing of the skin and an immensely pleasurable sensation in the lower abdomen lasting for about 45 seconds and is known as 'high', 'rush' or 'kick'. The person loses rational thinking and is lost in colorful day dreams. It also produces drowsiness, a calming effect, inability to concentrate, feeling of detachment and indifference to surroundings.
   The effects of morphine may not be pleasurable in all. A person has to learn to experience its pleasurable effects. It may produce dysphoria in some.
   c. **Respiration:** Morphine produces significant respiratory depression. It directly depresses the respiratory center in the brainstem. This action is dose dependent. All phases of respiration, rate and tidal volume are depressed. Death from morphine poisoning is almost always due to respiratory arrest.

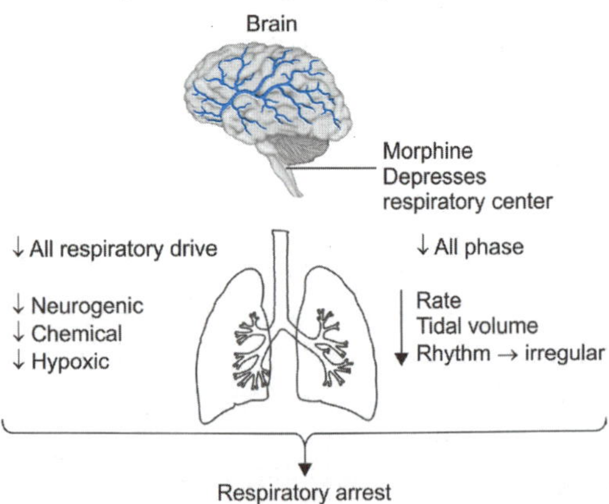

Sedation and indifference to surroundings add to the respiratory depression.

d. **Cough center:** It directly depresses the cough center and thereby suppresses cough.
However, opioids should be used as antitussives only in dry cough because in presence of respiratory secretions, suppression of cough causes accumulation of secretions in the lung leading to infection and other dangerous effects.

e. **Nausea and emesis:** Morphine directly stimulates the chemoreceptor trigger zone (CTZ) in the medulla causing nausea and vomiting. In higher doses it depresses the vomiting center and hence there is no vomiting in poisoning. Therefore, emetics should not be tried in poisoning.

f. **Pupils:** Morphine produces constriction of pupil. In higher doses a characteristic pinpoint pupil is seen by a central effect.

g. **Truncal rigidity:** Higher doses of some opioids like fentanyl increase the tone of the large muscles of the trunk. This may interfere with breathing. It can be overcome by a neuromuscular blocker.

2. **Cardiovascular system:** Morphine produces postural hypotension.

3. **GIT:** Opioids decrease the motility of the gut.
   - **Stomach:** Gastric motility is decreased and gastric acid secretion is reduced. Opioids increase the tone of the antrum and first part of the duodenum which also result in delayed emptying by as much as 12 hours.
   - **Intestines:** Morphine reduces all intestinal secretions, delays digestion of food in the small intestine; resting tone is increased. There can be spasms of the intestine. The tone of the sphincters is increased leading to spasm. The intestinal motility is markedly diminished. Thus, reduced secretions and motility result in constipation (Fig. 7.1).

4. **Other smooth muscles**
   - **Biliary tract:** Morphine causes spasm of the sphincter of Oddi and may cause biliary colic.
   - **Urinary bladder and ureter:** Tone and contractions of the ureter is increased; tone of external sphincter and volume of the bladder are increased. Opioids inhibit urinary voiding reflex. All these result in urinary retention especially in elderly male with prostatic hypertrophy.
   - **Bronchi:** Morphine causes release of histamine from the mast cells leading to bronchoconstriction. This can be dangerous in asthmatics.

Pharmacokinetics

Given orally, absorption of morphine is slow and incomplete and undergoes extensive first pass metabolism. Bioavailability is 20 to 40 percent.

Given subcutaneously, onset of action is within 15–20 minutes, duration of action is 3–5 hours. Morphine is metabolized in the liver by glucuronide conjugation.

Adverse Effects

Morphine can produce a wide range of adverse effects like—nausea, vomiting, dizziness, mental clouding, respiratory depression,

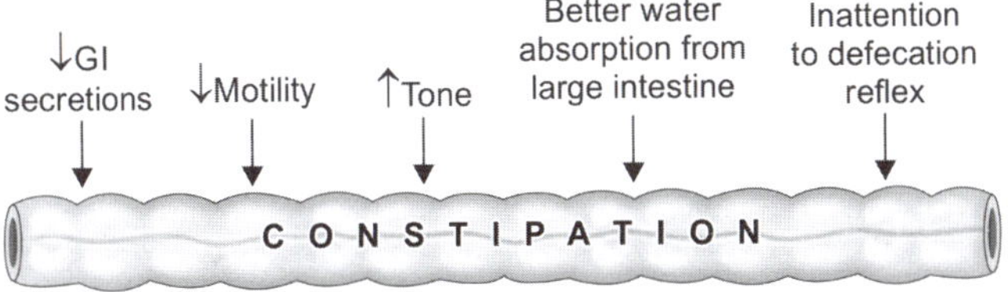

Fig. 7.1: Effect of opioids on gut.

constipation, dysphoria, urinary retention and hypotension.

Allergic reactions including skin rashes, pruritus and wheal at the site of injection and rarely anaphylaxis may be seen. This is because morphine liberates histamine.

Tolerance: Repeated administration of morphine results in the development of tolerance to some of its effects including respiratory depression, analgesia, sedation and euphoriant effects and other CNS depressant effects. Constipation and miosis show no tolerance. Though lethal dose of morphine is about 250 mg, addicts can tolerate morphine in grams. An addict needs progressively higher doses to get his 'kick' or 'rush'. Patients in pain can also tolerate a higher dose of morphine. Cross-tolerance is seen among different opioids.

Dependence: Opium has been a drug of addiction for many centuries. Its ability to produce euphoria makes it a drug of addiction. Opioids produce both psychological and physical dependence. Sudden withdrawal of opioids or administration of opioid antagonists produce significant withdrawal symptoms in such dependent individuals. **Signs and symptoms** of opioid withdrawal—*see* Flowchart 7.2.

The word 'cold turkey' is used for sudden withdrawal because skin resembles that of a plucked turkey. Goose flesh is due to pilomotor activity. Withdrawal symptoms are generally not fatal. Administration of a suitable opioid, dramatically and completely reverses the symptoms of withdrawal. Without treatment, symptoms disappear in 7–10 days.

Withdrawal in the newborn: Babies born to mothers who were addicts prior to delivery—will also be dependent. Withdrawal symptoms seen are irritability, excessive crying, tremors, frantic suckling of fists, diarrhea, sneezing, yawning, vomiting and fever. Tincture of opium is started and gradually withdrawn.

Management of Addiction

Morphine is slowly withdrawn over several days and oral methadone is given.

Advantages of methadone administration are:

- Methadone is effective orally and by this route no 'kick' is experienced.
- It is more potent, long-acting and prevents withdrawal symptoms.

The dose is adjusted based on the degree of dependence. Methadone is then slowly withdrawn.

Clonidine a central α_2 agonist can suppress some of the autonomic withdrawal symptoms like anxiety, nausea, vomiting and diarrhea. It is given for 7–10 days and withdrawn over 3–4 days. Night time sedation with a hypnotic like **diazepam** is helpful.

Most addicts can be completely withdrawn from opioids in about 10 days though mild withdrawal symptoms still remain. Symptoms like insomnia, restlessness, irritability, fatigue and GI hyperactivity may last up to several months.

Flowchart 7.2: Signs and symptoms of opioid withdrawal.

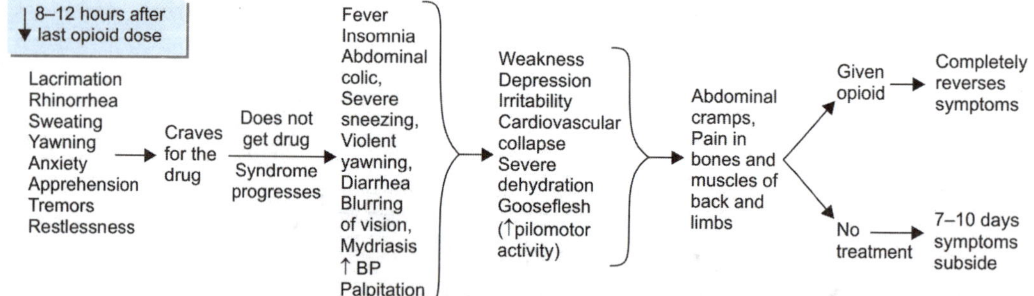

Precautions and Contraindications

1. Avoid opioids in patients with respiratory insufficiency—chronic obstructive pulmonary disease (COPD); it should also be avoided in infants.
2. Acute **bronchial asthma** can be precipitated by morphine.
3. **Head injury**—morphine is contraindicated because:
   - Morphine increases cerebrospinal fluid (CSF) pressure.
   - Causes respiratory depression.
   - Vomiting, miosis and mental clouding produced by morphine makes it difficult to treat head injuries.
4. In hypovolemic shock, morphine further decreases the BP.
5. Opioids potentiate CNS depressants-avoid concurrent use of CNS depressants.
6. Undiagnosed acute abdomen—morphine relieves pain, may cause vomiting and constipation. All these may interfere with the diagnosis. Hence it can be administered only after the diagnosis is made.
7. In the elderly respiratory depression can be more. Opioids can also cause urinary retention in men with prostatic hypertrophy-hence they should be used cautiously in the elderly.

Acute morphine poisoning may be accidental, suicidal or homicidal. Lethal dose in non-addicts is about 250 mg but addicts can tolerate grams of morphine. Signs and symptoms include respiratory depression with shallow breathing, pin point pupils, hypotension, shock, cyanosis, flaccidity, stupor, hypothermia, coma and death due to respiratory failure and pulmonary edema.

Treatment

- Positive pressure respiration.
- Maintenance of BP.
- Gastric lavage with potassium permanganate to remove unabsorbed drug.
- Specific **antidote is naloxone**—0.4-0.8 mg IV repeated every 10-15 minutes.

Other Opioids

Heroin is converted to morphine in the body. It has higher lipid solubility because of which euphoric effects are faster and greater resulting in **higher abuse potential**. It has a strong smell of vinegar. Though it is an analgesic, it is a banned drug.

Codeine is a naturally occurring opium alkaloid.

- Codeine depresses the cough center even in low doses.
- It is effective orally and is well-absorbed.
- It produces less respiratory depression and is less constipating.
- Codeine has less addiction liability and less chances of tolerance. It is well absorbed on oral administration.

Constipation is the most common side effect.

Uses codeine is used as an antitussive and analgesic. Duration of action is 4-6 hours.

It is also available in combination with paracetamol for analgesia.

Noscapine, pholcodine and **dextromethorphan** have no other actions on the CNS except for antitussive effects. Hence no disadvantages of opioids. They are highly effective and safe and the only adverse effect is nausea. They are used as cough suppressants.

Tramadol and **tapentadol** are synthetic analgesics They are weak opioid agonists. In addition, they inhibit the re-uptake of noradrenaline and serotonin in the CNS. The mechanism of action is not clear.

Adverse effects include drowsiness, dryness of mouth and nausea. Respiratory depression is mild. They may precipitate seizures. They too are drugs of dependence.

They should be avoided in patients with MAO inhibitors because these drugs also increase serotonin levels by inhibiting serotonin uptake into the synapses.

Uses:

Both are used in acute and chronic pain, like postoperative pain and neuralgias.

Pethidine (Meperidine)

Pethidine is a derivative of morphine and many of its actions resemble that of morphine. When compared to morphine:

- Pethidine is one-tenth as potent as morphine (100 mg pethidine = 10 mg morphine). However, as an analgesic pethidine is equal to morphine.
- The onset of action is more rapid and duration of action is shorter.
- It produces corneal anesthesia.
- It is not a good antitussive.
- It is less constipating.
- In some patients, it may cause dysphoria.
- In toxic doses, pethidine sometimes produces CNS stimulation and convulsions instead of sedation.

Adverse effects are similar to morphine except that constipation and urinary retention are less common.

Uses

Dose: 25–100 mg IM/SC is the analgesic dose.

1. **In pain:** Pethidine is used as an analgesic in visceral pain and also for other indications of morphine. Because of efficacy and less spasmogenic effect, it is preferred to morphine.
2. **During labor:** Given during labor, pethidine produces less respiratory depression in the newborn when compared to morphine and is therefore preferred to morphine for obstetric analgesia.
3. Preanesthetic medication - can be used.

Derivatives of Pethidine

Fentanyl is a pethidine congener about 100 times more potent than morphine as an analgesic and is faster acting.

- Epidural fentanyl is used for postoperative and obstetric analgesia.
- Fentanyl is also used for chronic pain.

Transdermal patches of fentanyl are available.

Other derivatives of pethidine **alfentanil, sufentanil** and **ramifentanil** are similar to fentanyl.

Methadone a synthetic opioid, has actions similar to morphine. It's main features are:

- It is an effective analgesic.
- It is also effective by oral route.
- It is more effective than morphine in some neuropathic and cancer pain - hence preferred.
- It has a long duration of action and therefore effectively suppresses withdrawal symptoms in addicts.
- Methadone is firmly bound to proteins in various tissues, including brain. After repeated administration, it accumulates in tissues. When administration is stopped, it is slowly released from these binding sites. Hence, its withdrawal symptoms are mild.
- As euphoric effects are less intense, risk of abuse is less. Tolerance develops more slowly. Even in addicts, withdrawal symptoms are gradual in onset, less intense, but prolonged.

Uses

1. **In opioid dependence:** In morphine addicts oral methadone is given and morphine is stopped. Methadone prevents withdrawal symptoms in them.
2. **Opioid maintenance:** Gradually increasing doses of methadone is given orally to produce a high degree of tolerance. Such subjects do not experience the pleasurable effects of IV morphine, because of tolerance, i.e., opioids are not pleasurable in them and they give up the habit.
3. **Analgesic**—in some neuropathic and cancer pain

Dextropropoxyphene a congener of methadone produces effects similar to morphine. It is less constipating and is orally effective. It is used in mild to moderate pain. It is marketed in combination with aspirin.

Dextropropoxyphene 32 mg + aspirin 600 mg.

Uses of Morphine and Other Opiods

1. **Analgesic:** Morphine is one of the most potent analgesics available. It provides **symptomatic relief of pain** without affecting the underlying disease. It is an excellent analgesic for severely painful conditions such as acute myocardial infarction, fractures, burns, pulmonary embolism, terminal stages of cancer, acute pericarditis, spontaneous pneumothorax and postoperative pain. In excruciating pain, morphine can be given IV.

In **myocardial infarction**, morphine relieves pain and thereby anxiety. As a result reflex sympathetic stimulation is reduced.

- Morphine is given with atropine to relieve **renal and biliary colic.** Atropine relieves spasm.
- Since opiate receptors are present in the spinal cord, epidural morphine can be used to produce **epidural analgesia.** There is no interference with motor function or autonomic changes and no systemic adverse effects.
- **Obstetric analgesia:** Pethidine is preferred to morphine for this condition.
- Opioids can be given to control pain of **cancers**.

However, opioids should *not be* freely used in case of other chronic pain because of the risk of addiction.

2. **Acute left ventricular failure:** Morphine relieves the dyspnea of LVF and pulmonary edema. The mechanism is not clear. The relief may be due to:

- Reduction in the work of the heart due to decreased anxiety. Reduced anxiety decreases sympathetic stimulation which in turn decreases cardiac work.
- Cardiovascular effects like decreased PVR reduces the cardiac workload.

3. **Diarrhea:** Opioids are effective for the symptomatic treatment of diarrhea. Synthetic opioids—diphenoxylate and loperamide are preferred as antidiarrheals.

4. **Cough:** Codeine, pholcodine, noscapine and dextromethorphan are antitussives used for the treatment of cough.

5. **Special anesthesia:**

- High doses of morphine can be used IV to produce general anesthesia
- Morphine can be used epidurally for the relief of postoperative and chronic pain.

6. **As preanesthetic medication:** Though morphine and pethidine reduce anxiety, provide analgesia, allow smoother induction and reduce the dose of the anesthetic required, they have certain disadvantages:

- Opioids depress respiration.
- Morphine may cause bronchospasm and is dangerous in patients with poor respiratory reserve.
- They cause vasomotor depression.
- They may induce vomiting.
- Postoperative urinary retention and constipation may be troublesome.

7. **Sedative:** Morphine relieves anxiety in threatened abortion without affecting uterine motility. It is an useful sedative in the presence of pain.

Mixed Agonists and Antagonists

Pentazocine: In an attempt to develop an analgesic with less risk of addiction and low adverse effects, pentazocine was developed. Pentazocine is a κ receptor agonist.

- CNS effects of pentazocine are similar to morphine. Euphoria is seen only in low doses. With higher doses—dysphoria can occur due to κ receptor stimulation.
- Sedation and respiratory depression are less.
- It has weak antagonistic properties at μ receptors.
- Tolerance and dependance develop on repeated use.

- CVS—in contrast to morphine, pentazocine causes ↑BP and ↑heart rate and thereby increases cardiac work. It is therefore not suitable in myocardial infarction.
- Biliary spasm and constipation are less severe.
- Pentazocine can be given both orally and parenterally. It undergoes first pass metabolism.
- Dose 50–100 mg oral; 30–60 mg IM.

Adverse effects: Sedation, sweating, dizziness, nausea, dysphoria with anxiety, nightmares and hallucinations, which are unpleasant are seen above 60 mg. As it is an irritant, IM injection can be painful and cause sterile abscesses.

Uses: Pentazocine is used as an analgesic especially in postoperative and chronic pain—abuse liability is less than morphine.

Nalbuphine and **butorphanol** are agonist-antagonists—like pentazocine. They are used as analgesics.

Buprenorphine is a highly lipid soluble synthetic opioid. It is a partial μ agonist, duration of analgesia is long.

Dose: 0.3–0.6 mg SC, IM or sublingual (oral not available).

Uses: Chronic pain like terminal cancer pain.

Nalorphine is also an agonist-antagonist. At low doses, it is a good analgesic but it causes dysphoria (κ agonist) and respiratory depression even in low doses. Hence it cannot be used as an analgesic. At high doses it acts as an antagonist and counters all the actions of opioids.

Uses: Nalorphine may be used in acute opioid poisoning. It can also be used for the diagnosis of opioid addiction.

Opioid Antagonists

Naloxone is a pure antagonist—acts as a competitive antagonist to all types of opioid receptors. In normal individuals, it does not produce any significant actions. However, in opium addicts, given IV, it promptly antagonizes all the actions including respiratory depression and sedation and precipitates withdrawal syndrome. It also blocks the action of endogenous opioid peptides—endorphins, enkephalins and dynorphins. **It blocks the analgesia produced by placebo and acupuncture.** This suggests that endogenous opioid peptides are responsible for analgesia by these methods.

Given orally it undergoes first pass metabolism and is metabolized by the liver. Duration of action is 3–4 hours.

Uses

1. Naloxone is the drug of choice for morphine overdosage.
2. Used to reverse neonatal asphyxia due to opioids used in the mother during labor.
3. Diagnosis of opioid dependence—naloxone precipitates withdrawal in addicts.
4. Hypotension seen during shock could be due to endogenous opioids released during stress and naloxone reverses such hypotension.

Naltrexone is another pure opioid antagonist. It is:

- Orally effective.
- Has a longer duration of action of 1–2 days.

Uses:

1. Naltrexone is used for **'opioid blockade'** therapy in post addicts so that even if such persons take an opioid, they do not experience the pleasurable effects and therefore lose the liking for opioids.
2. **Alcohol craving** is also reduced by naltrexone and is used to prevent relapse of heavy drinking.

Nalmefene is an orally effective and longer acting opioid antagonist. It has better bioavailability than naltrexone and is used in opioid overdosage.

DRUGS USED IN PSYCHIATRIC DISORDERS: ANTIPSYCHOTICS, ANTIDEPRESSANTS AND ANTIANXIETY AGENTS

Since ages, man has sought the help of drugs to modify behavior, mood and emotion. Psychoactive drugs were used both for recreational purposes and for the treatment of mental illnesses (Psyche = mind).

Psychiatric conditions are broadly divided into psychoses, neuroses and personality disorders.

1. **Psychoses** are the more severe psychiatric disorders of the three and involve a marked impairment of behavior, inability to think coherently, and to comprehend reality. Patients have no 'insight' into these abnormalities.

Psychoses could be due to:

- An organic cause, i.e., there is a definable toxic, metabolic or pathological change—as seen following head injury.
- Functional or idiopathic disorders—where there is no definable cause like in schizophrenia, paranoia and affective disorders.

Schizophrenia (split mind) affects about 1 percent of population, starts in an early age and is highly incapacitating. It is characterized by delusions, hallucinations, irrational conclusions, interpretations and withdrawal from social contacts. Patients with chronic schizophrenia have shrinkage of the brain.

2. **Neuroses** are the milder forms of psychiatric disorders and include anxiety, mood changes, panic disorders, obsessions, irrational fears and reactive depression as seen following tragedies.

3. **Personality disorders** include paranoid, schizoid, histrionic, avoidant, antisocial and obsessive compulsive personality types.

Drugs used in psychiatric illnesses may be grouped as:

- **Antipsychotics or neuroleptics**—used in psychoses.
- **Antidepressants or psychotropic drugs**—used in affective disorders.
- **Antianxiety drugs.**

Neuroleptic is a drug that reduces initiative, brings about emotional quietening and induces drowsiness. **Tranquilizer** is a drug that brings about tranquility by calming, soothing and quietening effects. This is the older terminology. Neuroleptics or antipsychotics were called 'major tranquilizers' and antianxiety drugs were called 'minor tranquilizers'. These terminologies are no longer used.

Antipsychotics (Neuroleptics)

Classification

1. **First generation/Classical/typical neuroleptics**
   - **Phenothiazines:** Chlorpromazine, triflupromazine, thioridazine, mesoridazine, trifluoperazine, fluphenazine.
   - **Butyrophenones:** Haloperidol, droperidol, trifluperidol.
   - **Thioxanthenes:** Thiothixene, chlorprothixene.
2. **Second generation/Atypical neuroleptics:** Clozapine, olanzapine, risperidone, quetiapine, ziprasidone, aripiprazole.
3. **Miscellaneous:** Loxapine.

First Generation Antipsychotics

Chlorpromazine is an antipsychotic with a wide range of actions.

Chlorpromazine (CPZ)

Mechanism of action: Chlorpromazine has a wide variety of actions because it blocks the actions of several neurotransmitters including dopamine, adrenaline, histamine, acetylcholine and serotonin (5-HT). Antipsychotic effects are due to the blockade of dopamine receptors (Flowchart 7.3).

Flowchart 7.3: Mechanism of action, pharmacological actions and adverse effects of chlorpromazine.

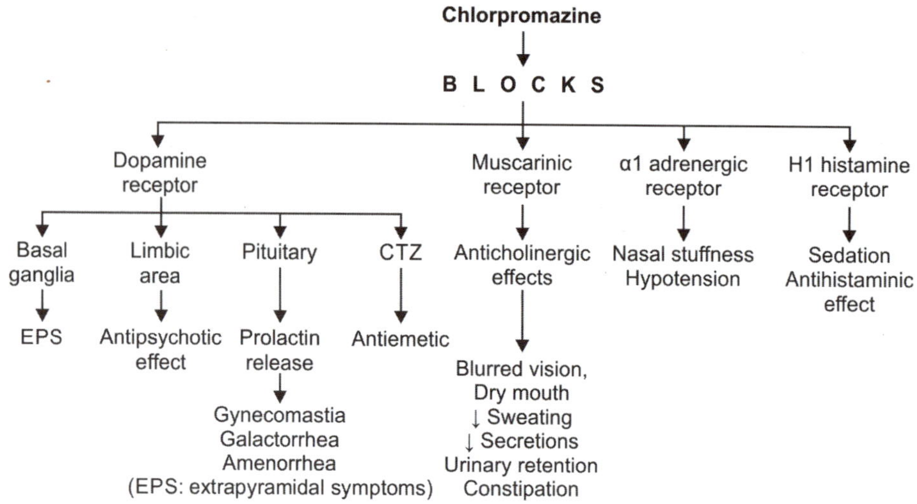

Pharmacological Actions

1. **CNS:** Behavioral effects—in normal subjects CPZ reduces motor activity, produces drowsiness and indifference to surroundings. In psychotic agitated patients, it reduces aggression, initiative and motor activity, relieves anxiety and brings about emotional quietening and drowsiness. It normalizes the sleep disturbances characteristic of psychoses.

Other CNS Actions

a. **Cortex:** CPZ lowers seizure threshold and can precipitate convulsions in untreated epileptics.
b. **Hypothalamus:** CPZ decreases gonadotrophin secretion and may result in amenorrhea in women. It increases the secretion of prolactin resulting in galactorrhea and gynecomastia.
c. **Basal ganglia:** CPZ acts as a dopamine antagonist and therefore results in extrapyramidal motor symptoms (drug induced parkinsonism).
d. **Brainstem:** Vasomotor reflexes are depressed leading to a fall in BP.
e. **CTZ:** Neuroleptics block the dopamine (DA) receptors in the CTZ and thereby act as antiemetics.

2. **Autonomic nervous system (ANS):** The actions on the ANS are complex. CPZ is an alpha blocker. The alpha blocking potency varies with each neuroleptic. CPZ also has anticholinergic properties which leads to side effects like dryness of mouth, blurred vision, reduced sweating, decreased gastric motility, constipation and urinary retention. The degree of anticholinergic activity also varies with each drug.

3. **CVS:** Neuroleptics produce orthostatic hypotension due to alpha blockade action and reflex tachycardia. CPZ also has a direct myocardiac depressant effect like quinidine.

4. **Local anesthetic:** CPZ has local anesthetic properties—but is not used for the purpose since it is an irritant.

5. **Kidney:** CPZ depresses antidiuretic hormone (ADH) secretion and has weak diuretic effects.

Tolerance develops to the sedative and hypotensive actions while no tolerance is seen to the antipsychotic actions.

Pharmacokinetics: CPZ is incompletely absorbed following oral administration and also undergoes significant first pass metabolism (bioavailability is 30%). It is highly protein bound; has a t½ of 20–24 hours and is therefore given once a day.

Adverse reactions: Antipsychotics have a high therapeutic index and are fairly safe drugs.

1. **Cardiovascular and autonomic effects:** Postural hypotension, palpitation, blurred vision, dry mouth, constipation, nasal stuffiness and urinary retention.
2. **CNS effects:** Drowsiness and mental confusion are common. A variety of neurological syndromes involving the **extrapyramidal system** including parkinsonism, dyskinesias, dystonias, akathesia, perioral tremors and malignant neuroleptic syndrome are troublesome side effects (due to dopamine blockade).
3. **Endocrine disturbances:** Gynecomastia, amenorrhea and galactorrhea.
4. **Hypersensitivity reactions:** Jaundice, agranulocytosis and skin rashes.

Drug interactions:

1. Neuroleptics + CNS depressants → ↑Sedation
2. Neuroleptics + α blockers → Additive effects
3. Neuroleptics + Anticholinergics → Additive effects
4. Neuroleptics + DA agonists/levodopa → antagonism (↓ effects)

Uses

1. **Psychiatric conditions:** Psychoses including schizophrenia and organic brain syndromes like delirium and dementia all respond to antipsychotics. Neuroleptics are given orally (chlorpromazine 100–800 mg). In acute psychosis they may be given intramuscularly and the response is seen in 24 hours. In chronic psychosis it takes 2–3 weeks of treatment to obtain the response.
2. **Nausea, vomiting:** CPZ is a good antiemetic and is used in vomiting due to radiation sickness and drug induced vomiting.
3. **Hiccough:** CPZ can control intractable hiccough though the mechanism of action is not known.
4. **Other neuropsychiatric syndromes:** Neuroleptics are useful in the treatment of several syndromes with psychiatric features like psychoses associated with chronic alcoholism, mania, bipolar mood disorders and Huntington's disease.

Haloperidol is a potent antipsychotic with actions similar to chlorpromazine. Advantages are—it has lesser incidence of autonomic side effects and is therefore preferred in older patients. It has a longer t½ of 24 hours.

Haloperidol is useful in acute schizophrenia, and is the drug of choice in Gilles de la Tourette's syndrome and Huntington's disease.

Second Generation/Atypical Antipsychotics

The second generation anipsychotics have weak dopamine blocking effects but prominent serotonin blocking properties.

Atypical antipsychotics have the following advantages over conventional antipsychotics:

- Very low incidence of extrapyramidal side effects.
- Sedation is low.
- No endocrine side effects, i.e., no galactorrhea and gynecomastia.
- They are effective in patients not responding to conventional antipsychotics.

Clozapine: In addition to blocking DA receptors, clozapine also blocks 5-$HT_{2,}$ α-adrenergic and muscarinic receptors. Clozapine is an effective antipsychotic.

Disadvantage: May cause agranulocytosis in some patients which can be fatal. Hence use should be restricted to patients who are not responding to other drugs. Clozapine can also cause sedation, weight gain and hypotension.

Olanzapine: It has the advantage that it causes no extrapyramidal symptoms and no agranulocytosis has been reported.

Risperidone: It blocks serotonin and dopamine receptors and is a commonly used antipsychotic.

Advantages:

- At low doses no EPS dysfunction.
- Low sedation.

ANTIDEPRESSANTS

Affective disorders are a group of psychoses associated with changes of mood, i.e., depression and mania.

Depression is a common psychiatric disorder and could be:

1. **Unipolar**
    - **Reactive:** Due to distressing circumstances in life.
    - **Endogenous:** Major depression due to a biochemical abnormality in the brain is thought to be due to deficiency of monoamine activity (NA, 5-HT) in the CNS.
2. **Bipolar mood disorder:** Mania and depression occur alternately causing cyclic mood swings.

Classification

1. **Tricyclic antidepressants (TCA):** Imipramine, desipramine, amitriptyline, nortriptyline doxepin.
2. **Selective serotonin reuptake inhibitors (SSRI):** Fluoxetine, fluoxamine, paroxetine, citalopram, escitalopram, sertraline.
3. **Atypical antidepressants:** Trazodone, nefazodone, bupropion, mirtazapine, atomoxetine, mianserine, venlafaxine, desvenlafaxine, duloxetine.
4. **Monoamine oxidase (MAO) inhibitors:** Phenelzine, tranylcypromine.

Tricyclic Antidepressants

Pharmacological Actions

1. **CNS:** In normal subjects, TCA cause dizziness, drowsiness, confusion and difficulty in thinking. In depressed patients, after 2–3 weeks of treatment, elevation of mood occurs; the patient shows more interest in the surroundings and the sleep pattern becomes normal.
2. **CVS:** Postural hypotension and tachycardia (due to blockade of α_1 adrenergic and muscarinic receptors) can be severe in overdosage.
3. **ANS:** TCAs have anticholinergic properties and cause dry mouth, blurred vision, constipation and urinary retention.

Mechanism of action: TCAs block the reuptake of amines (noradrenaline or 5-HT) into the presynaptic terminal, and thereby prolong their action on the receptors. Thus they potentiate amine neurotransmission in the CNS.

Pharmacokinetics

TCAs are rapidly absorbed, highly protein bound and metabolized in the liver. They have a long t½ and can be given once daily.

Adverse Effects

- Sedation, postural hypotension, tachycardia, sweating
- Anticholinergic side effects like dry mouth, constipation, blurred vision and urinary retention are relatively common.
- TCA may precipitate convulsions in epileptics; may cause hallucinations and mania in some patients.
- Many TCAs may also cause weight gain due to increased appetite.

Poisoning

Signs and Symptoms

Mimic symptoms of atropine poisoning—delirium, excitement, hypotension, convulsions, fever, arrhythmias, respiratory depression and coma.

Treatment: Physostigmine is given to overcome atropine-like effects; sodium bicarbonate for acidosis, phenytoin for seizures and arrhythmias—with other supportive measures.

Tolerance and dependence: Tolerance develops gradually to the sedative and anticholinergic effects over 2–3 weeks.

Following long-term treatment, TCAs should be gradually withdrawn as withdrawal symptoms like headache, anxiety and chills can occur due to physical dependence.

Drug Interactions

- Tricyclics potentiate sympathomimetics—even small amounts of adrenaline used with local anesthetics can cause serious hypertension.
- Highly protein bound drugs like phenytoin, aspirin and phenylbutazone displace TCAs from binding sites resulting in toxicity.
- TCAs potentiate the effects of alcohol and other CNS depressants.

Selective serotonin reuptake inhibitors (SSRIs): Fluoxetine, fluoxamine, paroxetine, citalopram, escitalopram and sertraline are SSRIs. They inhibit the reuptake of serotonin and thereby increase the levels of serotonin in the synapse. Since they have several advantages over TCAs, they are the preferred antidepressants now.

SSRIs have the following advantages:

1. Low cardiovascular side effects.
2. Anticholinergic side effects are less.
3. Less sedation.
4. Preferred in elderly (low anticholinergic side effects).
5. Safer in overdose.

Atypical antidepressants: Trazodone, nefazodone, bupropion, mirtazapine, atomoxetine, mianserine, venlafaxine, desvenlafaxine, duloxetine.

Advantages

- Fewer side effects—particularly sedation and anticholinergic effects.
- Safer in overdose.
- Effective in patients not responding to TCA.

MAO inhibitors: Tranylcypromine, phenelzine:

- Irreversibly inhibit the enzyme MAO and increase neuronal levels of noradrenaline, dopamine and 5-HT.
- Antidepressant actions develop slowly over weeks of treatment.
- Side effects are hypotension, weight gain, CNS stimulation and atropine-like effects.
- They interact with many drugs and food.
- **Food and drug interactions:** Patients on MAOI taking tyramine containing foods like cheese, beer, wines, yeast, buttermilk and fish—develop severe hypertension and is known as **cheese reaction**. Tyramine is normally metabolized by MAO in the gut wall. On inhibition of MAO by drugs, tyramine escapes metabolism and displaces noradrenaline (NA) from nerve endings leading to hypertension. Similar interaction with SSRIs can result in severe hypertension **(serotonin syndrome)**.

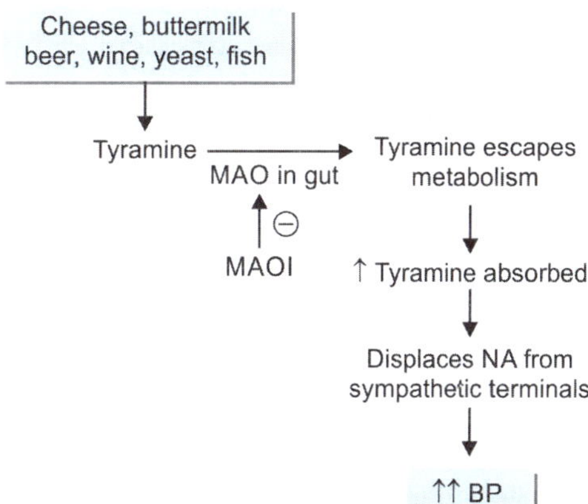

- Because of the side effects and drug interactions, MAO inhibitors are **not** the **preferred** antidepressants.

Uses of Antidepressants

1. **Endogenous depression:** Antidepressants are used over a long period. The response appears after 2–3 weeks of treatment. The choice of the antidepressant depends on the side effects and patient factors like age. In severe depression with suicidal tendencies, electroconvulsive therapy (ECT) is given.

2. **Panic attacks, post-traumatic stress disorders** and **other anxiety disorders**—all respond to antidepressants (acute episodes of anxiety are known as panic attacks).
3. **Obsessive compulsive disorders:** SSRIs and clomipramine are effective.
4. **Nocturnal enuresis** in children may be treated with antidepressants only when other measures fail and drugs are needed.
5. **Disorders of pain:** SSRIs and venlafaxine are effective in chronic pain including diabetic neuropathy, backache, and neuralgia.
6. **Smoking withdrawal:** Bupropion has been shown to reduce the urge in people who need to quit smoking.
7. **Psychosomatic disorders:** Newer antidepressants are tried in fibromyalgia, irritable bowel syndrome, chronic fatigue, tics, migraine and sleep apnea.
8. **Other indications:** Attention deficit hyperactivity disorder, chronic pain and chronic alcoholism—may result in depression—antidepressants are tried.

Mood Stabilizers

Mood stabilizers control the mood swings that are seen in bipolar mood disorders.

Mood stabilizers include:

- Lithium
- Sodium valproate
- Carbamazepine
- Lamotrigine
- Gabapentin

Lithium is a monovalent cation. On prophylactic use in bipolar mood disorder (manic-depressive illness), lithium acts as a mood stabilizer. It prevents swings of mood and thus reduces both the depressive and manic phases of the illness. Given in acute mania, it gradually suppresses the episode over weeks.

Mechanism of action of lithium is complex and not fully understood. It inhibits the synthesis of second messengers inositol triphosphate (IP_3) and diacylglycerol (DAG) and thereby blocks the respective receptor-mediated effects. This is the most accepted mechanism of action.

Pharmacokinetics: Lithium is a small ion and mimics the role of sodium in excitable tissues. Given orally it is well-absorbed. It is filtered at the glomerulus but reabsorbed like sodium. Steady state concentration is reached in 5–6 days. Since safety margin is narrow, **plasma lithium concentration needs to be monitored.**

Adverse Effects

Lithium has low therapeutic index and side effects are common.

- Nausea, vomiting, mild diarrhea, thirst and polyuria occur initially in most patients.
- As the plasma concentration rises, hypothyroidism, CNS effects like coarse tremors, drowsiness, giddiness, confusion, ataxia, blurred vision and nystagmus are seen.
- In severe overdosage, delirium, muscle twitchings, convulsions, arrhythmias and renal failure develop.

Precautions

- Minimum effective dose should be used.
- Patients should always use the same formulation/brand.
- Patients should be aware of the first symptom of toxicity.
- Lithium is contraindicated in pregnancy.

Drug Interactions

- Diuretics increase Na^+ loss and lithium absorption from the kidney. This increases plasma lithium levels resulting in toxicity.
- NSAIDs ↓ lithium elimination and increase toxicity.

Uses

1. **Mood swings and prophylaxis of bipolar mood disorder**—episodes of mania and depression are reduced.

2. **Acute mania**—the response to lithium is slow - hence, neuroleptics are preferred.
3. **Depression:** Lithium is given along with other antidepressants in recurrent depression.
4. **Other uses**—lithium is tried in recurrent neuropsychiatric disorders, hyperthyroidism and inappropriate ADH secretion syndrome.

Other mood stabilizers: Because of difficulty in using lithium, other less toxic drugs are being tried.

Carbamazepine is effective in preventing the relapses of bipolar mood disorder and in the treatment of acute mania. It can be used alone or can be combined with lithium for better therapeutic effects but lithium can increase the toxicity of carbamazepine.

Sodium valproate is effective in mild to moderate cases or along with lithium in refractory bipolar mood disorder.

Other antiepileptics: Lamotrigine, gabapentin, topiramate, some newer antiepileptics and a neuroprotective agent riluzole are being tried in the prophylaxis of bipolar mood disorder as alternatives to lithium.

Antianxiety Drugs (Anxiolytics)

Anxiety is tension or apprehension which is a normal response to certain situations in life. It is a universal human emotion. But when it becomes excessive and disproportionate to the situation, it becomes disabling and needs treatment.

Classification

Benzodiazepines: Diazepam, chlordiazepoxide, lorazepam, alprazolam.

5-HT agonist-antagonists: Buspirone, gepirone, ipsapirone.

β-blockers: Propranolol.

Others: Meprobamate, hydroxyzine.

Benzodiazepines have good antianxiety actions and are the most commonly used drugs for anxiety. They are CNS depressants. Alprazolam in addition has antidepressant properties.

Buspirone is an azapirone with good anxiolytic properties. It is a selective 5-HT_{1A} partial agonist and a weak D_2 antagonist. It is useful in mild to moderate anxiety. Antianxiety effect develops slowly over 2 weeks. Unlike diazepam, it is not a muscle relaxant, not an anticonvulsant, does not produce significant sedation, tolerance or dependence and is not useful in panic attacks.

Buspirone is rapidly absorbed and metabolized in the liver.

Dose: 5–15 mg OD or TDS.

Side effects are mild including headache, dizziness, nausea and rarely restlessness.

β-blockers In patients with prominent autonomic symptoms of anxiety like tremors, palpitation and hypertension, propranolol may be useful. β-blockers are also useful in anxiety inducing states like public speaking and stage performance. They can be used as adjuvants to benzodiazepines.

Meprobamate has anxiolytic property but is not preferred now as it is less effective and causes high sedation.

Hydroxyzine is an antihistaminic with anxiolytic actions. But due to high sedation it is not preferred.

CNS STIMULANTS

Drugs that have a predominantly stimulant effect on the CNS may be broadly divided into:

1. **Respiratory stimulants:** Doxapram, nikethamide.
2. **Psychomotor stimulants:** Amphetamine, cocaine and methylxanthines.
3. **Convulsants:** Leptazol, strychnine.

Respiratory stimulants are also called **analeptics**. These drugs stimulate respiration and are sometimes used to treat respiratory failure. Though they may bring about temporary improvement in respiration, the mortality is not reduced. They have a low safety margin and may produce convulsions.

Doxapram appears to act mainly on the brainstem and spinal cord and increase the activity of respiratory and vasomotor centers.

Adverse effects are nausea, cough, restlessness, hypertension, tachycardia, arrhythmias and convulsions.

Uses

1. Doxapram is occasionally used IV as an analeptic in acute respiratory failure.
2. Apnea in premature infants not responding to theophylline.

Nikethamide is not used because of the risk of convulsions.

Psychomotor stimulants: Amphetamine and dextroamphetamine are sympathomimetic drugs.

Cocaine is a CNS stimulant, produces euphoria and is a drug of abuse. It is also a local anesthetic.

Methylxanthines: Caffeine, theophylline and theobromine are the naturally occurring xanthine alkaloids. The beverages—coffee contains caffeine; tea contains theophylline and caffeine; cocoa has caffeine and theobromine.

Actions

CNS: Caffeine and theophylline are CNS stimulants. They bring about an increase in mental alertness, a reduction of fatigue, produce a sense of well being and improve motor activity and performance, with a clearer flow of thought. Caffeine stimulates the respiratory center. Higher doses produce irritability, nervousness, restlessness, insomnia, excitement, and headache. High doses can result in convulsions.

CVS: Methylxanthines increase the force of contraction of the myocardium and increase the heart rate and therefore increase the cardiac output. However, they also produce peripheral vasodilatation which tends to decrease the BP. The changes in BP are therefore not consistent. Caffeine causes vasoconstriction of cerebral blood vessels.

Kidneys: The xanthines have a diuretic effect and thereby increase the urine output.

Smooth muscle: Xanthines cause relaxation of smooth muscles especially the bronchial smooth muscle.

Skeletal muscle: Xanthines increase the power of muscle contraction and thereby increase the capacity to do muscular work by both a central stimulant effect and the peripheral actions.

GI tract: Xanthines increase the secretion of acid and pepsin in the stomach and are gastric irritants.

Adverse effects include nervousness, insomnia, tremors, tachycardia, hypotension, arrhythmias, headache, gastritis, nausea, vomiting, epigastric pain and diuresis. High doses produce convulsions. Tolerance develops after sometime. Habituation to caffeine is common.

Uses

1. **Headache:** Because of the effect of caffeine on cerebral blood vessels, it is combined with ergotamine for the relief of migraine headache. Caffeine is also combined with aspirin/paracetamol for the treatment of headache.
2. **Bronchial asthma:** Theophylline is used in the treatment of bronchial asthma.
3. **Apnea in premature infants:** Episodes of prolonged apnea (>15–20 sec) may be seen in premature infants which if too frequent may result in neurologic and other tissue damage due to hypoxia. When no primary cause can be detected, methylxanthines may be used orally or iv. Theophylline or caffeine may be used for 1–3 weeks to reduce the duration of episodes of apnea which may be seen in premature babies.

Nootropics are drugs that improve memory and cognition (cognition enhancers).

Piracetam – described as a 'nootropic agent' is thought to protect cerebral cortex from hypoxia and improve learning and memory. In higher doses it also inhibits platelet aggregation. Adverse effects include insomnia, weight gain, nervousness, depression and gastrointestinal disturbances.

Piracetam has been tried in dementia, myoclonus, stroke and other cerebrovascular accidents; alcoholism, behavioral disorders and learning problems in children and in vertigo. The beneficial effects in all these is not proved.

OTHER DRUGS ACTING ON THE CNS

GENERAL ANESTHETICS

Anesthetics

Anesthetics are agents that bring about reversible loss of sensation. They may be general or local anesthetics.

General anesthetics are agents that bring about reversible loss of sensation and consciousness. Before 1846, alcohol, opium, packing a limb with ice and concussion, i.e., making the patient unconscious by a blow on the head were used to relieve surgical pain. Dr Horace Wells a dentist, tried to demonstrate the effect of nitrous oxide as an anesthetic in 1844 but was unsuccessful as he removed the gas bag too early. Dr William Morton who was present at the demonstration, worked on it and in 1846 demonstrated ether anesthesia successfully. Since then several anesthetics have been synthesized over the decades.

Classification

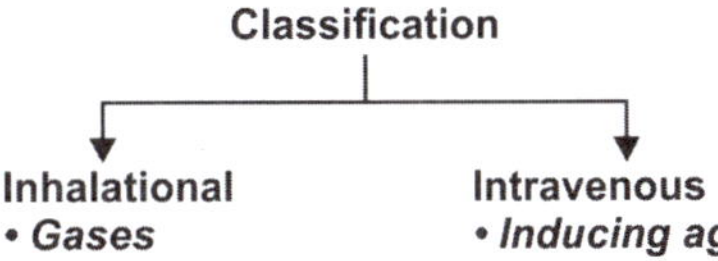

Inhalational
- ***Gases***
  - Nitrous oxide
  - Xenon
- ***Liquids***
  - Ether
  - Halothane
  - Enflurane
  - Isoflurane
  - Desflurane
  - Sevoflurane

Intravenous
- ***Inducing agents***
  - Thiopentone sodium
  - Propofol
  - Etomidate
- ***Dissociative anesthesia***
  - Ketamine
- ***Opioid analgesic***
  - Fentanyl
- ***Benzodiazepines***
  - Diazepam
  - Lorazepam
  - Midazolam

Inhalational Anesthetics

Nitrous oxide is a gas with a slightly sweetish odor. It produces light anesthesia without significant depression of respiration or vasomotor center.

Advantages

- Strong analgesic.
- Induction is rapid and smooth.
- It is non-irritating and non-inflammable.
- Recovery is rapid.
- Postoperative nausea is not significant.
- Has little effect on respiration and cardiovascular functions, hence ideal for combination.
- It is non-toxic to liver, kidney and brain and is quickly removed from lungs.

Disadvantages

- It produces light anesthesia and should be used with other agents.
- Poor muscle relaxant.

Status in anesthesia: Nitrous oxide is used along with oxygen (30%).

Xenon is an inert gas and has properties close to an ideal anesthetic.

Advantages

- Rapid induction
- Rapid recovery
- Potent anesthetic
- No effect on hepatic, renal or pulmonary function.

Disadvantages

Currently xenon cannot be manufactured but can only be extracted from air. This makes it **very expensive**. If this problem is taken care of, xenon could be considered the best anesthetic.

Ether is a colorless volatile liquid. It is highly inflammable and vapors are irritating. Though a good anesthetic, analgesic and a muscle relaxant, it is now not used because of flammability and irritant property.

Halothane is a colorless volatile liquid with a sweet odor. It is non-irritant and non-inflammable.

Advantages

- Potent, non-inflammable anesthetic.
- Induction is smooth and rapid—in 2-5 minutes anesthesia can be produced.
- Non-irritant—therefore does not increase salivary or bronchial secretions.
- Recovery is rapid.
- Postoperative nausea and vomiting is of low incidence.

Disadvantages

- Not a good analgesic; not a muscle relaxant.
- Halothane is a direct cardiac depressant. Cardiac output and BP start falling and heart rate may decrease. It sensitizes the heart to the actions of adrenaline.
- It also causes some respiratory depression.
- Severe hepatitis which may be fatal occurs rarely.
- Malignant hyperthermia—a genetically determined reaction occurs rarely. Succinylcholine adds to this effect of halothane. It is due to intracellular release of calcium which causes muscle contraction and increased heat production. It is treated with dantrolene.

Status in anesthesia: Halothane was one of the most popular anesthetics. Analgesics and muscle relaxants are used along with it. Non-flammability, non-irritant property, rapid induction and recovery made halothane an important and preferred anesthetic and was most widely used. However the newer derivatives **enflurane, isoflurane** and **sevoflurane** are now used due to certain advantages like—

- They are safer regarding the liver toxicity.
- They do not sensitize the heart to adrenaline.

Desflurane and sevoflurane are newer agents which allow very rapid induction and recovery but they too have some disadvantages. Desflurane is pungent—may induce coughing and sometimes laryngospasm. A special vaporizer is required for its administration. Sevoflurane is chemically unstable and its metabolite may cause renal damage. If these disadvantages of sevoflurane could be overcome, we may have found an ideal anesthetic.

Oxygen in anesthesia: Oxygen should be added routinely to inhalational agents to protect against hypoxia (especially when halothane is used). When O_2 is not available, ether is the safest agent for maintenance of anesthesia.

Intravenous Anesthetics

Intravenous anesthetics allow an extremely rapid induction because the blood concentration can be raised rapidly—in one arm-brain circulation (~ 11 sec) there is loss of consciousness. These are used for induction because of the rapid onset of action and anesthesia is maintained by an inhalational agent.

Inducing Agents

Thiopentone sodium is an ultrashort-acting barbiturate which when administered IV, rapidly induces anesthesia in 20-30 sec, duration of action is 4-7 minutes and induction is smooth, rapid and pleasant.

Disadvantages: Not a good analgesic nor muscle relaxant. Thiopentone sodium cannot be used alone as the dose required results in respiratory depression and hypotension.

Uses: For induction of anesthesia prior to administration of inhalational anesthetics.

Propofol is an oily liquid; quick induction (30 sec) and recovery (4 min) is possible from a single dose. It is used for induction and maintenance for short procedures of up to 1 hour duration.

Dissociative Anesthesia

Ketamine: In anesthetic doses, it produces a trance-like state known as *dissociative anesthesia* characterized by intense analgesia, immobility, amnesia (loss of memory) and a feeling of dissociation from one's own body and surroundings within 3–5 minutes which lasts for 10–15 minutes after a single injection. Amnesia lasts for 1–2 hours. Return to consciousness is gradual. If diazepam is administered pre and postoperatively, delirium can be avoided. Heart rate, CO and BP are increased due to sympathetic stimulation.

Advantages

- Provides profound analgesia and can be used as a single agent for minor procedures.
- Respiration is not depressed, does not induce hypotension.
- It is particularly useful in children and poor-risk patients and also in asthmatic patients since it does not induce bronchospasm.

Disadvantages

- Hallucinations and involuntary movements may occur during recovery.
- May be dangerous in hypertensives as it raises the BP.

Opioid Analgesic

Fentanyl is a short-acting (30–50 min) and potent opioid analgesic (*See* page 168) used to supplement inhalational anesthetics. It can be used for short surgical procedures.

Neuroleptanalgesia

Droperidol is a rapidly acting, potent neuroleptic related to haloperidol.

When the combination of droperidol with fentanyl is given IV, a state of 'neuroleptanalgesia' is produced. This is characterized by calmness, psychic indifference and intense analgesia without loss of consciousness. It lasts for 30–40 minutes. Patient is drowsy but cooperative. Respiratory depression is present. There is a slight fall in BP and HR. During recovery extrapyramidal symptoms may be seen—due to droperidol. It is employed for endoscopies, burn dressing, angiographies and other diagnostic and minor surgical procedures but not preferred now.

Benzodiazepines

Benzodiazepines like diazepam, lorazepam and midazolam are used to induce or supplement anesthesia. They cause sedation, amnesia and reduce anxiety which are beneficial in such patients. BZD may be employed alone in procedures like endoscopies, reduction of fractures, cardiac catheterization and cardioversion. IV midazolam is particularly preferred as it is faster and shorter-acting, more potent and does not cause pain or irritation at the injection sites. BZDs are also used as preanesthetic medication.

Preanesthetic Medication

Prior to anesthesia, certain drugs are administered in order to make anesthesia safer and more pleasant and is known as preanesthetic medication. It is given in order to:

- Decrease anxiety.
- Provide amnesia for the preoperative period.
- Relieve preoperative pain if present.
- Make anesthesia safer.
- Reduce side effects of anesthetics.
- Reduce gastric acidity.

To achieve the above purpose, more than one drug is required. An informative, supportive, preoperative visit by the anesthesiologist is very much essential.

Benzodiazepines are used to reduce anxiety and produce sedation. It also produces amnesia.

Antihistamines have sedative, antiemetic and anticholinergic properties and are useful, e.g., promethazine.

Antiemetics: Metoclopramide, domperidone or ondansetron may be used. Antihistamines with antiemetic properties may also be used for this purpose.

Anticholinergic drugs: Some anesthetics increase the salivary and respiratory secretions. The secretions from the oral cavity may enter into the larynx causing various problems including laryngospasm and aspiration pneumonia. Hence we need drugs that reduce these secretions. Atropine, scopolamine or glycopyrrolate can be used. They

- Reduce the secretions.
- Prevent bradycardia due to vagal stimulation.
- Prevent laryngospasm which is due to excessive secretions.

Scopolamine produces more sedation. **Glycopyrrolate** is a derivative of atropine. As compared to atropine glycopyrrolate is longer acting, and is less likely to cause significant tachycardia. It also produces less sedation than scopolamine.

Drugs that reduce acidity: H_2 blockers like ranitidine decrease gastric acid secretion and are given on the night before surgery. Decrease in gastric secretions reduces the damage to lungs if aspiration occurs when the patient is on anesthesia.

Gastrokinetic agents: Metoclopramide is a dopamine antagonist that promotes gastrointestinal motility and increases the tone of esophageal end of the stomach. This speeds up gastric emptying. The combination of an H_2 blocker + metoclopramide provides best protection against aspiration.

Balanced anesthesia: Since it is not possible to achieve ideal anesthesia with a single drug, multiple drugs are employed—preanesthetic medication, IV anesthetics for induction, inhalational agents for maintenance, oxygen, skeletal muscle relaxants and analgesics to attain *balanced anesthesia.*

LOCAL ANESTHETICS

Local anesthetics (LAs) are drugs that block nerve conduction when applied locally to nerve tissue in appropriate concentrations. Their action is completely reversible. They act on every type of nerve fiber and can cause both sensory and motor paralysis in the innervated area. They act on axons, cell body, dendrites, synapses and other excitable membranes that utilize sodium channels as the primary means of action potential generation.

Cocaine was the first agent to be isolated by Niemann in 1860. In spite of its addiction potential, cocaine was used for 30 years as a surface anesthetic. In an effort made to improve the properties of cocaine, procaine was synthesized in 1905. It ruled the field for the next 50 years. In 1943, lignocaine was synthesized and it continues to dominate the field of local anesthetics till today.

Classification of local anesthetics (LAs) based on the route of administration and duration of action:

- **Injectable**
  - **Short-acting**
    - Procaine, chloroprocaine
  - **Intermediate-acting**
    - Lignocaine, prilocaine
  - **Long-acting**
    - Tetracaine, bupivacaine
    - Dibucaine, ropivacaine, etidocaine.
- **Surface anesthetics:** Lignocaine, cocaine, tetracaine, benzocaine, oxethazaine, dibucaine, dyclonine

Mechanism of Action

Local anesthetics prevent the generation and the conduction of nerve impulses. The primary mechanism of action is **blockade of voltage-gated sodium channels**.

With increasing concentration, impulse conduction slows, rate of rise of action potential (AP) declines, AP amplitude decreases and finally the ability to generate an AP is abolished. Thus, it prevents the generation of an AP and its conduction.

Sensory and motor fibers are equally sensitive. Non-myelinated fibers are blocked more readily than the myelinated when they are of smaller diameter.

Addition of a vasoconstrictor like adrenaline (1:1,00,000 to 1:2,00,000) or phenylephrine (1:20,000):

- Prolongs the duration of action of LAs by slowing the rate of absorption from the site of administration.
- Reduces systemic toxicity of LAs since the absorption rate is reduced and as it gets absorbed, it gets metabolized.

In presence of **inflammation or infection**, LA are less effective which could be due to the following:

1. Inflamed tissue has acidic pH because of which LA penetration may be low.
2. Presence of products of inflammation at the site may counter the action of LA.

Systemic Actions

Depending on the concentration attained in the plasma, any LA can produce systemic effects. LAs interfere with the function of all organs in which conduction or transmission of impulses occur. Thus CNS, autonomic ganglia, neuromuscular junction (NMJ) and all muscles are affected.

CNS: Local anesthetics depress the inhibition from the cerebral cortex. This loss of inhibition results in unopposed excitatory activity which is manifested as restlessness, tremors and may proceed to convulsions. This central stimulation is followed by generalized CNS depression and death may result from respiratory failure.

CVS: The primary site of action is the myocardium—lignocaine decreases excitability, conduction rate and force of contraction (quinidine like effects). It also causes arteriolar dilatation. Bupivacaine is more cardiotoxic than other LAs.

Smooth muscle: LAs depress contractions in the intact bowel. They also relax vascular and bronchial smooth muscles.

Pharmacokinetics

Local anesthetics are rapidly absorbed from the mucous membranes and abraded skin. Ester-linked LAs are rapidly hydrolyzed by plasma pseudocholinesterase and in the liver. Amide linked LAs are metabolized by the liver. They undergo extensive first pass metabolism.

Adverse Effects

LA can cause adverse effects as given below (Table 7.2).

Table 7.2: Adverse effects of local anesthetics.

CNS	Dizziness, confusion, anxiety, tremors, occasionally convulsions and respiratory depression
CVS	Hypotension, bradycardia, arrhythmias
Hypersensitivity reactions	Rashes, dermatitis, asthma, rarely anaphylaxis
Local	Irritation at the injection site

Lignocaine: Most widely used LA. It is faster and longer-acting. Action is seen in 3 minutes for nerve block. It is useful for all types of blocks. In contrast to other LAs, lignocaine causes drowsiness and mental clouding (Table 7.3).

Lignocaine (xylocaine) is available as 4% topical solution, 2% jelly, 5% ointment, 1% and 2% injection, 5% for spinal anesthesia.

Uses of Local Anesthetics

Local anesthesia is the loss of sensation without the loss of consciousness or impairment of central control of vital functions. Depending on the site and technique of administration, LA can be:

1. **Surface anesthesia:** Anesthesia of mucous membrane of the eyes, nose, mouth, tracheobronchial tree, esophagus and genitourinary tract can be produced by direct application of the anesthetic solution. Tetracaine 2%, lignocaine 2–10% are most often used. Surface anesthesia is useful in the eye for tonometry, surgery, nasal lesions, stomatitis, sore throat, tonsillectomy, endoscopies, intubation, gastric ulcer, burns and proctoscopy. Proparacaine is used on the eye for surface anesthesia.
2. **Infiltration anesthesia:** Injection of a local anesthetic solution directly into the tissue can be (i) superficial—only into

Table 7.3: Preparations and uses of some local anesthetics.

Drugs	*Preparations*	*Uses*
Tetracaine	1–2% ointment, eye drops, cream, powder	Topical, spinal anesthesia
Lignocaine	2–4% drops, spray, jelly, ointment, cream, 1–10% Inj	Topical, infiltration, nerve block, spinal, epidural and IV regional anesthesia
Benzocaine	1–2% dusting powder, 5% suppository, cream, gels, ointments, 20% spray	Topical anesthesia
Oxethazaine	0.2% suspension	Topical anesthesia (used in peptic ulcer)
Prilocaine	5% cream, 4% Inj	Topical, nerve block anesthesia
Dibucaine	0.5–1% cream	Topical anesthesia
Mepivacaine	1–3% Inj	Nerve block, epidural anesthesia
Bupivacaine	0.25–0.75% Inj	Infiltration, nerve block, spinal, epidural anesthesia
Ropivacaine	2–10% Inj	Infiltration, nerve block, spinal, epidural anesthesia
Etidocaine	1% Inj	Epidural anesthesia

the skin, or (ii) into deeper structures including intra-abdominal organs. Duration of anesthesia can be increased by adrenaline (1:2,00,000). Adrenaline should not be used (i) around end arteries to avoid necrosis, and (ii) intradermally to avoid sloughing.

Uses: For minor procedures like incisions, drainage of an abscess, excision, etc.

3. **Field block:** Subcutaneous injection of a LA solution proximal to the site to be anesthetized, interrupts nerve transmission in the region distal to the injection. Sites such as forearm, scalp, anterior abdominal wall and lower limbs are used for field block. Knowledge of the neuroanatomy of the area is essential.
4. **Nerve block:** Injection of a solution of a LA around individual peripheral nerves or nerve plexuses produces larger areas of anesthesia with a smaller amount of the drug than the above techniques. Anesthesia starts a few centimeters distal to the injection.

   Nerve block anesthesia is useful for:
   - Blocks of brachial plexus for procedures on the arm (distal to deltoid).
   - Intercostal nerve blocks to anesthetize anterior abdominal wall.
   - Cervical plexus block for surgery of the neck.
   - Sciatic and femoral nerve blocks for surgeries distal to the knee.
   - Blocks of nerves at wrist and ankle.
   - Radial and ulnar nerve block at the elbow.
   - Sensory cranial nerve blocks.
   - Facial and lingual nerve blocks.
   - Inferior alveolar nerve block for extraction of lower jaw teeth.
5. **Spinal anesthesia (SA):** Local anesthetic solution is injected into the subarachnoid space between L2–3 and L3–4. The drug acts on nerve roots. Lower abdomen and lower limbs are anesthetized and paralyzed. Duration depends on the concentration, dose and the drug itself.

   Uses: Surgical procedures on the lower limb, pelvis, lower abdomen, obstetric procedures, cesarean section and other operations are done on spinal anesthesia.

   Complications of SA:
   - **Hypotension and bradycardia** due to sympathetic blockade.

- **Respiratory paralysis:** Hypotension and ischemia of the respiratory center results in respiratory failure. Due to paralysis of the abdominal muscles, cough reflex is less effective resulting in stasis of respiratory secretions → respiratory infections.
- **Headache** due to seepage of CSF, can be treated with analgesics.
- **Cauda equina syndrome** is uncommon—control over bladder and bowel sphincters is lost because of damage to nerve roots.
- **Infection:** Resulting in meningitis.
- **Nausea and vomiting:** Premedication can be given to prevent this.

6. **Epidural anesthesia:** LA is injected into the spinal extradural space and it acts on the nerve roots. It is technically more difficult and comparatively larger volumes of the anesthetic are needed.

   Advantages:
   - Sensory blockade is 4–5 segments higher than motor blockade. This is useful in childbirth, as the mother has no labor pain and can still cooperate in the process of labor and is conscious throughout.
   - As there is no risk of injecting into SA space, there are no chances of infection.

7. **Intravenous regional anesthesia:** This type of anesthesia is useful for rapid anesthetization of an extremity. A rubber bandage is used to force the blood out of the limb (veins) and a tourniquet is applied to prevent the re-entry of the blood. A dilute solution of the local anesthetic is then injected intravenously. It diffuses into extravascular tissues. Onset of anesthesia is in 2 minutes. Because of the pain produced by the tourniquet, this type of anesthesia is used for procedures lasting less than one hour. About 25 percent of the drug enters into the systemic circulation. This type of anesthesia is commonly used on the upper limbs though it can also be used on the legs and the thighs.

ALCOHOLS

Ethyl Alcohol (Ethanol)

Ethyl alcohol is manufactured by fermentation of sugars. It is a colorless, volatile, inflammable liquid. The ethanol content of various alcoholic beverages ranges from 4–55%.

Actions

- **Local:** On topical application, ethanol evaporates quickly and has a cooling effect. It is an astringent—precipitates surface proteins and hardens the skin. 40–50% alcohol is rubefacient causes redness and counter irritant. Alcohol is also an antiseptic. At 70%, it has maximum antiseptic properties which decrease above that. It is not effective against spores.
- **CNS:** Alcohol is a CNS depressant. Small doses cause euphoria, relief of anxiety and loss of social inhibitions. Moderate doses impair muscular coordination and visual acuity making driving dangerous. With higher doses mental clouding, impaired judgment, drowsiness and loss of self control result. High doses cause coma. Death is due to respiratory depression.

Alcohol may precipitate convulsions in epileptics. Tolerance develops on long-term use.

Other effects:

- Chronic consumption of moderate amounts of alcohol results in accumulation of fat in the liver, liver enlargement, followed by fatty degeneration and cirrhosis.
- Alcohol induces microsomal enzymes leading to drug interactions.
- Alcohol causes vasodilation in the skin causing warmth. But this increases heat

loss and should not be used in cold weather.

- Alcohol also increases gastric secretion. It is an appetizer.
- Low doses taken over a long-time increases high-density lipoprotein (HDL) and lowers low-density lipoprotein (LDL) cholesterol.
- Alcohol is a diuretic (↓ADH secretion).
- Food value is 7 calories/gram.

Uses

1. **Antiseptic:** 70% alcohol is applied topically.
2. **Bed sores:** When rubbed onto the skin, alcohol hardens the skin and prevents bed sores.
3. Alcoholic sponges are used for reduction of body temperature *in fevers.*
4. **Appetite stimulant:** About 50 mL of 6–10 percent alcohol given before meals is an appetite stimulant.
5. **Neuralgias:** In severe neuralgias like trigeminal neuralgia, injection of alcohol around the nerve causes permanent loss of transmission and relieves pain.
6. In methanol poisoning.

Disulfiram

Disulfiram inhibits the enzyme aldehyde dehydrogenase. If alcohol is consumed after taking disulfiram, acetaldehyde accumulates and within few minutes it can produce flushing, throbbing headache, nausea, vomiting, sweating, hypotension and confusion called **the antabuse reaction**. The effect lasts for 7-14 days after stopping disulfiram. The reactions can sometimes be very severe and therefore treatment should be given in a hospital.

Other drugs that cause antabuse reaction are: **metronidazole, chlorpropamide, tolbutamide, griseofulvin, cephalosporins and phenylbutazone**.

Contraindications: Patients with liver disease, patients physically dependent on alcohol.

Methyl Alcohol/Methanol

Methanol is used to denature ethyl alcohol. Ingestion results in methanol poisoning.

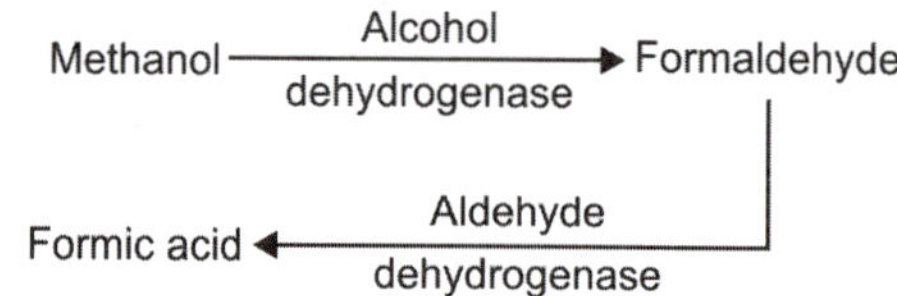

Toxic effects are due to formation of formic acid.

Signs and symptome: vomiting, headache, vertigo, severe abdominal pain, hypotension, delirium, acidosis and coma. Formic acid has affinity for optic nerve and causes retinal damage resulting in blindness. Death is due to respiratory failure.

Treatment

- **Correction of acidosis:** As acidosis speeds up retinal damage, immediate correction of acidosis with IV sodium bicarbonate infusion helps in preventing blindness.
- Patient should be kept in a dark room to **protect the eyes**.
- **Antidote:** Fomepizole specifically inhibits the enzyme alcohol dehydrogenase and thereby prevents the formation of toxic compounds—formaldehyde and formic acid. Fomepizole thus acts as an antidote in methanol poisoning. Moreover, it has the advantage over ethyl alcohol that it does not cause any intoxication by itself.
- **Hemodialysis** should be started at the earliest possible.
- **Stomach wash** should be given.
- **BP** and **ventilation** should be maintained.
- **Ethyl alcohol** is given as infusion. It competes with methanol for alcohol dehydrogenase, slows the metabolism of methanol and thus prevents the formation of toxic metabolites.

8

CHAPTER

Autacoids and Respiratory System

CHAPTER HIGHLIGHTS

- Histamine and Antihistamines
- 5-Hydroxytryptamine, Ergot Alkaloids, Angiotensin and Kinins
- Eicosanoids
- Drugs Used in the Treatment of Bronchial Asthma
- Drugs Used in the Treatment of Cough
- Drugs Used in Allergic Rhinitis

AUTACOIDS

Autacoids are substances formed in various tissues, have complex physiological and pathological actions and act locally at the site of synthesis. They have a brief action and are destroyed locally. Hence they are called *local hormones* and differ from true hormones which are produced by specific cells and reach their target tissues through circulation. The word autacoid is derived from Greek: *autos*-self, *akos*-remedy. Histamine, 5-hydroxytryptamine (serotonin), endogenous peptides like bradykinin and angiotensin; prostaglandins and leukotrienes are autacoids.

HISTAMINE AND ANTIHISTAMINES

Histamine

Histamine (tissue amine) (*Histos* = tissue) is a biogenic amine formed in many tissues. It is also found in the venoms of bees, wasps and other stinging secretions.

Synthesis, storage, distribution and degradation: In humans, histamine is formed from the amino acid histidine. Large amounts are found in the lungs, skin and intestines. Histamine is stored in the granules of the mast cells and basophils in an inactive form. Histamine found in brain serves as a neurotransmitter. Degranulation of the mast cells release histamine which is quickly degraded at the site.

Mechanism of Action

Histamine produces its effects by acting on the histamine receptors. Four subtypes are known.

- H_1—present in lungs, gut, blood vessels, nerve endings and brain.
- H_2—stomach (gastric glands), heart, blood vessels and brain.
- H_3—CNS.
- H_4—Leukocytes, CD4 cells.

Actions

1. **CVS:** Histamine dilates small blood vessels resulting in hypotension accompanied by reflex tachycardia. Cerebral blood vessels dilate—producing severe throbbing headache.

   Triple response: Intradermal injection of histamine produces triple response comprising of flush, flare and wheal.
   - *Flush: Red spot at the site*—due to local capillary dilation.
   - *Flare:* Redness surrounding the 'flush' due to arteriolar dilatation.
   - *Wheal:* Local edema due to the escape of fluid from the capillaries.

   This response is accompanied by pain and itching.
2. **Smooth muscle:** Histamine causes contraction of the nonvascular smooth

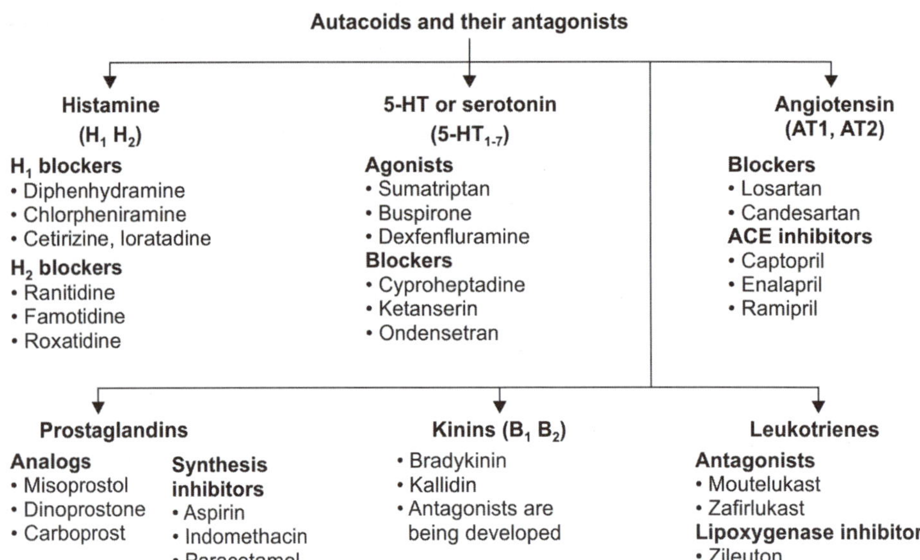

Some autacoids with examples of agonist and antagonists. Receptor types are given in brackets

muscles. Thus bronchospasm and increased intestinal motility are produced.

3. **Glands:** Histamine is a powerful stimulant of the gastric acid secretion-acts through H_2 receptors. It also stimulates pepsin and intrinsic factor secretion.
4. **CNS:** Histamine is a neurotransmitter in the CNS.
5. **Nerve endings:** Histamine stimulates sensory nerve endings causing pain and itching.

Adverse reactions include hypotension, flushing, tachycardia, headache, wheal, bronchospasm and diarrhea.

Uses

Histamine is of no therapeutic value. It is occasionally used in some diagnostic tests like to test the acid secreting ability of the stomach, diagnosis of pheochromocytoma, and to test for bronchial hyperreactivity.

Histamine Substitutes

Betazole is a H_2 agonist and can be used in gastric function tests. *Betahistine* is a H_1 agonist used to control vertigo in Meniere's disease.

Antihistamines

Antihistamines are histamine receptor antagonists.

Drugs that competitively block H_1 histamine receptors are conventionally called the *antihistamines*. H_2 blockers are used in the treatment of peptic ulcer.

Classification of H_1 Blockers

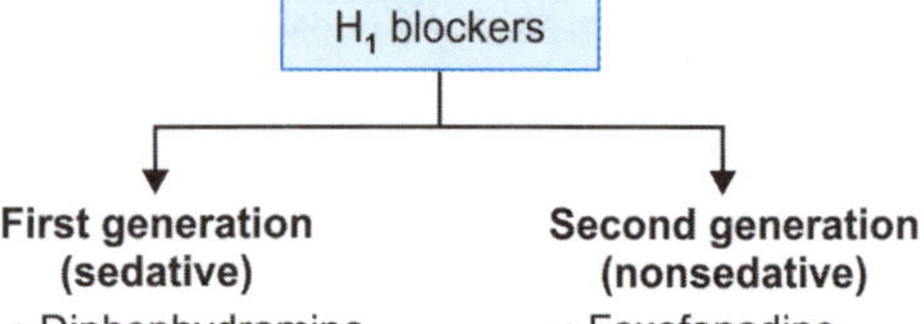

- Diphenhydramine
- Dimenhydrinate
- Promethazine
- Pheniramine
- Chlorpheniramine
- Cyclizine
- Meclizine
- Buclizine
- Mepyramine
- Tripelennamine

- Fexofenadine
- Loratadine
- Desloratadine
- Cetirizine
- Levocetirizine
- Acrivastine
- Azelastine
- Mizolastine
- Levocabastine
- Mequitazine

Actions

- **Blockade of actions of histamine:** H_1 receptor antagonists block the actions of histamine on H_1 receptors. They block the histamine induced effects on smooth muscles of the gut, bronchi, blood vessels and triple response.
- **Sedation:** Antihistamines cause CNS depression; sedation, dizziness, inability to concentrate and disturbances of coordination are common. Alcohol and other CNS depressants potentiate this action. Some patients may experience CNS stimulation resulting in tremors, restlessness and insomnia.
- **Antimotion sickness effects:** Several antihistamines prevent motion sickness and vomiting due to other labyrinthine disturbances. Some of them also control vomiting of pregnancy.
- **Antiparkinsonian effects:** Some of them suppress tremors, rigidity and sialorrhea probably due to their anticholinergic properties.
- **Anticholinergic actions:** Many of the H_1 blockers have anticholinergic property.
- **Other actions:** Antihistamines also have local anesthetic effects in high doses. Some of them also block α_1 adrenergic and 5-HT receptors.

Pharmacokinetics: Antihistamines are well-absorbed, widely distributed in the body, metabolized in the liver and are excreted in the urine. Route of administration and preparations are given in Table 8.1.

Table 8.1: Dose and route of administration of some antihistamines.

Antihistamine	*Route*	*Brand name*
First generation (sedative) antihistamines		
Diphenhydramine HCl	Oral IM	Benadryl cap, syr
Dimenhydrinate	Oral, IM	Dramamine tab, syr inj
Promethazine	Oral, IM	Phenergan tab, syr, inj
Promethazine chlortheophyllinate	Oral	Avomine tab
Pheniramine maleate	Oral, IM	Avil tab, syr, inj
Chlorpheniramine	Oral, IM	Zeet tab, syr, inj
Cyclizine HCl	Oral	Marezine tab
Meclizine HCl	Oral	Ancolan tab
Buclizine	Oral	Longifene tab, syr
Cinnarizine	Oral	Stugeron tab
Second generation (non-sedative) antihistamines		
Loratadine	Oral	Lorfast, tab, syr
Desloratadine	Oral	Deslor tab
Cetirizine	Oral	Alerid, tab, syr
Levocetirizine	Oral	Levocet tab

Mnemonic for uses

PHC CAMPs use Antihistamines Very Dearly
P—Preanesthetic medicine
H—Hypnotic
C—Common cold
C—Cough
A—Alllergies
M—Motion sickness
P—Parkinsonism
A—Antiemetic
V—Vertigo
D—Dystonia

Adverse reactions are mild and on continued use tolerance develops.

Sedation, dizziness, motor incoordination, inability to concentrate make driving dangerous while on antihistamines.

Anticholinergic effects like dryness of mouth, blurred vision, constipation and urinary retention may be troublesome. Epigastric distress and headache can also occur. Many of them are teratogenic.

Second generation (non-sedative) antihistamines have the following advantages over classical antihistamines:

- No sedation because they poorly cross the blood-brain barrier.
- No anticholinergic side effects as these are pure H_1 blockers and do not block cholinergic receptors.

However, the therapeutic uses of these agents are limited to allergic disorders like allergic rhinitis and chronic urticaria. They are more expensive.

Uses

1. **Allergic reactions:** Antihistamines are useful for the prevention and treatment of symptoms of allergic reactions. They are effective in allergic rhinitis, conjunctivitis, hay fever, urticaria, pruritus, some allergic skin rashes and pollinosis.
2. **Common cold:** Antihistamines reduce rhinorrhea and afford symptomatic relief in common cold.
3. **Motion sickness:** Given 30–60 minutes before journey, antihistamines prevent motion sickness. They are also useful in treating vertigo of Meniere's disease and other vestibular disturbances. Cinnarizine is preferred.
4. **Antiemetic:** Promethazine is used to prevent drug induced and postoperative vomiting. It has also been used in 'morning sickness.'
5. **Preanesthetic medication:** For its sedative, anticholinergic and antiemetic properties, promethazine has been used as preanesthetic medication.
6. **Hypnotic:** The sedative antihistamines are sometimes used to induce sleep. Hydroxizine has been used as an anxiolytic.
7. **Parkinsonism:** Some of them are useful in drug induced parkinsonism due to their anticholinergic action.
8. **Cough** due to postnasal drip can be controlled by antihistamines like diphenhydramine.
9. **Vertigo:** Antihistamines, like dimenhydrinate are useful in vertigo.
10. **Dystonia:** Promethazine is useful to relieve acute dystonia due to antipsychotic drugs.

5-HYDROXYTRYPTAMINE, ERGOT ALKALOIDS, ANGIOTENSIN AND KININS

5-Hydroxytryptamine

5-Hydroxytryptamine (serotonin) is of great pharmacological interest. It is found in various plant and animal tissues. In human body, 5-HT is present in the intestines, platelets and brain. It is synthesized from the amino acid tryptophan and stored in granules. It is degraded mainly by monoamine oxidase (MAO).

5-HT Receptors: The actions of serotonin are mediated through its receptors. Seven types of 5-HT receptors (5-HT_{1-7}) with further subtypes of 5-HT_1 and 5-HT_2 receptors are presently known. Many receptor selective agonists and antagonists are being developed.

Actions

- **CVS:** The action on blood vessels is complex. Large vessels are constricted while arterioles dilate. A characteristic triphasic response is seen on blood pressure following IV injection.
  Initial fall in BP is followed by a rise and then fall.
- **GI tract:** 5-HT increases gastrointestinal motility and contraction resulting in diarrhea.
- **Other actions:** Weak bronchoconstriction, platelet aggregation; stimulation of sensory nerve endings—causes pain if injected into the skin. 5-HT is a neurotransmitter in the CNS.

Physiological and pathophysiological role: 5-HT has a role in peristalsis, vomiting, platelet aggregation, homoeostasis and inflammation. It is also thought to initiate the vasoconstriction in migraine.

Drugs acting on 5-HT receptors: Serotonin has no therapeutic uses. However its receptor agonists and antagonists have been used in various conditions.

Serotonin Agonists

Sumatriptan—a 5-HT_{1D} agonist is effective in the treatment of acute migraine and cluster headache. Given at the onset of a migraine attack, sumatriptan relieves headache and also suppresses nausea and vomiting of migrane. It is short-acting.

Buspirone (*See* page 177) is a 5-HT_{1A} agonist-antagonist used as an antianxiety agent.

Serotonin Antagonists

Cyproheptadine blocks 5-HT_2, H_1 histamine and cholinergic receptors. It increases appetite and is used to promote weight gain especially in children.

Ketanserin blocks 5-HT_2 receptors and antagonizes vasoconstriction and platelet aggregation promoted by 5-HT. It is used in hypertension.

Ondansetron is a 5-HT_3 antagonist (*See* page 206) used in the prevention and treatment of vomiting.

Many other drugs including some antihistamines also block serotonin receptors.

Table 8.2: Serotonin agonists, antagonists and their therapeutic uses.

	Uses
Agonists	
Sumatriptan	• Acute migraine • Cluster headache
Buspirone	Anxiolytic
Antagonists	
Cyproheptadine	• Appetite stimulant • Carcinoid tumors
Ketanserin	Hypertension
Ondansetron	Antiemetic
Ergot alkaloids	
Ergotamine	Acute migraine
Ergometrine	Postpartum hemorrhage

Ergot Alkaloids

Ergot alkaloids are produced by a fungus *Claviceps purpurea*. Consumption of such grains results in 'ergotism' manifested as gangrene of the hands and feet, hallucinations and other CNS effects.

Natural ergot alkaloids include **ergometrine, ergotamine** and **ergotoxine**. The semisynthetic ones are also available.

Actions: Ergot alkaloids have agonist, partial agonist and antagonistic actions at 5-HT and alpha adrenergic receptors and agonistic actions at CNS dopamine receptors. Thus their actions are complex. Some of them are powerful hallucinogens, e.g., lysergic acid diethylamide (LSD). They cause stimulation of smooth muscles—some mainly vascular smooth muscles and others mainly uterine smooth muscles. The vasoconstrictor effect is responsible for gangrene.

Adverse effects like nausea, vomiting and diarrhea are common. Prolonged use results in gangrene due to persistent vasospasm.

Uses (Table 8.2)

- Migraine.
- Postpartum hemorrhage (after child birth)—ergometrine is used for the prevention and treatment.

Drugs Used in the Treatment of Migraine

Migraine is a common disorder characterized by severe, throbbing, unilateral, headache often associated with nausea, vomiting and fatigue lasting for several hours. In the classical migraine, a brief 'aura' of visual disturbances occurs prior to the headache. An attack is triggered by factors like stress, anxiety, excitement, food (like chocolate and cheese) and hormonal changes. These triggering factors stimulate the release of vasoactive substances from nerve endings which are responsible for the events that follow. However the exact pathophysiology is not understood and several hypotheses have been put forward.

Acute migraine: Aspirin, paracetamol or other NSAIDs, **ergotamine** and **sumatriptan** are effective in acute attacks. Drug should be taken at the initiation of an attack.

Prophylaxis: When the attacks are frequent and severe, prophylaxis is needed. Drugs used for the prophylaxis are: **propranolol, flunarizine, cyproheptadine** and **amytriptyline**.

Angiotensin

Angiotensins are peptides synthesized from the precursor angiotensinogen. Angiotensin

II, the most potent angiotensin, acts through angiotensin receptors (AT_1 and AT_2) present on the tissues.

Actions

Angiotensin II causes vasoconstriction resulting in increased blood pressure. It stimulates the synthesis of aldosterone by the adrenal cortex which increases sodium reabsorption by the kidneys. By these actions, renin-angiotensin system regulates the fluid and electrolyte balance and blood pressure.

Inhibitors of ACE and blockers of angiotensin II receptors are now used in the treatment of hypertension, congestive heart failure and other conditions that are due to excess of angiotensin II activity.

Kinins

Kinins are vasodilator peptides formed from the precursor kininogen by the action of the enzymes called kallikreins. The most important of kinins is bradykinin.

Kinins are potent vasodilators and cause a brief fall in BP. They stimulate contraction of other smooth muscles—thus they induce bronchospasm in asthmatics, slow contraction of intestines (*Brady*=slow) and uterus. Kinins mediate inflammation, and stimulate the pain nerve endings. Kinins produce their actions by acting through B_1 and B_2 receptors.

Drugs affecting the kallikrein-kinin system—B_1 and B_2 antagonists are now being developed.

EICOSANOIDS

Eicosanoids are 20-carbon (eicosa referring to the 20-C atoms) unsaturated fatty acids derived mainly from arachidonic acid in the cell walls. The principal eicosanoids are the **prostaglandins** (PG), the **thromboxanes** (TX), and the **leukotrienes** (LT).

Biosynthesis: Eicosanoids are synthesized locally in most tissues from arachidonic acid. The pathway for synthesis is shown in Figure 8.1.

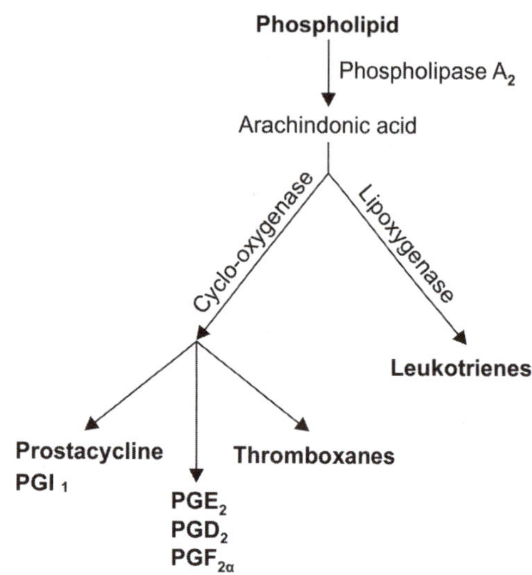

Fig. 8.1: Biosynthesis of eicosanoids.

The cyclo-oxygenase (COX) pathway generates PGs and TXs while lipoxygenase (LOX) pathway generates LTs. There are 2 cyclo-oxygenase isozymes *viz.* COX-1 and COX-2. Eicosanoids produced by COX-1 mainly take part in physiological functions while those produced by COX-2 result in inflammatory and pathological changes.

Prostaglandins and Thromboxanes

In 1930s it was found that human semen contains a substance that contracts uterine smooth muscle. As this substance was thought to originate in the prostate, they called it 'prostaglandin'. However, it was later found to be produced in many tissues.

Actions

The eicosanoids act through their specific receptors present on the tissues.

CVS: Prostacycline (PGI_2) causes vasodilation while TXA_2 causes vasoconstriction. PGE_2 and $PGF_{2\alpha}$ are weak cardiac stimulants.

Other actions: PGs (TXA_2, $PGF_{2\alpha}$) contract gastrointestinal and bronchial smooth muscles. TXA_2 induces platelet aggregation while PGI_2 inhibits it. PGE_2 and $PGF_{2\alpha}$ contract uterus. PGs also stimulate bone turnover and sensitize the nerve endings to pain.

Adverse effects depend on the type of PG, dose and route. Diarrhea, nausea, vomiting, fever, hypotension and pain due to uterine contractions are common.

Uses

1. **Gynecological and obstetrical**
   - **Abortion:** For I and II trimester abortion and ripening of cervix during abortion, PGE_2 and $PGF_{2\alpha}$ are used. They are also used with mifepristone to ensure complete expulsion of the products of conception.
   - **Facilitation of labor:** As alternative to oxytocin in patients with renal failure.
   - **Cervical priming:** Intravaginal PGE_2 is used.
   - **Postpartum hemorrhage:** Intramuscular $PGF_{2\alpha}$ is used as an alternative to ergometrine.
2. **Gastrointestinal:** *Peptic ulcer* PGE_1 (misoprostol) and PGE_2 (enprostil) are used for the prevention of peptic ulcer in patients on high dose NSAIDs.
3. **Cardiovascular**
   - **Patent ductus arteriosus:** Patency of fetal ductus arteriosus depends on local PG synthesis. In neonates with some congenital heart diseases, patency of the ductus arteriosus is maintained with PGs until surgery is done.
   - To prevent platelet aggregation during hemodialysis.
4. **Other uses:** PGs are used in pulmonary hypertension and some peripheral vascular diseases. They can also be used in open angle glaucoma to lower intraocular pressure.

Leukotrienes

Leukotrienes (LT) are products of arachidonic acid metabolism synthesized by the lipoxygenase pathway and are found in the lungs, platelets, mast cells and white blood cells. ('Leuko'—because they are found in white cells; 'trienes'—they contain triene system of double bonds). LTA_4 is the precursor from which LTB_4, LTC_4, LTD_4, LTE_4 and LTF_4 are derived. LTC_4, LTD_4 and LTE_4 are together known as slow reacting substances (SRS-A) of anaphylaxis. The LTs produce their effects through specific receptors.

Actions

Leukotrienes cause vasoconstriction, increase vascular permeability leading to edema, increase airway mucous secretion and are potent bronchiolar spasmogens. Given subcutaneously they cause wheal and flare. Leukotrienes have a role in inflammation including rheumatoid arthritis, psoriasis and ulcerative colitis. They also contribute to bronchial hyper-responsiveness in bronchial asthma.

Leukotriene receptor antagonists montelukast and zafirlukast are used in the treatment of bronchial asthma (see below).

Platelet Activating Factor (PAF)

PAF is an important mediator in acute and chronic, allergic and inflammatory phenomena. PAF is released from inflammatory cells and acts on specific receptors. It causes local vasodilatation resulting in edema, hyperalgesia and wheal formation. It is a potent chemotaxin for leukocytes and a spasmogen on bronchial and intestinal smooth muscles.

RESPIRATORY SYSTEM

DRUGS USED IN THE TREATMENT OF BRONCHIAL ASTHMA

Bronchial asthma is characterized by dyspnea and wheeze due to increased resistance to the flow of air through the bronchi. Bronchospasm, mucosal congestion and edema result in increased airway resistance. The bronchial smooth muscle is hyperresponsive to various stimuli like dust, allergens, cold air, infection and drugs. These trigger factors—trigger an acute attack. Antigen-antibody interaction on the surface of mast cells cause (Fig. 8.2):

- Degranulation of mast cells releasing stored mediators of inflammation.
- Synthesis of other inflammatory mediators which are responsible for bronchospasm, mucosal congestion and edema.
- **Inflammation is the primary pathology.**

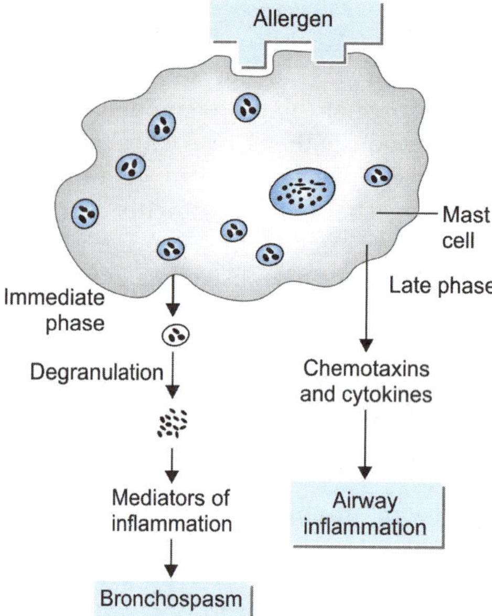

Fig. 8.2: Immediate and late responses of mast cell activation by antigen.

Classification

1. **Bronchodilators**
   - **Sympathomimetics:** Salbutamol, terbutaline, salmeterol, isoprenaline adrenaline, ephedrine.
   - **Methylxanthines:** Theophylline, aminophylline.
   - **Anticholinergics:** Ipratropium bromide, atropine, tiotropium bromide.
2. **Anti-inflammatory agents**
   - **Systemic glucocorticoids:** Hydrocortisone, prednisolone.
   - **Inhalational:** Beclomethasone, budesonide, fluticasone, mometasone, ciclesonide, triamcinolone.
3. **Mast cell stabilizers**
   - Disodium cromoglycate, nedocromil, ketotifen.
4. **Leukotriene receptor antagonists**
   - Montelukast, zafirlukast.
5. **Anti-IgE antibody**
   - Omalizumab.

BRONCHODILATORS

Sympathomimetic Drugs

These drugs are potent bronchodilators and are the most useful drugs to relieve bronchospasm.

Salbutamol and terbutaline are selective β_2 agonists.

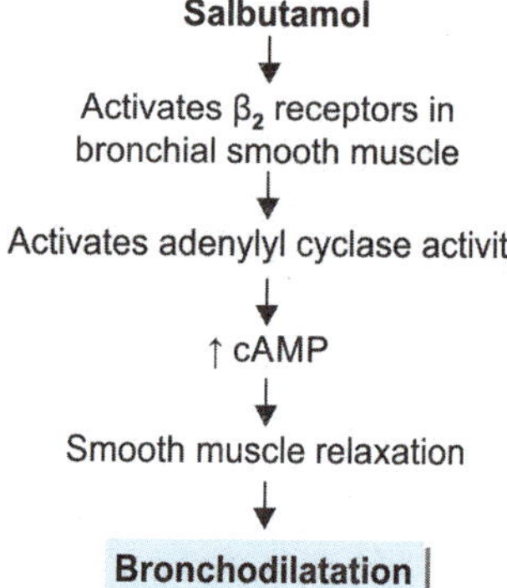

Mechanism of action: Adrenergic agonists stimulate β_2 receptors in bronchial smooth muscles resulting in increased cyclic adenosine monophosphate (cAMP) levels (Fig. 8.3). This increased cAMP leads to bronchodilatation. The increased cAMP in mast cells inhibit the release of inflammatory mediators. They also reduce bronchial secretions and congestion (by acting on α receptors).

Salbutamol and terbutaline are selective β_2 agonists. Given by inhalation, they are fastest-acting bronchodilators with peak effect in 10 minutes. The action lasts for 6 hours. Adverse effects to β_2 agonists include muscle tremors, palpitation and nervousness.

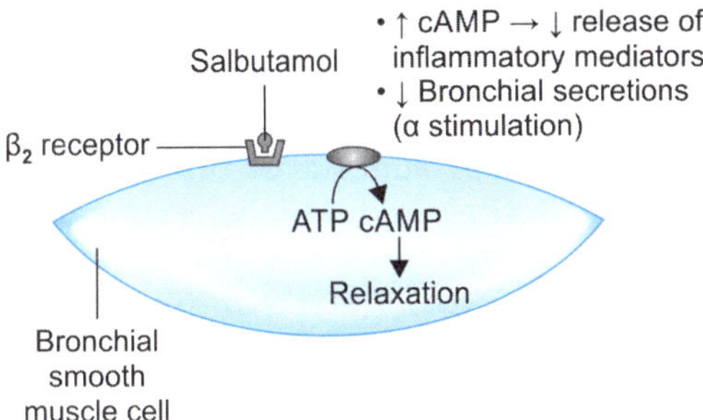

Fig. 8.3: Mechanism of action of β_2 agonists in bronchial asthma.

Selective β_2 agonists are the first line bronchodilators as they are the most effective, fast-acting, convenient and relatively safe bronchodilators. They are available as metered dose inhalers, nebulizers and also tablets for oral use. The proper technique of using the inhaler should be taught. 'Spacers' can be used in children and adults who cannot follow the right technique of inhalation.

Oral β_2 agonists have higher adverse effects and are used only in small children who cannot use inhalers and have occasional wheezing (1-4 mg 6 hourly).

Longer-acting β_2 agonists like salmeterol have a slow onset of action (hence not useful in acute attacks) but the effect remains for 12 hours. They are therefore, used for long-term maintenance and for prevention of nocturnal asthmatic attacks.

Newer agents like **fenoterol, formoterol bambuterol, pirbuterol, indacaterol** are similar to salmeterol.

Long-term use of β_2 agonists may result in the development of tolerance.

Others

Adrenaline, **ephedrine** and **isoprenaline** produce prompt bronchodilation through β2 stimulation. However, they are not preferred due to the risk of adverse effects as they are non-selective in their action.

Methylxanthines (See page 178)

Theophylline and its derivatives like *aminophylline* are good bronchodilators.

Mechanism of action: Phosphodiesterase (PDE) is the enzyme that degrades cyclic AMP. Methylxanthines inhibit PDE and thereby cAMP levels which brings about bronchodilation. cAMP also inhibits the release of mediators of inflammation.

cAMP
↓ PDE ←——— Methylxanthines
5'AMP

Adverse effects: Theophylline is a drug of low therapeutic index. Gastric irritation, vomiting, insomnia, tremors, diuresis, palpitation, and hypotension are quite common. Higher doses cause restlessness, delirium, convulsions and arrhythmias. Children may develop behavioral abnormalities on prolonged use—should be avoided in children.

Uses

1. **Bronchial asthma:** Theophylline is a second line drug in bronchial asthma.
   - **Chronic asthma:** Oral theophylline can be used to control mild to moderate asthma. Etophylline + 80% theophylline (Deriphylline) injections (IM) are used to relieve acute attacks.
   - **Acute severe asthma (status asthmaticus):** Intravenous aminophylline was tried when sympathomimetics fail to relieve bronchospasm—but are found to be less effective and not safe. Rapid IV injection may cause collapse and death due to hypotension and arrhythmias. Convulsions can also occur.
2. **Apnea in premature infants:** Theophylline or caffeine may be used for 1-3 weeks to reduce the duration of episodes of apnea.

***Anticholinergics*—Ipratropium bromide** and **tiotropium bromide** are atropine derivatives and act by blocking the muscarinic receptors in the airways. They are given by inhalation and their actions are largely limited to the respiratory tract. They are more effective in chronic bronchitis, are safe and well-tolerated.

Use in Bronchial Asthma

- **Acute bronchospasm:** Along with β_2 agonists or as alternatives.
- As bronchodilators in chronic bronchitis.

Anti-inflammatory Drugs

1. **Leukotriene antagonists:** Leukotrienes are one of the important mediators of inflammation. They bring about bronchospasm, mucosal edema, increase the influx of inflammatory cells and respiratory mucous production, by their actions on leukotriene receptors. **Montelukast** and **Zafirlukast** are highly selective and competitive antagonists of leukotriene receptors. They block the effects of leukotrienes and thereby reduce mucosal edema and relieve bronchospasm. They decrease the response to allergens. They inhibit exercise induced and aspirin-induced bronchospasm.

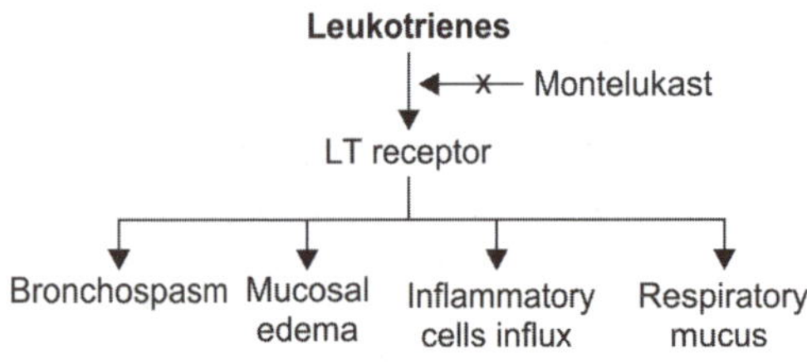

Adverse effects are rare—headache, rashes and gastrointestinal disturbances.

Uses: Prophylaxis of mild to moderate asthma as alternatives or as add-on drugs. They also reduce the dose of the steroid required. Bronchodilator effect is additive with beta 2 agonists.

2. **Glucocorticoids:** Since inflammation is the primary pathology in bronchial asthma, anti-inflammatory agents provide significant benefit.

Mechanism of action: Glucocorticoids are **not bronchodilators**. They suppress the inflammatory response to antigen-antibody reaction and thereby reduce mucosal edema and hyperirritability. They restore response to β_2 agonists if tolerance has developed. Oral prednisolone is commonly used.

Inhaled steroids: The use of inhalational steroids largely minimizes their adverse effects because of the small dose required. However, they are not effective in acute attacks and are only of prophylactic value. They prevent episodes of acute asthma and bronchial hyperreactivity and effectively control symptoms. The effect develops after 1 week of treatment.

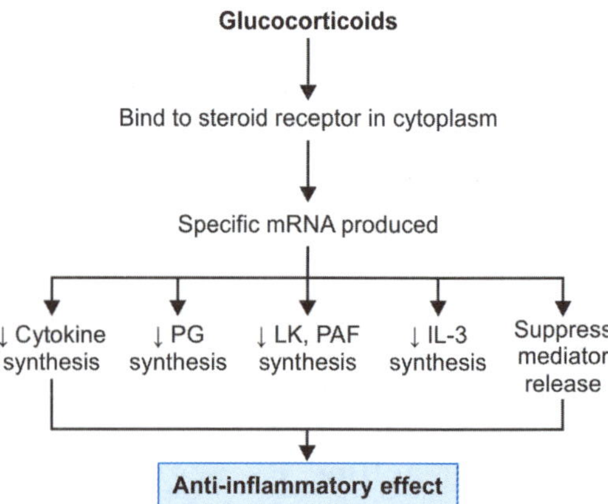

Side effects of inhaled glucocorticoids include hoarseness of voice, sore throat and oropharyngeal candidiasis. Rinsing the mouth and throat with water after each use can reduce the incidence of candidiasis and sore throat. No HPA axis suppression is seen in the recommended doses.

Beclomethasone dipropionate, budesonide, fluticasone and ***mometasone*** are used as inhalers.

Dose: Beclomethasone: BECLATE INHALER 50, 100 and 200 μg per metered dose → 1–2 Puffs 3–4 times a day.

Use of Glucocorticoids in Asthma

1. **Acute exacerbation:** A short course (5–7 days) of oral prednisolone is given in addition to β_2 agonists.

2. **Chronic asthma:** Budesonide/fluticasone inhalation for a long period as prophylaxis.
3. **Status asthmaticus:** IV hydrocortisone hemisuccinate followed by oral prednisolone.

Mast Cell Stabilizers

Cromolyn sodium (disodium cromoglycate) was synthesized in 1965.

Mechanism of action: Cromolyn inhibits the degranulation of mast cells and thereby inhibits the release of mediators of inflammation. It thus prevents bronchospasm and inflammation following exposure to allergens. It is therefore used for *prophylaxis*. It is **not a bronchodilator**—hence not useful in acute episodes.

Cromolyn sodium is used as an inhaler; it takes 2–4 weeks of treatment for the beneficial effects to develop.

Adverse effects are rare. Throat irritation, cough and sometimes bronchospasm can occur on inhalation due to the fine powder.

Uses

1. **Prophylaxis of bronchial asthma:** Cromolyn sodium used prophylactically over a long period—2 puffs—3–4 times a day, reduces the frequency and severity of episodes of acute asthma. Young patients are more likely to be benefitted. It is not useful in acute bronchospasm.
2. **Allergic rhinitis:** Prophylactic nasal spray is used.
3. **Allergic conjunctivitis:** Eyedrops are used prophylactically.

Nedocromil is similar to cromolyn sodium in its actions and uses. It is given twice daily.

Ketotifen is an antihistaminic with actions like cromolyn sodium. It inhibits airway inflammation but it is not a bronchodilator. It is given orally. Beneficial effects are seen after 6–12 weeks of use. It is used for the prophylaxis of bronchial asthma and other allergic disorders like allergic rhinitis and conjunctivitis. **Drowsiness** and dry mouth are common side effects.

Anti-IgE Antibody

Omalizumab is a monoclonal antibody against IgE antibodies. It binds to IgE antibodies and prevents the development of allergic response. Omalizumab is given subcutaneously once in 2–4 weeks for prophylaxis in moderate to severe asthmatics and in allergic rhinitis. It is expensive. It is well tolerated. It reduces the frequency and severity of acute attacks. Omalizumab is also useful in allergic rhinitis, chronic urticaria and food allergy.

Others

Roflumilast is a phosphodiesterase 4 inhibitor (PDE4) effective orally. It has anti-inflammatory properties and may be used in COPD.

Treatment of Asthma

Mild asthma: Occasional episodes of bronchospasm need inhaled β_2 stimulants like salbutamol at the onset of bronchospasm.

Moderate asthma: Regular prophylaxis with inhaled steroids is given. Acute episodes are managed with inhaled β_2 agonists.

Severe asthma:

- Regular inhaled steroids.
- Inhaled β_2 agonists 3–4 times a day.
- Oral steroids may be considered.
- Additional inhaled ipratropium bromide or oral theophylline may be given.

Status asthmaticus or acute severe asthma is an acute exacerbation. It is a medical emergency; may be triggered by an acute respiratory infection, abrupt withdrawal of steroids, drugs, allergens or emotional stress.

Treatment

- Nebulization of β_2 agonist and ipratropium alternately—every 30 minutes. Additional salbutamol injection (IM/SC) may be given. Severe tachycardia should be watched for.

- Hydrocortisone hemisuccinate (100 mg) IV followed by a course of oral prednisolone.
- Oxygen inhalation - may be given.
- Antibiotics if required.
- IV fluids to correct dehydration.
- Artificial ventilation may be required in extreme cases.

DRUGS USED IN THE TREATMENT OF COUGH

Cough is a protective reflex that removes the irritant matter and secretions from the respiratory tract. It could be due to infection, allergy, pleural diseases and malignancy. Since it is a protective mechanism, undue suppression of cough can cause more harm than benefit. Only in some conditions as in dry annoying cough, it may serve no useful purpose. In such situations, **antitussives** or cough suppressants may be used. Antitussives only provide symptomatic relief and do not alter the cause.

Drugs for Cough

1. **Central cough supressants (Antitussives):** Codeine, noscapine, dextromethorphan, antihistamines, benzonatate
2. **Pharyngeal demulcents:** Lozenges, cough drops, linctuses
3. **Expectorants:** Potassium iodide, guaiphenesin, ammonium chloride, ipecacuanha
4. **Newer drugs:** Cloperastine and levocloperastine
5. **Bronchodilators:** Salbutamol, terbutaline
6. **Mucolytics:** Bromhexine, ambroxol, acetylcysteine, carbocysteine.

Central Cough Suppressants

Central cough suppressants act by inhibiting cough center in the medulla.

Codeine is a good antitussive with less addiction liability; nausea, constipation and drowsiness are common. *Dose:* 10–15 mg every 6 hours.

Noscapine is a potent antitussive; no other CNS effects are prominent in therapeutic doses. Nausea is the only occasional side effect. *Dose:* 15–30 mg every 6 hours.

Dextromethorphan and pholcodeine are synthetic opioid derivatives with antitussive actions like codeine but with less side effects. Pholcodeine is longer-acting—given twice daily.

Benzonatate is chemically related to the local anesthetic procaine. It acts on the cough receptors in the lungs and also has a central effect. It is given orally.

Antihistamines are useful in cough due to allergy except that due to bronchial asthma.

Newer drugs: Cloperastine and levocloperastine are novel antitussives with dual action—mild bronchodilator and antihistaminic activity. They are not opioids but act centrally at the cough center and peripherally on the receptors in the tracheobronchial tree. Advantages are—

- they do not depress the respiratory center,
- do not cause drowsiness,
- rapid acting,
- non-addicting
- well tolerated.

They significantly reduce night time cough. However, they have the disadvantage of being short acting.

Cloperastine and levocloperastine are useful in the treatment of dry cough particularly chronic cough.

Pharyngeal Demulcents

These drugs increase the flow of saliva which produces a soothing effect on the pharyngeal mucosa (*demulcere* = to caress soothingly—in Latin) and reduce afferent impulses arising from the irritated mucosa. Dry cough due to irritation of the pharyngeal mucosa is relieved. Candy sugar or a few drops of lemon also serve this purpose.

Expectorants

Expectorants (Latin—*expectorate* = to drive from the chest) increase the production of respiratory tract secretions which cover the irritated mucosa. As the secretions now become thin and less viscid, they can be easily coughed out. Expectorants may increase the secretions directly or reflexly.

Direct stimulants: Volatile oils like eucalyptus oil; creosotes, alcohol, cidar wood oil—when administered by inhalation with steam can increase respiratory secretions.

Reflex expectorants are given orally, they are gastric irritants and reflexly increase respiratory secretions.

Potassium iodide acts both directly and reflexly. **Ipecacuanha** is an emetic. In sub-emetic doses it is used as an expectorant.

Bronchodilators

Bronchodilators like salbutamol and terbutaline relieve cough that is resulting from bronchospasm.

The antitussive preparations generally have a combination of a central cough suppressant, an expectorant, an antihistaminic and sometimes a bronchodilator and a mucolytic agent.

Mucolytics

Normally the respiratory mucus is watery. The glycoproteins in the mucus are linked by disulfide bonds to form polymers making it slimy. In respiratory diseases, the glycoproteins form larger polymers with plasma proteins present in the exudate and the secretions become thick and viscid. Mucolytics liquefy the sputum making it less viscid so that it can be easily expectorated.

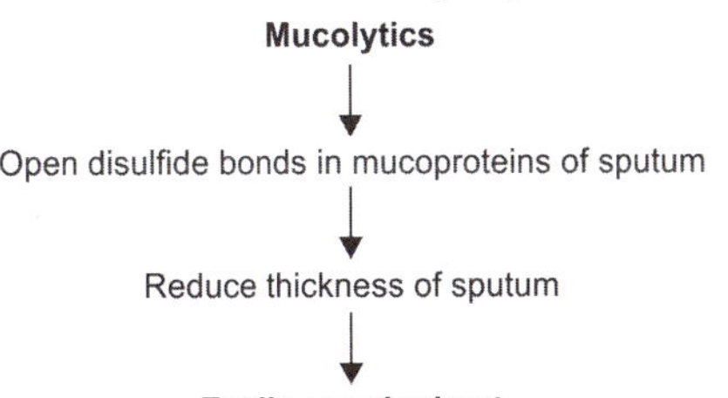

Bromhexine obtained from the plant *Adhatoda vasica* is a good mucolytic. It depolymerizes the mucopolysaccharides in the mucus. It is given orally (8-16 mg thrice daily). Side effects are minor—may cause rhinorrhea.

Ambroxol is a metabolite of bromhexine with actions similar to it. Ambroxol may be given orally by inhalation. It can be used as an alternative to bromhexine.

Acetylcysteine opens disulfide bonds in the mucoproteins of the sputum reducing its viscosity. It is given by aerosol. Side effects are common and hence not preferred.

Carbocysteine is similar to acetylcysteine and is used orally.

Pancreatic dornase—deoxyribonucleoprotein is a major component of the purulent respiratory tract secretions. Pancreatic dornase is a deoxyribonuclease obtained from the bovine pancreas. It breaks the deoxyribonucleic acid (DNA) into smaller parts thus making the secretions thin and less viscid. It is administered by inhalation.

Pancreatic dornase can cause allergic reactions.

Steam inhalation offers an effective and inexpensive alternative to drugs. In presence of dehydration, just rehydrating the patient is found to be beneficial.

DRUGS USED IN ALLERGIC RHINITIS

Allergic rhinitis is a common allergic condition with inflammation of the nasal mucous membrane due to allergic etiology. Rhinitis is triggered when allergens like dust, pollen or animal dander are inhaled. Hay fever is allergy to pollen. Typical symptoms include itching in the nose, eyes and throat, sneezing, nasal stuffiness, headache and rhinorrea (running nose).

Treatment

When the allergen is known, it is best to be avoided. Nasal wash with warm saline helps by washing away mucous and also prevents infection. Drugs used include:

Acute episode

1. **Antihistamines:** Like azelastine nasal spray twice a day relieves symptoms and can also be used prophylactically. Orally antihistamines are needed only in more severe cases for 2–3 days.
2. **Decongestants:** Oxymetazoline or xylometazoline nasal drops quickly relieve nasal blocks. However they should not be used over prolonged periods.
3. **Leukotriene antagonists:** Like montelukast and zafirlukast effectively relieve symptoms.

Prophylaxis

4. Cromolyn sodium nasal spray can be used for the prophylaxis of allergic rhinitis. Continued use over prolonged periods is needed.
5. **Glucocorticoids:** Budesonide or flunisolide nasal spray taken over several weeks effectively prevents allergic rhinitis.

9

CHAPTER

Gastrointestinal Tract

CHAPTER HIGHLIGHTS

- Drugs Used in Peptic Ulcer
- Prokinetic Agents
- Emetics and Antiemetics
- Drugs Used in the Treatment of Constipation
- Drugs Used in the Treatment of Diarrhea

DRUGS USED IN PEPTIC ULCER

Acid-peptic disease is common in the present days that are full of tension and anxiety. Peptic ulcer results from an imbalance between acid-pepsin secretion and mucosal defense. The factors that protect the mucosa are its ability to secrete mucous, bicarbonate and prostaglandins.

Gastric acid secretion is controlled by three pathways—vagus (ACh), gastrin and local release of histamine—each acting through its own receptors (Fig. 9.1). Histamine acts through H_2 receptors on parietal cells while acetylcholine through M_1 muscarinic and gastrin through G receptors on the parietal cells. These activate H^+ K^+ ATPase (proton pump) on the parietal cells resulting in the secretion of H^+ into the gastric lumen. This H^+ combines with Cl^- (drawn from plasma) and HCl is secreted.

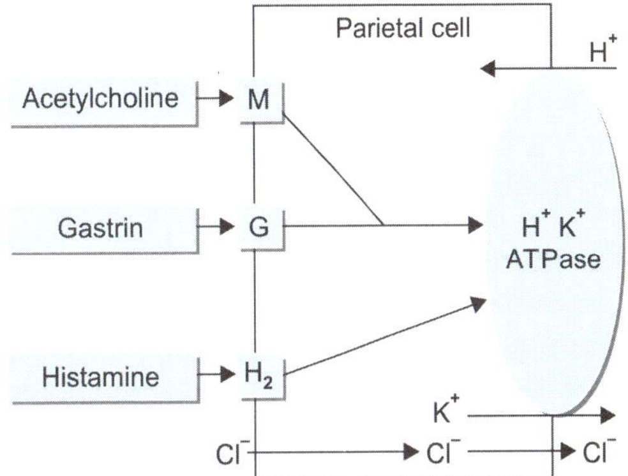

Fig. 9.1: Regulation of gastric secretion: M—Muscarinic receptor (M2/3); G—Gastrin receptors; H_2—Histamine H_2 receptor.

Classification

Drugs used in peptic ulcer may be classified as given in Flowchart 9.1.

Antacids

Antacids are basic substances. Given orally they neutralize the gastric acid and raise the pH of gastric contents. Peptic activity is also reduced because, pepsin is active only above pH 4. Antacids are of two types:

1. **Systemic:** Sodium bicarbonate
2. **Nonsystemic:** Aluminium hydroxide, magnesium trisilicate, magnesium hydroxide, calcium carbonate.

Systemic Antacids

Sodium bicarbonate is rapid but short-acting. CO_2 that is released in the stomach escapes as eructation. Sodium bicarbonate gets absorbed from the intestines leading to systemic alkalosis. There is 'rebound' hyperacidity as gastrin levels increase due to raised gastric pH. Sodium load may increase. It is not preferred because of the above disadvantages.

Uses

1. Sodium bicarbonate is used with other antacids in peptic ulcer.
2. To alkalinize the urine in poisoning
3. To treat metabolic acidosis.

Flowchart 9.1: Classification.

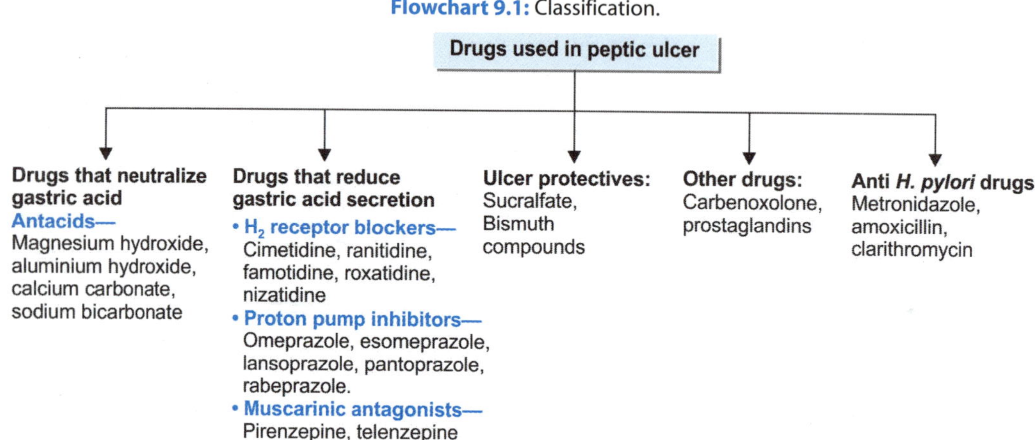

Non-systemic Antacids

Non-systemic antacids are insoluble compounds that react in the stomach with HCl to form a chloride salt and water. They are not absorbed.

Aluminium hydroxide is slow acting. Food further slows its neutralizing capacity. It is also an astringent and demulcent—forms a protective coating over the ulcers. The aluminium ions relax the smooth muscles resulting in delayed gastric emptying and constipation. Aluminium hydroxide binds phosphate and prevents its absorption resulting in hypophosphatemia on prolonged use.

Magnesium salts: The action is quick and prolonged. Rebound acidity is mild. Magnesium salts are osmotic purgatives and the dose used as antacids may cause mild diarrhea.

Calcium carbonate acts quickly and has prolonged action but liberates CO_2 which may cause discomfort. It may also cause constipation and hypercalcemia.

Combination of Antacids

Antacids are given in combination to obtain maximum effects with least adverse effects as follows:

- **Quick and prolonged effect:** Fast-acting [$Mg(OH)_2$] and slow acting [$Al(OH)_3$] are combined.
- **Neutralizing side effects:** Magnesium salts cause diarrhea while aluminium salts are constipating—combination neutralizes each other's side effects.
- **Gastric emptying:** Magnesium salts hasten while aluminium salts delay gastric emptying.

All antacid tablets should be chewed and swallowed as they do not disintegrate well in the stomach. Gels are more effective than tablets. One dose given 1 hr after food neutralizes the acid for 2 hours (Table 9.1).

Uses: Antacids are used in hyperacidity, peptic ulcer and reflux esophagitis.

Drug interactions: Antacids form complexes with iron, tetracyclines, digoxin, ranitidine, fluoroquinolones, sulfonamides and antimuscarinic drugs. To avoid these, antacids should be taken 2 hours before or 2 hours after other drugs.

H_2 receptor blockers: *Cimetidine, ranitidine, famotidine, roxatidine.*

Table 9.1: Some antacid combination preparations.

Brand name	*Combination*
Gelusil liquid, tablet	Aluminium hydroxide gel + Magnesium trisilicate
Digene gel, tablet	Magnesium hydroxide + Aluminium hydroxide gel + Carboxymethyl cellulose sodium + Methylpolysiloxane

These drugs bind to H_2 receptors and competitively inhibit the action of histamine on H_2 receptors and thereby reduce gastric secretion. Both volume and acidity of basal, nocturnal and food induced secretion are reduced. They can cause 60–70% reduction in gastric secretion by a single dose. Gastrin induced HCl secretion and pepsin are also reduced. Due to these actions, healing of peptic ulcers is faster.

Pharmacokinetics: H_2 blockers are well-absorbed. Cimetidine acts for 5–8 hours, ranitidine and famotidine for 12 hours.

Adverse effects: The H_2 blockers are well-tolerated with minor side effects like dizziness, diarrhea, muscle pain and headache. Because the H_2 receptors do not have any significant functions in other tissues except stomach, H_2 receptor blockers other than cimetidine are fairly selective and thereby safe drugs.

Cimetidine has antiandrogenic actions, it increases plasma prolactin levels and inhibits estrogen metabolism in the liver. On prolonged use it may result in gynecomastia, impotence and loss of libido. CNS effects include confusion, delirium and hallucinations in the elderly. Headache, dizziness, rashes and diarrhea can result. Cimetidine inhibits microsomal enzymes and interferes with the metabolism of many drugs.

Ranitidine is the preferred H_2 blocker as it has several advantages over cimetidine.

- Ranitidine is more potent
- Longer acting
- Has no antiandrogenic effects
- No CNS effects as it does not cross BBB
- Does not inhibit microsomal enzymes significantly.

Only adverse effects are headache and dizziness.

Famotidine and **Roxatidine** are similar to but more potent and longer-acting than ranitidine. Headache and rashes can occur.

Uses of H_2 Blockers

H_2 blockers are used in the treatment of:

1. **Peptic ulcer:** H_2 blockers bring about rapid relief from pain and ulcers heal in 6–8 weeks of treatment.
2. **Gastritis:** H_2 blockers are first-line drugs.
3. **GERD:** H_2 blockers are alternatives to PPIs.
4. **Preanesthetic medication:** To reduce gastric acid secretion and prevent damage to the respiratory mucosa if aspiration occurs during surgery.
5. **Zollinger-Ellison syndrome:** High doses of H_2 blockers are used as alternatives to PPIs.

Ranitidine is the most preferred. It is given for 4–8 weeks (300 mg daily) in peptic ulcers. It may be continued for 6 months to prevent recurrence.

Proton Pump Inhibitors

Proton pump inhibitors (PPI) are the most powerful inhibitors of gastric acid secretion.

Omeprazole was the first proton pump inhibitor (PPI) to be developed.

Mechanism of action: The parietal cells of the stomach secrete H^+ with the help of an enzyme $H^+ K^+$ ATPase (proton pump) present in the plasma membrane. This is the final step in gastric acid secretion. Proton pump inhibitors specifically inhibit this $H^+ K^+$ ATPase enzyme and thereby inhibit gastric secretion. Omeprazole is a **prodrug**,

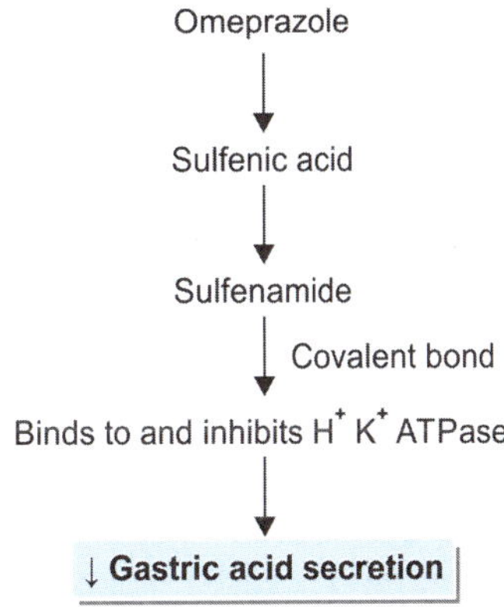

gets activated in the acidic environment of the stomach and a single dose can totally inhibit gastric secretion. Acid secretion starts only after new $H^+ K^+$ATPase enzyme is synthesized. Ulcer heals rapidly even in resistant cases.

Adverse effects: Omeprazole is well-tolerated. Prolonged acid suppression may allow bacterial overgrowth in the stomach. Dizziness, headache, arthralgia, nausea and rashes are rare.

Long-term administration may result in:

- Vitamin B_{12} deficiency due to its reduced absorption.
- ↑ gastrin levels.
- Also reduced absorption of calcium and iron
- Atrophic changes in the stomach—have been noticed after 3–4 years of use.
- Increased risk of osteoporosis.

Lansoprazole and esomeprazole are similar to omeprazole and are longer-acting.

Pantoprazole is more acid stable and an IV formulation is also available. It is the most commonly used PPI.

Rabeprazole has the fastest onset of action.

Uses of PPIs

- **Peptic ulcer:** Proton pump inhibitors are the drugs of choice in peptic ulcers. Ulcers heal fast and pain is relieved. They are given for 4–8 weeks.
- **Dyspepsia:** For non-ulcer dyspepsia including gastritis and hyperacidity, H_2 blockers are preferred but PPIs may also be used.
- **GERD:** Responds well to PPIs but require long-term use.
- ***H. pylori:*** PPIs also form a component in *H. pylori* treatment regimen.
- **Preanesthetic medication:** To reduce gastric acid secretion in the perioperative period, PPIs may be used.
- In **Zollinger-Ellison syndrome** - PPIs effectively reduce gastric acidity.

Anticholinergics: Though atropine reduces gastric secretion, the dose needed results in several adverse effects. A derivative of atropine—pirenzepine selectively blocks muscarinic (M_1) receptors present in the stomach and inhibits gastric secretion without much side effects. It also inhibits the secretion of gastrin, mucus and bicarbonate. It is used as an adjuvant.

Ulcer Protectives

Sucralfate: In acidic medium ($pH < 4$), sucralfate polymerizes to form a sticky, viscid gel which firmly sticks to the base of the ulcers and covers the ulcers. It remains there for over 6 hours acting as a physical block and prevents contact with acid and pepsin. It also stimulates the PG synthesis in gastric mucosa. It thus promotes healing by protecting the ulcer. Sucralfate is not absorbed and is well-tolerated.

One tablet is given 1 hr before each meal and one at bed time for 4–8 weeks and then it is continued for 6 months to prevent recurrence.

Side effects are rare and include constipation and dryness of mouth.

Drug Interactions

- Sucralfate needs acidic pH for activation. Hence antacids should not be given with it.
- Sucralfate adsorbs and interferes with the absorption of tetracyclines, digoxin, phenytoin and cimetidine.

Bismuth salts: Colloidal bismuth subcitrate on oral administration forms complexes with proteins in the ulcer base and forms a protective coating over the gastric mucosa. It also inhibits the growth of *H. pylori* on gastric mucosa and stimulates the mucus production and PG synthesis. By these actions it promotes ulcer healing in 4–8 weeks. It may cause constipation and black stools.

Other Drugs

Prostaglandins: PGE_2 and PGI_2 synthesized by the gastric mucosa inhibits gastric secretion, enhances mucous production and exerts a protective effect. PG analogs misoprostol and enprostil are of special value in preventing drug induced (e.g. NSAIDs) gastric ulceration. Diarrhea and muscle cramps are common.

Treatment of H. pylori Infection

Infection with *H. pylori* is associated with gastroduodenal disease including gastritis and peptic ulcer. It is also thought to be responsible for recurrence of peptic ulcer disease. Eradication of *H. pylori* along with reduction of acid secretion has shown to reduce the relapse rate.

Various combination regimens are tried with clarithromycin, amoxicillin or tetracycline; metronidazole and omeprazole for 1-2 weeks.

One week regimen:

1. Clarithromycin 250 mg + Metronidazole 400 mg + Omeprazole 20 mg—All BD.
2. Amoxicillin 1000 mg + Tinidazole 500 mg + Lansoprazole—30 mg—All OD.

Two weeks regimen:

1. Amoxicillin 750 mg + Tinidazole 500 mg + Omeprazole 20 mg—All BD.
2. Amoxicillin 1000 mg + Clarithromycin 500 mg + Lansoprazole 30 mg—All BD.

PROKINETIC AGENTS

Drugs that increase gastroduodenal motility and the rate of gastric emptying are called **prokinetic agents. Metoclopramide, domperidone, cisapride mosapride, itopride** and **prucalopride** are some prokinetic agents.

Metoclopramide

Actions GIT: Metoclopramide tightens the lower esophageal sphinter, promotes forward movement of contents of the upper GI tract, speeds up gastric emptying, prevents reflux esophagitis and also slightly increases intestinal peristalsis.

CNS: Metoclopramide acts as an antiemetic by its actions on the CTZ and by speeding up gastric emptying.

Mechanism of action: Metoclopramide acts

- By blocking the dopamine receptors in the gut.
- By increasing acetylcholine release from the cholinergic neurons in the gut.
- By blocking the D_2 receptors in the CTZ—responsible for antiemetic actions.

Adverse effects are sedation, dystonia and diarrhea; gynecomastia, galactorrhea and parkinsonism (extrapyramidal symptoms) can occur on long-term use due to blockade of dopamine receptors.

Uses

1. **Reflux esophagitis**—'heart burn' due to reflux of acid into the esophagus is benefited by prokinetic agents.
2. **As antiemetics**—in postoperative period and vomiting due to anticancer drugs.
3. **As preanesthetic medication** to promote gastric emptying before induction of general anesthesia in emergency.
4. **In endoscopy**—to assist passage of tubes into the duodenum.

Domperidone is similar to metoclopramide and has the advantage that it does not cross the blood-brain barrier and hence does not cause extrapyramidal side effects. Side effects include headache, dryness of mouth, diarrhea and rashes.

Domperidone can be used in place of metoclopramide.

Cisapride increases gastric and colonic motility by promoting the release of acetylcholine in the gut wall. It is now **banned** due to cardiac adverse effects.

Mosapride and **itopride** are similar to cisapride but does not cause cardiac adverse effects.

They are used as prokinetic agents n reflux esophagitis.

Gastroesophageal reflux disease (GERD): Reflux of acidic gastric contents into the esophagus results in 'heart burn' due to esophagitis. Based on severity, it may be treated with antacids, metoclopramide or drugs that reduce acid secretion like ranitidine and proton pump inhibitors. Omeprazole is the most effective agent. Avoiding—heavy meals, late night dinner, smoking and alcohol—all help.

EMETICS AND ANTIEMETICS

Stimulation of the vomiting center in the medulla oblongata results in vomiting. The vomiting center receives afferents from the chemoreceptor trigger zone (CTZ), vestibular apparatus, GI tract and centers in the brain. CTZ is not protected by the blood-brain barrier and is stimulated by various drugs, chemicals and radiation.

Emetics are drugs that produce vomiting. When a noxious or poisonous substance is swallowed, vomiting has to be induced. Mustard powder (1 teaspoon) with water or hypertonic salt solution can evoke vomiting.

Apomorphine is a derivative of morphine. Given SC/IM, it produces vomiting in 5–10 minutes. It acts by stimulating the CTZ.

Ipecacuanha contains an alkaloid emetine. Given as a syrup (15–20 mL), it produces vomiting in 15 minutes. It is safe even in children.

Antiemetics

Vomiting is a protective mechanism which tries to eliminate the unwanted harmful material from the stomach. But in some situations, vomiting may not serve any useful purpose and may only be troublesome. In such circumstances, vomiting needs to be suppressed with drugs.

Antiemetics are drugs that are used to prevent or control vomiting.

Classification

1. **5HT$_3$ antagonists:** Ondansetron, granisetron, dolasetron, tropisetron.
2. **Dopamine D$_2$ antagonists—prokinetics:** Metoclopramide, domperidone.
3. **Antimuscarinics:** Hyoscine, H$_1$ antihistamines like cyclizine, promethazine, diphenhydramine.
4. **Neuroleptics:** Chlorpromazine, prochlorperazine, haloperidol.
5. **Other agents**
   Cannabinoids: Dronabinol
   Neurokinin receptor antagonists: Aprepitant, fosaprepitant
   Glucocorticoids: Prednisolone.

5-HT$_3$ Antagonists

Ondansetron 5-hydroxytryptamine released in the gut is an important transmitter of emesis. Ondansetron blocks 5-HT$_3$ receptors in the GI tract and CTZ and prevents vomiting. It is a powerful antiemetic and can be given orally or intravenously (4–8 mg).

Adverse effects: All 5-HT$_3$ antagonists are well tolerated with minor adverse effects like headache, constipation, abdominal discomfort and rashes.

Granisetron and **dolasetron** are more potent than ondansetron as antiemetics and are longer-acting.

Uses

1. **Anticancer drug-induced vomiting**—to control vomiting induced by anticancer drugs and radiotherapy.
2. **Postoperative nausea and vomiting**—ondensetron is used as preanesthetic medication. It can also be used to treat postoperative vomiting.
3. **Drug induced vomiting**—many drugs can cause vomiting and ondensetron is useful But it is not effective in traveling sickness.
4. **Morning sickness**—Ondensetron has been used in the treatment of nausea and vomiting during pregnancy and studies have shown it to be safe.

Dopamine D$_2$ Antagonists

Metoclopramide acts centrally by blocking the dopamine D$_2$ receptors in the CTZ.

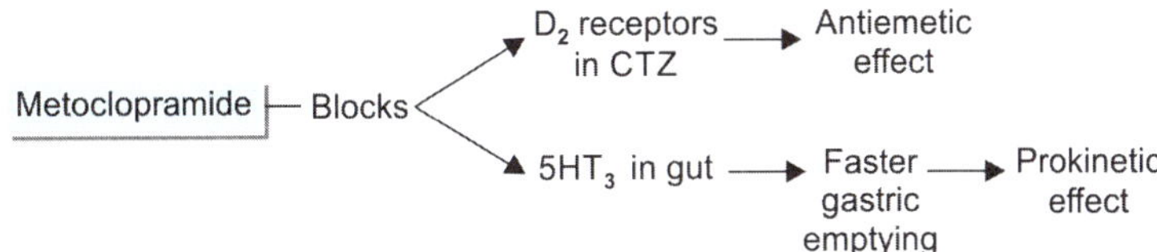

In higher doses, it also blocks the $5HT_3$ receptors in the gut. It increases the tone of the lower esophageal sphincter and increases gastric peristalsis (prokinetic). It is used in nausea and vomiting due to gastrointestinal disorders, migraine, in postoperative period and vomiting due to anticancer drugs and radiotherapy.

Domperidone acts like metoclopramide with less side effects because it does not cross the blood brain brain.

Antimuscarinics

Hyosine is very effective in motion sickness. Motion sickness or traveling sickness is due to overstimulation of the vestibular apparatus along with psychological and environmental factors. Taken 30 minutes before journey, hyoscine (0.4–0.6 mg oral) acts for 6 hours and the dose should be repeated if the journey is longer than that. A transdermal patch delivers hyoscine constantly over 3 days and is to be applied behind the ear. Sedation and dry mouth are common side effects.

Dicyclomine is used to control vomiting in morning sickness and motion sickness (Table 9.2).

Table 9.2: Preferred drugs for vomiting due to various causes.

Conditions	*Drugs*
Motion sickness	Hyoscine, cyclizine, promethazine, cinnarizine
Vomiting due to anticancer drugs	Ondansetron + Dexamethasone + Aprepitant
Vomiting due to other drugs	Chlorpromazine, metoclopramide
Postoperative vomiting	Ondansetron, metoclopramide
Vomiting in pregnancy	Dicyclomine, pyridoxine, cyclizine, meclizine, metoclopramide

H_1 antihistamines like promethazine, diphenhydramine, cyclizine and cinnarizine have anticholinergic properties. They may act both centrally and on the GI tract. They are useful in motion sickness and postoperative vomiting.

Neuroleptics

Neuroleptics block D_2-receptors in the CTZ (*See* page 171) are useful in vomiting due to most causes except motion sickness. Sedation and extrapyramidal symptoms are the common side effects. **Prochlorperazine** is mainly used as an antiemetic in vomiting and is also effective in vertigo associated with vomiting.

Other Drugs

Cannabinoids-dronabinol, a cannabinoid acts as an antiemetic by stimulation of cannabinoid receptors in the vomiting center. Dronabinol is used in combination with other antiemetics for prevention of anticancer drugs-induced vomiting.

Neurokinin receptor antagonists: *Aprepitant* and *fosaprepitant* bind to and block neurokinin receptors in the area postrema and act as antiemetics. They are used for prevention of chemotherapy-induced vomiting in combination with other drugs.

Glucocorticoids are used as adjuvants along with other antiemetics like ondansetron or metoclopramide.

DRUGS USED IN THE TREATMENT OF CONSTIPATION

Purgatives are drugs that promote defecation. They are also called **laxatives** and **cathartics**. Laxatives have milder action while cathartics or purgatives have more powerful action.

Classification

1. **Bulk laxatives**
   Bran, plantago seeds, agar, methylcellulose, ispaghula husk.
2. **Fecal softeners**
   Docusate sodium, liquid paraffin (emollients).
3. **Osmotic purgatives**
   Magnesium sulfate, Magnesium hydroxide, Sodium sulfate, Sodium phosphate, Lactulose, Polyethylene glycol.
4. **Stimulant purgatives**
   Phenolphthalein, bisacodyl, castor oil, anthraquinones—cascara sagrada, senna.

Bulk Laxatives

Bulk laxatives include vegetable fiber and other substances that are not digested but increase the volume of intestinal contents forming a large, soft, solid stool. Dietary fiber consists of cell walls and other parts of fruits and vegetables that are unabsorbable. Adding fiber to the diet is a safe and natural way of treating constipation in persons who are on low-fiber diet.

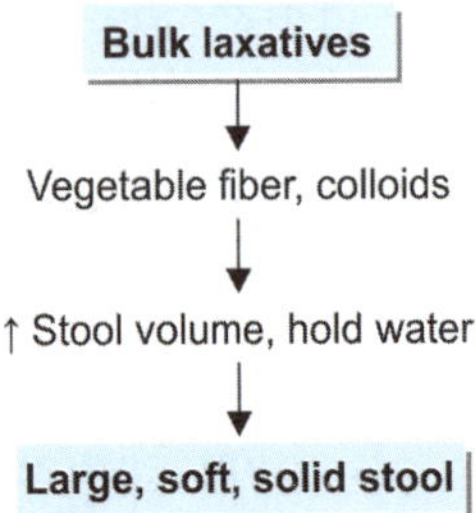

Bran is the residue left when flour is made from cereals and contains 40 percent fiber—but is unpalatable.

Ispaghula and **plantago seeds** contain natural mucilage which absorbs water to form a gelatinous mass and are more palatable than bran. **Methylcellulose** is a semisynthetic derivative of cellulose. Adequate water should be taken along with bulk laxatives.

Fecal Softeners

Docusate sodium (dioctyl sodium sulfosuccinate) softens feces by lowering the surface tension of the intestinal contents. This allows more water to be retained in the feces which becomes soft.

Liquid paraffin is a mineral oil that is not digested. It lubricates and softens feces. It is unpalatable; aspiration may cause lipoid pneumonia; it may leak out of the anus causing discomfort. Hence not preferred.

Osmotic Purgatives

Osmotic purgatives are solutes that are not absorbed in the intestine, osmotically retain water and increase the bulk of intestinal contents. They increase peristalsis and expel a fluid stool. Magnesium hydroxide, magnesium sulfate, sodium potassium tartrate, sodium sulfate and phosphate are some inorganic salts used as osmotic or saline purgatives. They are used to prepare the bowel before surgery and in food poisoning.

Osmotic purgatives (solutes)
↓
Not absorbed in intestine
↓
Retain water by osmosis
↓
↑ Bulk of intestinal contents
↓
↑ Peristalsis
↓
Soft stools

Lactulose is a synthetic disaccharide that is not absorbed (nonabsorbable sugar), holds water and acts as an osmotic purgative. Flatulence and cramps may be accompanied. In the colon, lactulose is fermented to lactic and acetic acids which inhibit the growth of ammonia-producing bacteria in the colon. It also inhibits the absorption of ammonia by lowering pH and thus lowers blood ammonia levels. It is used in hepatic coma for this effect (hepatic coma is worsened by ammonia).

Polyethylene glycol is a nonabsorbable sugar which is taken with water for chronic constipation. It has the advantage that there are no abdominal cramps or flatulence.

Stimulant Purgatives

Stimulant purgatives increase intestinal motility and increase the secretion of water and electrolytes by the mucosa. They may cause abdominal cramps.

When **cascara sagrada** and **senna** (source: plants) are given orally, active anthraquinones are liberated in the intestines which stimulate the myenteric plexus in the colon. Evacuation takes 6–8 hours. Long-term use causes melanotic pigmentation of the colon.

Phenolphthalein: Phenolphthalein an indicator used in laboratories, acts on the colon after 6–8 hours to produce soft, semiliquid stools. It undergoes enterohepatic circulation which prolongs its actions. Allergic reactions including pink colored skin eruptions and colic limit its use.

Bisacodyl: Bisacodyl related to phenolphthalein is converted to the active metabolite in the intestines. It can be given orally (5 mg) but usually is used as rectal suppositories (10 mg) which results in defecation in 15–30 minutes. It is safe except that prolonged use may cause local inflammation.

Opioid Antagonists

Opioid induced constipation can be troublesome in cancer patients and other terminally ill patients who are receiving opioids for pain relief. **Methylnaltrexone** and **alvimopan** are opioid antagonists which block the opioid receptors in the gut. They do not cross the BBB and therefore do not antagonize the analgesic effects of opioids.

Enema

Enema produces defecation by softening stools and distending the bowel. Evacuant enema is used to prepare the gut for surgery, endoscopy and radiological examination (*See* page 5).

Use of Laxatives in Constipation

Fiber rich diet, adequate fluid intake and physical activity are the best measures to prevent and treat mild constipation. If these measures are inadequate, a laxative may be given (Table 9.3).

Table 9.3: Choice of purgatives.

Conditions	*Preferred laxative*
Functional constipation	Increasing dietary fiber and adequate fluid intake
Elderly patients	Increasing dietary fiber and adequate fluid intake
Pregnancy	Dietary fiber
To avoid straining at stools—as in hernia, piles, fissure, cardiovascular diseases like myocardial infarction	Bulk laxatives or fecal softeners
Irritable bowel syndrome—chronic constipation	Bulk laxatives
Food or drug poisoning	Osmotic purgatives
Bowel preparation before surgery, endoscopy and radiological examination	Bisacodyl, osmotic purgatives

Drug Induced Constipation

Drugs like anticholinergics, NSAIDs, opioids, clonidine, iron, calcium channel blockers and antihistamines can cause constipation. When withdrawal of the causative drug is not possible, a laxative may be used.

Laxative Abuse

Habitual use of laxatives, especially stimulant laxatives may lead to various gastrointestinal disturbances like irritable bowel syndrome, loss of electrolytes, loss of calcium in the stool and malabsorption. Misconceptions regarding bowel habits should be cleared. The patient should be convinced that normal bowel habits may vary between 3 motions daily and 2 motions per week.

DRUGS USED IN THE TREATMENT OF DIARRHEA

Diarrhea is the frequent passage of liquid stools. It can be due to a variety of causes like infection, toxins, anxiety and drugs. Acute diarrhea is one of the major causes of death in infants specially in the developing countries. Death is due to dehydration.

In diarrhea, there is an increase in motility and secretions in the gut with absorption of water and electrolytes. Hence the approaches in the treatment of diarrhea include:

1. Replacement of fluid and electrolytes.
2. Treatment of the cause.
3. Antidiarrheal agents.

1. **Replacement of fluid and electrolytes:** Can be life saving in most cases especially infants. Oral rehydration with sodium chloride, glucose and water is useful. In the ileum, glucose increases sodium absorption and water follows. Oral rehydration powders are available. They are to be mixed with water and given in small amounts every 15–20 minutes for mild to moderate cases. When ready ORS powders are not available, a pinch (5g) of table salt and 1 tablespoon (20 grams) of sugar dissolved in 1 litre of boiled and cooled water may be used. In severe degrees of dehydration, prompt intravenous rehydration is necessary (Table 9.4).

2. **Treatment of the cause:** Acute diarrhea could often be due to viral, bacterial or protozoal infection. The pathogen should be identified whenever possible and treated accordingly.

Gastroenteritis is often due to virus and does not require antibiotics. Mild bacterial gastroenteritis also subsides by itself but some infections like typhoid, cholera and amoebic dysentery need antibiotics. Antimicrobials like norfloxacin, furazolidone are effective.

Table 9.4: Composition of oral rehydration salt/solution (ORS).

Sodium chloride	—	3.5 g
Potassium chloride	—	1.5 g
Sodium citrate	—	2.9 g
Glucose	—	20 g
To be dissolved in 1 liter of boiled and cooled water		

WHO–ORS New Formula

ORS with lower osmolality has improved efficacy with reduction in the incidence of vomiting and stool volume. WHO and UNICEF have therefore recommended new modified ORS solution with 245 mOsm/L osmolarity in place of the standard preparation (310 mOsm/L) with a decreased concentration of sodium and glucose.

Disadvantage: It can cause hyponatremia in adults suffering from cholera.

The contents are as follows:

New formula		
Sodium chloride	:	2.6 g
Potassium chloride	:	1.5 g
Trisodium citrate	:	2.9 g
Glucose	:	13.5 g
Water	:	1 L
Total osmolarity	:	245 mOsm/L

Super ORS: Amino acids are added which could promote sodium absorption. They are expensive and the benefit provided is marginal. Studies have shown that boiled rice powder 40–50 g/L is a good and simple glucose supplement. Since the rice also has some proteins (7%), it is a source of amino acids which stimulates the absorption of salt and water. The starch content adds to the calories. Rice is easily available, relatively inexpensive and has good efficacy—rice based ORS may be preferred particularly in developing countries. Wheat, maize or potato may be used instead of rice.

Uses of ORS

i. Diarrhea
ii. For rehydration as in heatstroke
iii. Burns
iv. Following surgery or trauma

3. **Antidiarrheal drugs** afford symptomatic relief and include:

i. **Adsorbants**

Kaolin, pectin, chalk, activated charcoal

ii. **Antimotility drugs**
Opioids—codiene, diphenoxylate, loperamide
iii. **Others**
Racecadotril, lactobacillus preparations, octreotide
iv. **Antispasmodics**
Dicyclomine (atropine derivatives), drotaverine.

Adsorbents

They include kaolin, pectin, chalk and activated charcoal. These adsorb intestinal toxins and microorganisms by coating them. They are not absorbed and have not many side effects.

Antimotility Drugs (Table 9.5)

Codeine an opium alkaloid, stimulates the opioid receptors on the gastrointestinal smooth muscles to reduce peristalsis. This delays passage of intestinal contents and facilitates absorption of water. Nausea and vomiting may occur.

Diphenoxylate is an opioid related to pethidine. It is given with a small dose of atropine in order to discourage abuse. In therapeutic doses CNS effects are not prominent-hence no risk of abuse. It is used only in diarrheas. Nausea, drowsiness and abdominal pain may occur.

Loperamide is an opiate. It has selective action on GI tract with additional antisecretory action. CNS effects are negligible. It is less sedating, less addicting and is the most commonly used antimotility drug. Its low solubility in water discourages abuse by injection.

Loperamide may cause nausea, vomiting and abdominal cramps. Loperamide use has resulted in paralytic ileus and several fatalities are reported in children. Hence loperamide is contraindicated in children below 4 years of age.

Uses of antimotility drugs:
- Symptomatic treatment of non-infective diarrhea
- For traveller's diarrhea (as adjuvant).

Table 9.5: Antimotility drugs—some preparations and dosage.

Drugs	*Trade names*	*Doses*
Diphenoxylate 2.5 mg + Atropine 0.025 mg	LOMOTIL	2–4 tablets stat; 1 every 6 hours
Loperamide	LOPESTAL	4 mg stat; 2 mg every 6 hours

Other Drugs

Racecadotril: Enkephelins are endogenous opioids which have antisecretory activity in the intestines. Racecadotril, a newly introduced antidiarrheal agent, is a prodrug and the active metabolite selectively inhibits enkephelinase which degrades enkephalins. Racecadotril, thereby enhances the activity of enkephelins in the gut and the peripheral tissues. It is well tolerated with minor adverse effects like drowsiness, skin rashes, nausea and flatulence. Racecadotril, is useful in the symptomatic treatment of acute secretory diarrhea.

Lactobacillus acidophilus and **lactobacillus sporogenes** are available as powders and tablets and are useful in some diarrheas. They promote the growth of saccharolytic flora and alter the gut pH so that the growth of pathogenic micro organisms is inhibited. They are called 'probiotics' and are found to be useful in reducing the incidence of antibiotic induced diarrhea. Curds and buttermilk are cheaper alternatives.

Antispasmodics

Dicyclomine and propantheline are atropine derivatives which relax gastrointestinal smooth muscles and relieve abdominal colics.

Drotaverine relaxes gastrointestinal and other smooth muscles and therefore can be used as an antispasmodic in renal, biliary and intestinal colic and in dysmenorrhea.

Traveler's diarrhea: Infection is the most common cause of traveller's diarrhea and should be treated with suitable antimicrobials. Oral rehydration salts and loperamide may also be used.

10

CHAPTER

Hormones

CHAPTER HIGHLIGHTS

- Hypothalamus and Anterior Pituitary Hormones
- Thyroid Hormones and Antithyroid Drugs
- Insulin and Oral Antidiabetics
- Androgens and Anabolic Steroids
- Estrogens, Progestins and Hormonal Contraceptives

HYPOTHALAMUS AND ANTERIOR PITUITARY HORMONES

The pituitary gland, under the influence of the hypothalamus secretes many hormones which either control the secretion of other glands or directly act on the target tissues. These are peptides and act by binding to specific receptors present on the target cells (Table 10.1).

Hypothalamic Hormones

Growth hormone releasing hormone (GHRH): It stimulates the anterior pituitary to secrete growth hormone. **Somatostatin** is growth hormone release inhibiting hormone and it inhibits the secretion of growth hormones (GH), thyroid stimulating hormone (TSH), prolactin, insulin, glucagon and the gastrointestinal (GI) secretions.

Octreotide is the synthetic somatostatin which is useful in acromegaly, some hormone secreting tumors and in bleeding esophageal varices.

Thyrotropin releasing hormone (TRH) secreted by the hypothalamus stimulates the release of TSH from the anterior pituitary.

Gonadotropin releasing hormone (GnRH) regulates the secretion of gonadotropins - FSH and LH. GnRH is used in infertility and delayed puberty.

GnRH antagonists: Cetrorelix, ganirelix, abarelix, degarelix suppress the secretion of LH, FSH and delay ovulation. They are used in *in vitro* fertilization and are also useful in prostatic cancer and in reducing uterine fibroids and endometriosis.

Anterior Pituitary Hormones

Growth hormone (GH) stimulates the growth of all organs except brain and eye. It increases the uptake of amino acids by the tissues, promotes protein synthesis and positive nitrogen balance. It causes lipolysis and reduces glucose uptake by skeletal muscles. It brings about linear growth. These anabolic actions are mediated by *somatomedins* or *insulin-like growth factors* (IGF) produced in the liver.

The secretion of growth hormone is regulated by growth hormone-releasing hormone (GHRH) and somatostatin [growth hormone release-inhibiting hormone (GHRIH)].

GH deficiency in children results in *dwarfism* while excessive production results in *gigantism* in children and *acromegaly* in adults.

Uses

- **GH deficiency:** Replacement therapy with GH in deficient children brings about normal growth. It can also be used in GH deficient adults.
- **Other conditions:** GH has been tried in chronic renal failure and in catabolic states like severe burns and AIDS. It is

Table 10.1: Hormones secreted by the hypothalamus and anterior pituitary and their chief functions.

Hypothalamic hormone	*Anterior pituitary hormone*	*Chief actions*
1. a Growth hormone releasing hormone (GHRH)	Growth hormone (GH)	Regulates growth
b. Growth hormone release-inhibiting hormone (GHRIH) (somatostatin)	—	Inhibits GH release
2. Corticotropin releasing hormone (CRH)	Corticotropin (ACTH)	Stimulates adrenal cortex to secrete glucocorticoids, mineralocorticoids and androgens
3. Thyrotropin–releasing hormone (TRH)	Thyroid-stimulating hormone (TSH, thyrotropin)	Stimulates release of T_3 and T_4
4. Gonadotrophin releasing hormone (GnRH, gonadorelin)	• Follicle stimulating hormone (FSH) • Luteinizing hormone (LH) or interstitial cell stimulating hormone (ICSH)	Stimulates growth of ovum and graafian follicle in the female and gametogenesis in the male; stimulates ovulation in females and regulates testosterone secretion in males
5. Prolactin–releasing factor	Prolactin (PRL)	Development of breast and lactation
6. Prolactin-release inhibiting factor (dopamine)	—	Inhibits prolactin-release
7. Melanocyte stimulating hormone releasing factor	Melanocyte stimulating hormone	Promotes melanin synthesis causing darkening of skin, also regulates feeding

liable for abuse in athletes to promote growth.

Corticotropin (Adrenocorticotropic hormone, ACTH)—controls the synthesis and release of glucocorticoids, mineralocorticoids, and androgens from the adrenal cortex. It is used in the diagnosis of adrenocortical insufficiency.

Thyroid-stimulating hormone (TSH, Thyrotropin) Thyrotropin stimulates the production and secretion of thyroid hormones and thus regulates the thyroid function. It is used to test thyroid function and to increase the uptake of radioactive iodine in thyroid carcinoma.

Gonadotropins: Follicle stimulating hormone (FSH) and **luteinizing hormone (LH)**—produced by the anterior pituitary regulate gonadal function. They stimulate follicular development in women and also stimulate ovarian steroidogenesis (estrogens and progesterone synthesis). In men they promote spermatogenesis.

Uses: 'Menotropins' is the combination of FSH and LH obtained from urine of postmenopausal women (Table 10.1).

Prolactin

This peptide hormone promotes the growth and development of breast during pregnancy. It stimulates milk production along with other hormones like estrogens and progestins. Deficiency results in lactation failure while excess prolactin results in galactorrhea.

Regulation of secretion: Suckling is the principal stimulus for prolactin secretion. Suckling stimulates the release of prolactin-releasing factor from hypothalamus. Estrogens and dopamine antagonists also stimulate prolactin-release. Prolactin is not used clinically.

Dopamine agonists like bromocriptine inhibit prolactin-release.

Bromocriptine is an ergot derivative with dopamine agonistic properties.

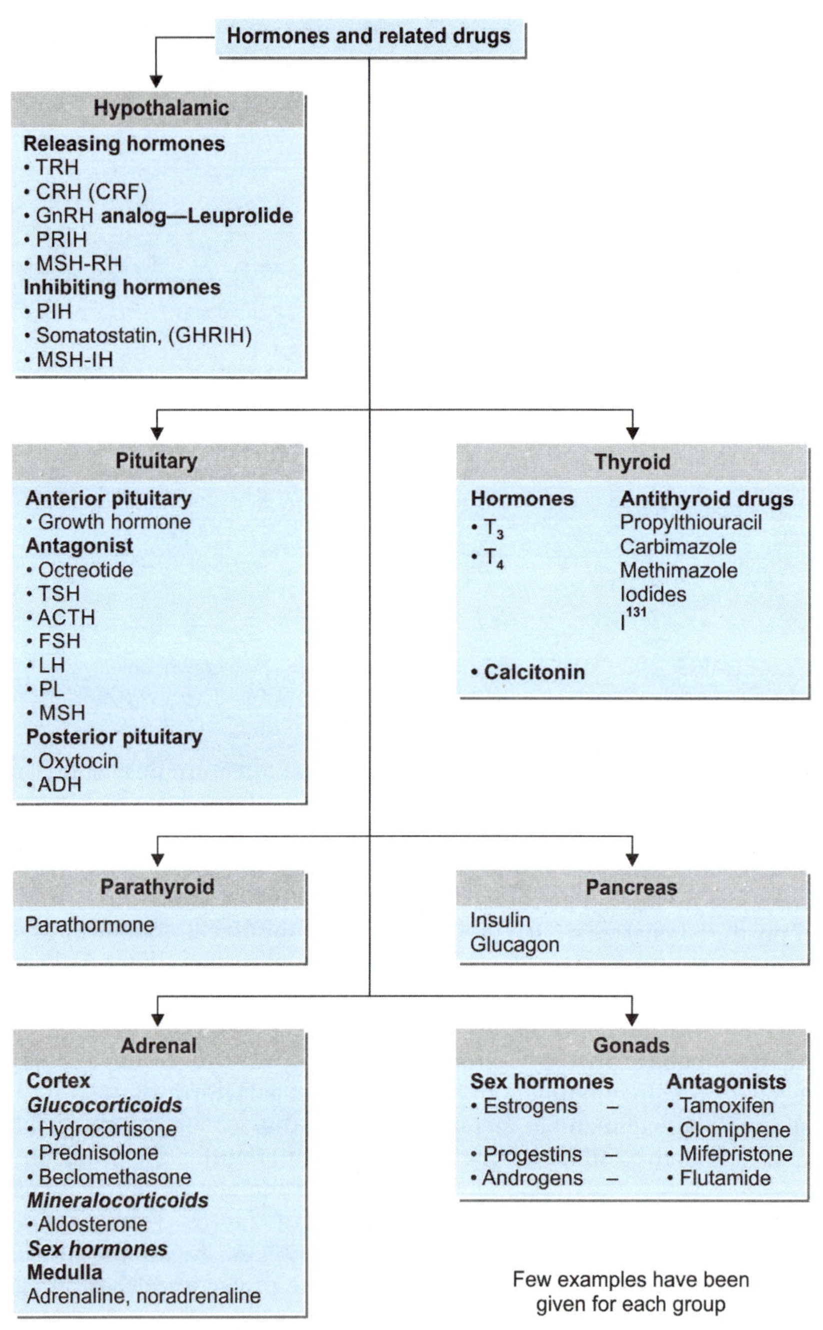

Bromocriptine uses:

1. To suppress lactation and breast engorgement after delivery (like in stillbirth) and following abortion.
2. In galactorrhea—due to excess prolactin.
3. Prolactin secreting tumors.
4. Parkinsonism—bromocriptine is used with levodopa.

THYROID HORMONES AND ANTITHYROID DRUGS

Thyroxine (T_4) and triiodothyronine (T_3) are the hormones secreted by the thyroid gland. T_4 is a less active precursor of T_3.

Synthesis, storage and secretion: The thyroid hormones are synthesized and stored in the thyroid follicles. The principle source of iodine is diet.

The hormones T_4 and T_3 are released into the circulation and the secretion is regulated by thyroid-stimulating hormone (TSH) secreted by the anterior pituitary and thyrotropin-releasing hormone (TRH) from the hypothalamus (Fig. 10.1). In the peripheral tissues, most of the secreted T_4 is converted to T_3 which is the active hormone.

Actions: Thyroid hormones are essential for normal growth, development, function and maintenance of all body tissues. Congenital deficiency results in cretinism. Thyroid hormones have important metabolic functions—they increase metabolic rate, enhance carbohydrate and protein metabolism and stimulate lipolysis. They facilitate erythropoiesis, are essential for normal functioning of the CNS (mental retardation is seen in cretinism), skeletal muscles, cardiovascular system, reproductive system and gastrointestinal system (hypothyroid patients are constipated while hyperthyroid have diarrhea).

Uses

1. **Replacement therapy:**
   a. **In cretinism,** treatment should be started immediately to avoid mental retardation. Replacement should be continued lifelong.
   b. **Hypothyroidism in adults** can be reversed by appropriate treatment.
   c. **Myxedema coma** is a medical emergency. IV thyroxine or liothyronine should be given with prophylactic corticosteroids to avoid adrenal insufficiency.

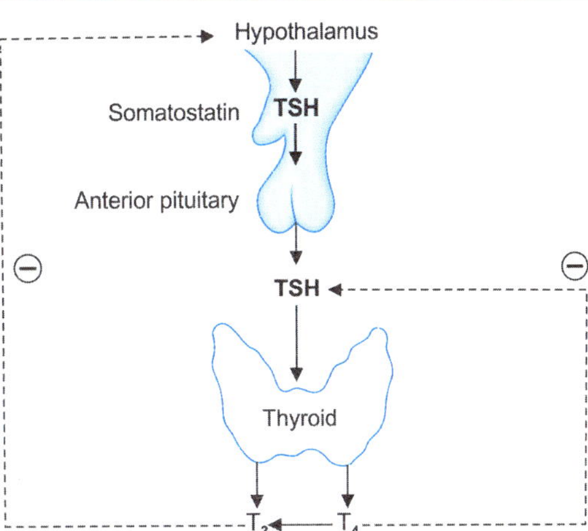

Fig. 10.1: Regulation of throid hormone secretion.

2. **Non-toxic goiter:** T_4 suppresses TSH production and the goiter regresses.
3. **Thyroid carcinoma:** T_4 induces temporary remission. It is used after surgery.
4. **Miscellaneous:** Thyroxine is tried in refractory anemias, infertility and non-healing ulcers.

Hyperthyroidism and Antithyroid Drugs

Hyperthyroidism is due to an excess of circulating thyroid hormones and could be due to various causes. Graves' disease, an autoimmune disorder, is the most common cause. It is characterized by hyperthyroidism, diffuse goiter and IgG antibodies that activate TSH receptors. Antithyroid drugs may act by interfering with the synthesis, release or actions of thyroid hormones.

Drugs used in Hyperthyroidism

1. **Antithyroid drugs:**
   Thionamides—Propylthiouracil, methimazole, carbimazole.
2. Iodine, Iodides and radioactive iodine.

Thionamides (thioureylenes)

Propylthiouracil, methimazole and carbimazole are thionamides or thioureylenes which act by inhibiting the synthesis of thyroid hormones. Propylthiouracil also inhibits peripheral conversion of T_4 to T_3. T_3 and T_4 levels fall. Adverse effects are allergic reactions, jaundice, headache and rarely granulocytopenia.

Uses: Hyperthyroidism—antithyroid drugs are used in hyperthyroidism.

1. **Graves' disease** or diffuse toxic goiter needs long term (1-15 years) treatment with antithyroid drugs.
2. **Toxic nodular goiter:** As an alternative—when surgery cannot be done as in case of the elderly patients.
3. **Preoperatively:** Hyperthyroid patients are made euthyroid with antithyroid drugs and then operated.

Iodides inhibit the release of thyroid hormones and in thyrotoxic patients the symptoms subside in 1-2 days. The gland becomes firm, less vascular and shrinks in size over a period of 10-14 days. These effects are transient and decrease after 15 days.

Adverse effects include allergic reactions like skin rashes, conjunctivitis, swelling of the lips and salivary glands, fever and lymphadenopathy. Chronic overdose can cause *iodism* with metallic taste, excessive salivation, lacrimation, running nose, sore throat, cough and rashes.

Uses

1. **Preoperative preparation for thyroidectomy:** Iodine is started just 10 days prior to surgery to make the thyroid gland firm and less vascular.
2. **Severe thyrotoxicosis/thyroid storm:** Iodides act rapidly to reduce the release of thyroid hormones.
3. **Prophylaxis:** Iodide or iodate is added to salt used in cooking to prevent endemic goiter.
4. **Antiseptic**
5. **Expectorant:** Iodine and potassium iodide are used in cough syrups.

Radioactive iodine ^{131}I given orally as a solution is rapidly absorbed and is concentrated by the thyroid in the follicles. It emits β rays which penetrate only 0.5 mm to 2 mm of the tissue so that it destroys only the thyroid tissue without damaging the surrounding structures.

It is used in the treatment of hyperthyroidism and in thyroid carcinoma. Small dose is also used for diagnostic purpose in thyroid function tests.

Advantages of ^{131}I are:

- Administration is simple
- Convenient
- Surgery and its associated risks can be avoided.

The disadvantages are:

- Long time (3 months) is needed for maximum response,
- Risk of hypothyroidism after some months or years
- Risk of thyroid cancer.

β-adrenergic blockers: Many of the symptoms of hyperthyroidism are of sympathetic overactivity as there is increased tissue sensitivity to catecholamines in hyperthyroidism. β-adrenergic blockers like propranolol relieve symptoms like palpitation, tremors, nervousness, sweating and myopathy. They only provide symptomatic relief.

DRUGS USED IN THE TREATMENT OF DIABETES MELLITUS

Diabetes mellitus is a chronic metabolic disorder characterized by hyperglycemia and altered metabolism of carbohydrates, lipids and proteins. It is a common condition affecting 1-2 percent of population and has a strong hereditary tendency.

Diabetes mellitus can be of four types:

Type I: (Previously called Insulin dependent diabetes mellitus/IDDM) is an autoimmune disorder where antibodies destroy the β cells of the islets of Langerhans. It usually occurs in young children and adolescents (hence called juvenile onset diabetes mellitus).

Type II: (Previously called Non-insulin dependent diabetes mellitus/NIDDM) is of maturity onset. Most patients are obese. There is both reduced sensitivity of tissues to insulin and impaired regulation of insulin secretion.

Type III: Secondary diabetes due to causes like pancreatectomy, drugs and nonpancreatic diseases.

Type IV: Gestational diabetes which may be due to placental hormones which promote insulin resistance.

Prolonged hyperglycemia results in various complications including premature atherosclerosis, retinopathy, nephropathy and gangrene of the limbs. This is thought to be due to reduced blood supply to these structures—because of thickening of the capillary walls. Hence, it is necessary to maintain normal blood glucose levels though diabetes mellitus as such does not cause significant troublesome symptoms. Treatment helps to prevent or delay the onset of complications of diabetes.

Insulin

In 1921 Banting and Best obtained insulin in the form of pancreatic extract. In 1922 the extract containing insulin was first used on a 14-year-old boy suffering from severe diabetes mellitus with excellent response. Insulin was then purified in a few years.

Chemistry, synthesis and secretion: Natural insulin is a polypeptide synthesized from the precursor proinsulin. Human insulin differs from bovine insulin by 3 amino acids and from porcine insulin by 1 amino acid. Hence porcine insulin is closer to human insulin. It is stored in granules in the β islet cells of the pancreas. Normal pancreas releases about 50 units of insulin everyday. The secretion is regulated by factors like food, hormones and autonomic nervous system. The islets of Langerhans are composed of 4 types of cells—β cells secrete insulin, α(A) cells glucagon, δ(D) cells somatostatin and P cells secrete pancreatic polypeptide.

Insulin is metabolized in the liver, kidney and muscle.

Actions of Insulin

- **Carbohydrate metabolism:** Insulin stimulates the uptake and metabolism of glucose in the peripheral tissues especially skeletal muscles and fat.
  It inhibits glucose production in the liver by inhibiting gluconeogenesis and glycogenolysis.
  By the above actions, insulin lowers the blood glucose concentration.
- **Lipid metabolism:** Insulin inhibits lipolysis in adipose tissue and promotes the synthesis of triglycerides. In diabetes, large amounts of fat are broken down. The free fatty acids so formed are converted by the liver to acetyl CoA and then ketone bodies. This results in ketonemia and ketonuria.
  Insulin indirectly enhances lipoprotein lipase activity resulting in increased clearance of very-low-density lipoprotein (VLDL) and chylomicrons. In insulin deficiency, there is hypertriglyceridemia.
- **Protein metabolism:** Insulin facilitates amino acid uptake and protein synthesis and inhibits protein break down—anabolic effect.
  In diabetes, there is increased catabolic effect and negative nitrogen balance.

Mechanism of action: Insulin binds to specific receptors present on the surface of the target cells and produces its effects.

Insulin receptors are present on almost all cells in the body.

Side Effects

1. **Hypoglycemia** is the most common complication of insulin therapy. It may be due to a large dose of insulin, inappropriate time of insulin administration, unusually small meal or vigorous exercise. Symptoms—sweating, palpitation, tremors, blurred vision, weakness, hunger and confusion. Severe hypoglycemia may result in convulsions and coma.
   Treatment: Glucose or fruit juice like orange juice can be given orally or in severe cases IV glucose promptly reverses the symptoms.

2. **Allergy:** This is due to the contaminating proteins in the insulin preparation. Urticaria, angiedema and rarely anaphylaxis can occur. It is rare with purified preparations and with human insulin.
3. **Lipodystrophy:** Atrophy of the subcutaneous fat at the site of injection may be due to immune response to contaminating proteins. **Lipohypertrophy** that is enlargement of subcutaneous tissue can also occur due to the local action of insulin. Lipodystrophy can be prevented by using different sites for injection.
4. **Edema:** Some severe diabetics develop edema which is self-limiting.

Preparations of Insulin

Older preparations of insulin were obtained from cattle and pig pancreas, but were antigenic. Highly purified insulins were then obtained which were less antigenic but now, human insulins and insulin analogs are available.

Human insulins are obtained by recombinant DNA technology. Human insulin is available as regular, neutral protamine Hagedorn (NPH), lente and ultralente preparations. They may be short, intermediate or long-acting (Table 10.2). Since insulins are destroyed when given orally, they are given parenterally. All preparations are given SC. Only regular (plain) insulin can be given IV in emergencies. Doses are expressed as units.

Mixtures of short-acting and intermediate/long-acting preparations are given for a rapid onset and long duration of action.

Insulin analogs

Analogs of insulin with favorable pharmacokinetic properties have been synthesized.

They are obtained by slightly altering the insulin structure. Insulin analogs have many advantages over human insulins.

- They are absorbed 3 times faster than human insulins—can be given subcutaneously 10 minutes before food.
- Have lesser chances of hypoglycemia.

Table 10.2: Preparations of insulin.

Type	*Onset action*	*Duration (hr)*
1. Rapid and short acting insulins		
Lispro	5–15 min	2–5
Aspart	5–15 min	1–2
Glulisine	5–15 min	1–2
Regular insulins (plain, soluble)	30–60 min	5–8
2. Intermediate-acting		
Insulin zinc suspension (lente)	1–2 hr	18–24
NPH* (isophane insulin)	1–2 hr	18–24
3. Long acting insulin analogs		
Insulin glargine	2–4 hr	20–24
Insulin detemir	1–4 hr	24
Insulin degludec	2–4 hr	>24
4. Insulin mixtures or premixed combinations: Combinations of 20–50% regular with 80–50% long acting insulins		

*NPH, i.e., Neutral Protamine Hagedorn insulin.

- Blood glucose control is better than with regular insulin.

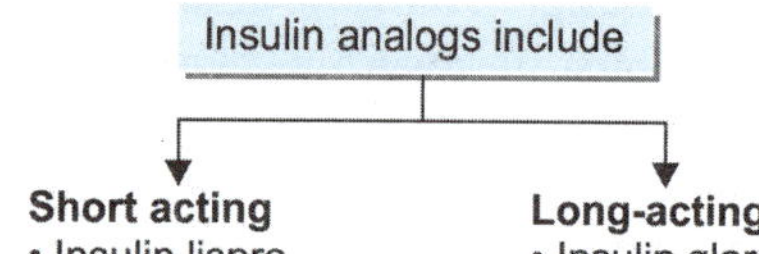

Insulin lispro, aspart and ***glulisine*** are rapid and fast acting insulin analogs. ***Insulin glargine, insulin detemir*** and ***insulin degludec*** are long-acting analogs which act for 24 hours.

Insulin delivery devices have been designed which make insulin administration more convenient. Portable *pen injectors* are small pen-size devices containing multiple doses of insulin and retractable needles. They can be easily carried (portable) while travelling. Insulin pumps deliver appropriate doses of insulin on the basis of self monitored blood glucose results. The set is inserted subcutaneously.

Alternative routes of insulin delivery have been tried—inhaled insulin and insulin nasal spray are being evaluated for use.

Drug Interactions

1. β-adrenergic blockers mask tachycardia, the important warning symptom of hypoglycemia. They also prolong hypoglycemia by inhibiting compensatory mechanisms acting through β_2 receptors.
2. Salicylates precipitate hypoglycemia by enhancing insulin secretion and β cell sensitivity to glucose.
3. Drugs that cause hypoglycemia, such as glucocorticoids, thiazide diuretics, diazoxide, phenytoin and adrenaline → reduce the effects of insulin and other antidiabetics.

Use of Insulin in Diabetes Mellitus

Insulin is effective in all types of diabetes mellitus. The dose should be adjusted as per the needs of each patient-guided by blood sugar levels.

Insulin resistance is said to be present when the insulin requirement is increased to >200 U/day. It is due to the antibodies to insulin which partly neutralize it. This is rare with human insulin. Antibodies may also develop to contaminants and other added constituents like protamine. In some patients, immunosuppression with corticosteroids like prednisolone may help.

Oral Antidiabetic Drugs

The main disadvantage of insulin is the need for injection. The introduction of oral antidiabetics is a boon to millions of Type II diabetes patients with early and mild diabetes mellitus. Sulfonylureas were the first oral antidiabetics (OAD) to be made available in 1950s. Oral antidiabetics may be classified as follows:

Classification

1. **Drugs that increase insulin secretion (Insulin secretagogues)**
   A. ***Sulfonylureas***
   Tolbutamide, glibenclamide, glipizide, gliclazide, glimepiride
   B. ***Meglitinides***
   Repaglinide, nateglinide
   C. ***GLP-1 agonists***
   Exenatide, liraglutide, albiglutide, dulaglutide, semaglutide
   D. ***DPP-4 inhibitor***
   Sitagliptin
2. **Biguanides**
   Metformin
3. **Thiazolidinediones**
   Pioglitazone, rosiglitazone
4. **Alpha glucosidase inhibitors**
   Acarbose, voglibose, miglitol
5. **Amylin analog (subcutaneous)**
   Pramlintide
6. **SGLT-2 inhibitors**
   Dapagliflozin, remogliflozin

Drugs that Increase Insulin Release

A. Sulfonylureas

A sulfonamide derivative used for its antibacterial effects in typhoid patients produced hypoglycemia. This observation led to the development of sulfonylureas.

Mechanism of action: Sulfonylureas reduce the blood glucose level by:

- Stimulating the release of insulin from the pancreatic β cells
- Increasing the sensitivity of peripheral tissues to insulin
- Increasing the number of insulin receptors
- Suppressing hepatic gluconeogenesis.

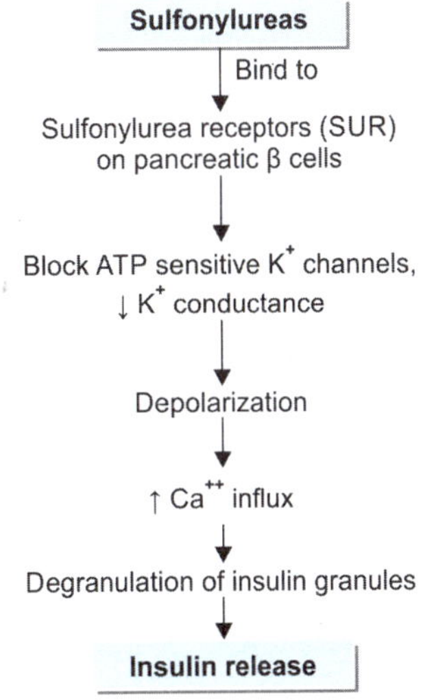

Sulfonylureas bind to receptors on pancreatic β cells, and block the ATP - sensitive K^+ channels. This reduced K^+ conductance causes depolarization and Ca^{++} influx leading to increased insulin secretion. Thus, some functional β-cells are essential for the action of sulfonylureas.

Tolbutamide is short-acting and is associated with several drug interactions - hence is not preferred.

Glibenclamide (Gliburide) is a commonly used sulfonylurea. It is longer acting—can be given once a day.

Glipizide has a short t½; food delays its absorption.

Glimepiride is longer acting and can be given as a single morning dose.

Gliclazide can be used in diabetes with renal dysfunction. It is found to delay the onset of retinopathy in diabetics.

Pharmacokinetics: Sulfonylureas are well-absorbed orally, extensively bound to plasma proteins, metabolized in the liver and some are excreted in the urine. Hence, they should be avoided in patients with renal or liver dysfunction. Dose (Table 10.3).

Adverse Effects

- Hypoglycemia is the most common adverse effect, least with tolbutamide due to short t½ and low potency
- Nausea, vomiting, jaundice, and allergic reactions can occur (Table 10.4)
- Patients on sulfonylureas may have an increase in the rate of cardiovascular

Table 10.3: Dose and duration of action of oral antidiabetics.

Drug	*Dose*	*Duration of action*
Glibenclamide	5 mg OD-BD	18–24 hours
Glipizide	5–15 mg OD-BD	12–18 hours
Gliclazide	40–240 mg OD	12–24 hours
Glimepiride	1–4 mg OD	12–24 hours
Metformin	500 mg OD-BD	6–8 hours
Repaglinide	0.5–4 mg BD-TID	4–5 hours
Nateglinide	60–120 mg BD-TID	3–4 hours
Pioglitazone	15–45 mg OD	12–24 hours
Acarbose	25–100 mg before each meal	–
Miglitol	25–100 mg before each meal	–

Table 10.4: Mechanism of action and prominent adverse effects of commonly used oral antidiabetics.

Oral antidiabetics	*Major mechanism*	*Adverse effects*
Sulfonylureas (e.g. tolbutamide, glibenclamide)	↑ insulin release from pancreas ↑ tissue sensitivity to insulin	Hypoglycemia, cholestatic jaundice
Biguanides (metformin)	↓ hepatic gluconeogenesis ↑ tissue sensitivity to insulin	Diarrhea, metallic taste, rarely lactic acidosis
Meglitinides (repaglinide, nateglinide)	↑ insulin release from pancreas	Hypoglycemia
Thiazolidinediones (pioglitazone)	PPAR γ agonist ↑ glucose transport into tissues ↓ hepatic gluconeogenesis	Weight gain, edema, may ppt CCF, risk of hepatotoxicity
α glucosidase inhibitors (acarbose, voglibose)	↑ glucose absorption ↓ hydrolysis of disaccharides	Flatulence, diarrhea, abdominal distension

death. However, this is still controversial and sulfonylureas continue to be used
- Sulfonylureas can precipitate a disulfiram like reaction on consumption of alcohol. Patients should be warned to abstain from alcohol while on sulfonylureas.

Drug Interactions

- Drugs that augment hypoglycemic effect
  - NSAIDs, warfarin, sulfonamides—displace sulfonylureas from protein binding sites
  - Alcohol, chloramphenicol, cimetidine—inhibit metabolism
- Drugs that decrease the action of sulfonylureas
  - Diuretics and corticosteroids—increase blood glucose levels.

B. Meglitinides

Repaglinide and **nateglinide** increase insulin secretion. Like sulphonylureas, meglitinides increase the release of insulin by blocking the ATP dependent K^+ channels in the pancreatic β cells.

Both repaglinide and nateglinide are rapidly absorbed from the gut; repaglinide has a t½ of 1 hour. Both drugs can cause hypersensitivity reactions and hypoglycemia, but the incidence is relatively lower with nateglinide. Gastrointestinal disturbances are common with repaglinide.

Meglitinides can be used in type 2 diabetes mellitus either alone or with metformin.

C. Glucagon Like Peptide 1 (GLP-1) Analogs

Glucagon like peptides (also called incretins) are released from the gut following oral glucose administration and GLP-1, in turn, increases insulin secretion (Fig. 10.2). Exenatide, liraglutide, semaglutide, albiglutide and dulaglutide are synthetic GLP-1 analogs which act by increasing glucose-1mediated insulin secretion, suppresses glucagon release, delays gastric emptying and reduces appetite. Studies have shown that they increase the beta cell mass.

Adverse effects: Cause nausea, vomiting (self-limiting), diarrhea and weight loss in some patients and rarely hemorrhagic pancreatitis which can be fatal. Albiglutide, dulaglutide and semaglutide are given once weekly subcutaneous.

Liraglutide is given once daily SC and is popular now.

D. Dipeptidyl Peptidase-4 (DPP-4) Inhibitors

Dipeptidyl peptidase is an enzyme which degrades incretins. **Sitagliptin** is a DPP-4 inhibitor and thereby increases incretin levels. It increases insulin secretion and decreases glucagon levels. Sitagliptin is orally effective and may be used alone or along with other antidiabetic drugs. Adverse effects include headache, upper respiratory infections and allergic reactions. **Dose:** 100 mg once daily.

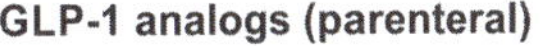

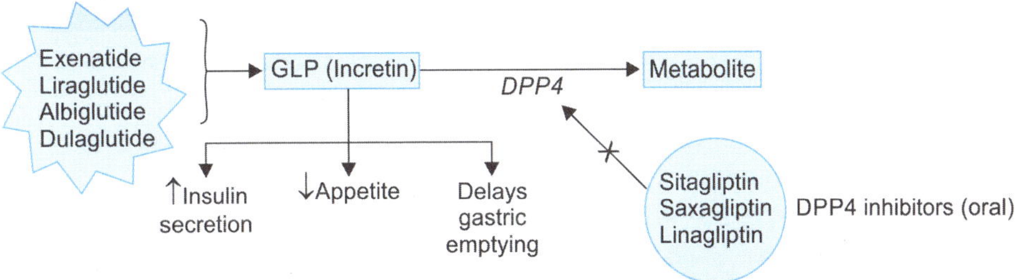

Fig. 10.2: Mechanism of action of GLP-1 analogs and DPP4 inhibitors.
(DPP4: dipeptidyl-peptidase 4; GLP: glucogon-like peptide)

Biguanides

Metformin lowers blood glucose level by insulin-like effects on the tissues (Box 10.1). Mechanism of action is not clear. It—

- Suppresses hepatic gluconeogenesis
- Inhibits glucose absorption from the intestines
- Stimulates the peripheral uptake of glucose in tissues in the presence of insulin.

Adverse effects: Metformin does not cause hypoglycemia because it is an euglycemic agent, that means, it does not reduce blood glucose levels below normal.

Nausea, diarrhea, and **metallic taste** are self-limiting. Rarely **lactic acidosis** can occur. It reduces appetite but **anorexia** is advantageous as it helps in reducing body weight. Long-term use may interfere with vitamin B12 absorption leading to **Vitamin B12 deficiency**.

Box 10.1: Biguanides (metformin).

- Have insulin-like effects
- Do not cause hypoglycemia
- Weight reduction—due to anorexia
- Nausea, diarrhea, metallic taste are transient
- Preferred in obese diabetics either alone or with sulfonylureas
- Contraindicated in renal, hepatic and cardiac diseases

Thiazolidinediones

Pioglitazone, a thiazolidinedione (TZDs) or glitazone is an agonist at the PPARγ-receptors (gamma subtype of peroxisome-proliferator activated receptors). TZDs activate the PPARγ receptors and induce the synthesis of genes which increase insulin action.

Advantages

- TZDs increase insulin-mediated glucose transport into muscle and adipose tissue
- Reduce hepatic gluconeogenesis
- Once a day administration
- Low potential for hypoglycemia
- ↑ HDL cholesterol
- No clinically significant drug interactions known so far.

Disadvantages

- 6–12 weeks of treatment is required to establish maximum therapeutic effect
- May cause weight gain and anemia
- Hepatotoxicity: Liver function should be monitored regularly
- Increase the risk of fractures
- May cause edema and precipitate or worsen CCF. **Rosiglitazone** is now **banned** due to cardiac adverse effects.

Uses: Pioglitazone is used along with sulfonylureas or biguanides in type II diabetes mellitus.

Rosiglitazone is now banned due to increased risk of cardiac problems.

α-Glucosidase Inhibitors

Acarbose, an oligosaccharide, **miglitol** and **voglibose** competitively inhibit the enzymes α-glucosidases which are present in the intestinal brush border and thereby prevent the absorption of carbohydrates. Monosaccharides like glucose and fructose are absorbed from the intestines while disaccharides and oligosaccharides are broken down into monosaccharides before being absorbed. This 'breaking down' is done by the enzymes α-glucosidases (e.g. sucrase, maltase, glycoamylase) and α-amylase present in the intestinal wall. α glucosidase inhibitors inhibit the hydrolysis of disaccharides and decrease carbohydrate absorption.

Acarbose, voglibose, miglitol
↓
Inhibit α glucosidases in intestinal brush border
↓
Prevent absorption and delay digestion of carbohydrates
↓
Reduce postprandial blood glucose

- Alpha glucosidase inhibitors reduce the glucose absorption from upper intestines thereby reducing post-prandial blood glucose levels.

- Alpha glucosidase inhibitors do not cause hypoglycemia. When used with other anti-diabetics if hypoglycemia occurs, glucose should be given and not sucrose because sucrase is inhibited

Adverse effects: They may cause gastrointestinal disturbances including abdominal distention, flatulence and diarrhea because of undigested carbohydrates reaching the colon and then getting fermented.

Uses: Alpha glucosidase inhibitors can be used alone in patients with predominantly postprandial hyperglycemia or in combination with other oral antidiabetics or insulin.

Amylin Analogs

Amylin is a polypeptide produced by the pancreatic beta cells. It inhibits glucagon secretion, delays gastric emptying and suppresses appetite. **Pramlintide** a synthetic amylin analog modulates postprandial glucose levels and has beneficial effects on HbA1C levels. Given subcutaneously it is rapidly absorbed and has a duration of action of around 2–3 hours. The concurrent dose of insulin or other antidiabetics may be reduced to avoid hypoglycemia. It should not be mixed with other drugs in the syringe. It can cause nausea, vomiting and anorexia. Pramlintide can be used in both type I and type II diabetes.

SGLT–2 Inhibitors

A large amount of glucose is reabsorbed from the proximal tubule by sodium-glucose cotransporter-2 (SGLT-2). Inhibition of SGLT-2 reduces the absorption of glucose and sodium (Fig. 10.3). **Dapagliflozin, remogliflozin** and **sergliflozin** are SGLT-2 inhibitors found to be useful in patients with diabetes. They are particularly useful when the patients also have hypertension. They do not cause hypoglycemia but could increase the risk of urinary infection due to the presence of glucose in the urine.

Treatment of Diabetes Mellitus

The aim of treatment is to keep the blood sugar within normal limits and prevent complications of diabetes. In type I diabetes, insulin is the only treatment.

Mild type II diabetes may be controlled by diet, exercise and weight reduction. When not controlled, an oral hypoglycemic should be given. Most type II diabetes patients may require insulin sometime later in life.

Status of Oral Antidiabetics

Uncomplicated Type II diabetes patients not controlled by diet and exercise are given OAD. Mild Type II diabetes patients with recent onset diabetes, age above 40 years

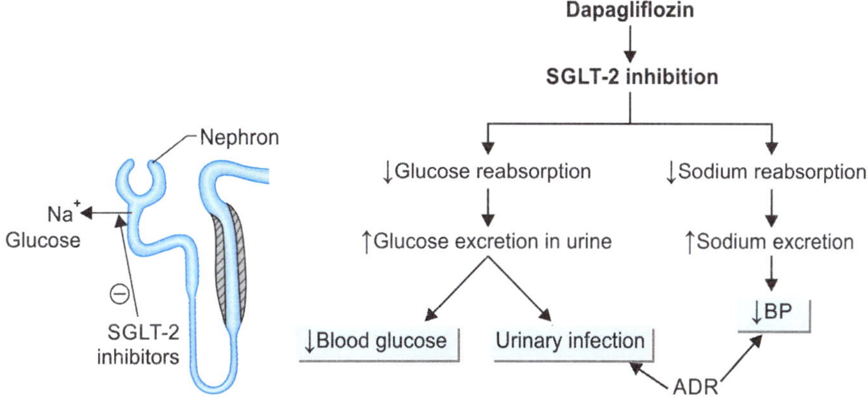

Fig. 10.3: Site, mechanism of action and ADR of SGLT-2 inhibitors.

Table 10.5: Preparations of some oral antidiabetics.

Drug	*Dose*	*Duration of action*
Tolbutamide	500 mg q 8–12 hr	6–8 hr
Glibenclamide	5 mg q 12–24 hr	18–24 hr
Metformin	500 mg q 12–24 hr	6–8 hr
Glipizide	5–15 mg OD/BD	12–18 hr
Gliclizide	40–240 mg OD	12–24 hr
Glimepiride	1–4 mg OD	12–24 hr
Repaglinide	0.5–4 mg TDS	4–5 hr
Nateglinide	60–120 mg	3–4 hr
Pioglitazone	15–45 mg OD	12–24 hr
Acarbose	25–100 mg TDS	2–4 hr
Canagliflozine	100–300 mg OD	12–24 hr

at the onset of diabetes, obese with fasting blood sugar < 200 mg/dL are candidates for oral antidiabetics. They are convenient to use. Sulfonylureas are first line drugs, but when blood sugar is not adequately controlled, metformin can be added. Metformin has the advantages of reducing appetite and being euglycemic. In conditions like stress, surgery or in any of the complications of diabetes, insulin should be used (Table 10.5). In some patients, insulin may be given along with sulfonylureas because the latter increase the tissue sensitivity to insulin. Many other oral antidiabetics are also available. They may be used depending on the requirement of the patient.

Treatment of diabetic ketoacidosis: Ketoacidosis may be precipitated by infection, trauma or stress and is more common in type 1 patients. Acidosis, dehydration, electrolyte imbalance, impaired consciousness, and hyperventilation are the common features seen. Treatment is with regular (plane) insulin by continuous IV infusion. Fluid and electrolyte replacement are important.

Glucagon

Glucagon is synthesized in the alpha (α) cells of the pancreatic islets of Langerhans; like insulin, the secretion of glucagon is regulated by nutrients—chiefly glucose, paracrine hormones and autonomic nervous system. Fasting stimulates glucagon secretion. It is degraded in the liver, kidney and plasma.

Actions: Glucagon increases blood glucose level by glycogenolysis and gluconeogenesis in the liver. It evokes insulin release. It mobilizes stored fat and carbohydrates. Glucagon increases heart rate and force of contraction. It also relaxes the intestinal smooth muscles.

Uses

- Severe hypoglycemia—glucagon can be used in the emergency treatment of severe hypoglycemia due to insulin.
- Diagnostic uses—for diagnosis of type 1.
- Radiology of the bowel—because glucagon relaxes intestines.

ANDROGENS AND ANABOLIC STEROIDS

Androgens are produced chiefly in the testis and small amounts in the adrenal cortex. In the females, small amounts of androgens are produced in the ovary and adrenal cortex. Testosterone is the most important natural androgen. In the adult male, 8–10 mg of testosterone is produced daily. Secretion is regulated by gonadotropins and GnRH.

Physiological actions: In the male, testosterone is essential for the development of secondary sexual characters and sex organs. It is necessary for normal spermatogenesis and is important for maintaining sexual function in men. Testosterone promotes bone growth, enhances the muscle mass, protein synthesis and positive nitrogen balance—has anabolic actions.

Mechanism of action of androgens is similar to other steroids. Androgens bind to androgen receptors on the target cells, the complex moves to the nucleus where it stimulates protein synthesis.

Adverse effects: Masculinization and acne in females, hepatotoxicity, increased libido and precocious puberty can occur in young boys. With large doses, salt and water retention, suppression of spermatogenesis resulting in infertility can be seen. Feminizing effects like gynecomastia in men can occur because some androgens are converted to estrogens.

Uses

- **Testicular failure:** Androgen replacement therapy in primary and secondary testicular failure.
- **Other uses:** Androgens may be used in senile osteoporosis and carcinoma of the breast in premenopausal women.

Anabolic Steroids

Anabolic steroids are synthetic androgens with higher anabolic and low androgenic activity. These are believed to enhance protein synthesis and increase muscle mass. However, with higher doses, the relative anabolic activity is lost and these drugs act like other androgens (Table 10.6).

Adverse effects are similar to those caused by androgens.

Table 10.6: Preparations of anabolic steroids.

Anabolic steroid	*Route*	*Dose*	*Trade name*
Methandienone	Oral	2–10 mg/day	Pronabol
Nandrolone phenylpropionate	IM	10–50 mg/wks	Durabolin
Nandrolone decanoate	IM	25–100 mg/ 3 wks	Decadura-bolin
Ethylestrenol	Oral	2–4 mg/day	Orabolin
Oxandrolone	Oral	5–10 mg/day	Anavar
Stanozolol	Oral	2–10 mg/day	Stromba

Uses

1. **Catabolic states:** Anabolic steroids may benefit patients following surgery, trauma, prolonged illness and debilitating conditions. Given during convalescence, the negative nitrogen balance is corrected, appetite improves and there is a feeling of well being.
2. **Osteoporosis:** In elderly males respond by formation of new bone tissue.
3. **Growth stimulation in children:** Anabolic steroids promote linear growth in prepubertal boys. They may be used only for short periods—but actual benefit on final height is not established.
4. **Chronic renal failure:** Anabolic steroids are tried in chronic renal failure to reduce nitrogen load on the kidneys.
5. **Anemias:** Androgens may be of benefit in refractory anemias with bone marrow failure.

Abuse in athletes: Anabolic steroids enjoy a reputation for improving athletic performance. When combined with adequate exercise, the muscle mass increases. But the dose used by athletes is very high and is associated with serious adverse effects like testicular atrophy, sterility and gynecomastia in men and virilizing effects in women; increased aggressiveness, psychotic symptoms and increased risk of coronary heart disease in both sexes. Moreover, there is no evidence that athletic performance improves. Hence the use of anabolic steroids by athletes has been banned and is medically not recommended.

Contraindications for the use of androgens.

- Pregnancy.
- Carcinoma of prostate/breast in males.
- Infants and children.
- Renal/cardiac/liver disease.

Antiandrogens

Cyproterone acetate—a derivative of progesterone competitively binds to androgen receptors and thus blocks the action of androgens. It also has progestational activity (Table 10.7).

Uses:

- To treat severe hypersexuality in males
- In carcinoma prostate
- In female hirsutism.

Flutamide and **bicalutamide** are potent competitive antagonists at androgen

Table 10.7: Antagonists of sex hormones and their uses.

Hormone	*Receptor antagonist*	*Uses of antagonist*
Estrogen	Tamoxifen Clomiphene citrate	Breast cancer • Infertility • *In vitro* fertilization
Progesterone	Mifepristone	Termination of pregnancy
Androgen	Flutamide Cyproterone	Carcinoma prostate • Carcinoma prostate • Hypersexuality in men • Female hirsutism

receptors. It is used in the treatment of carcinoma prostate.

Finasteride inhibits the enzyme 5-alpha reductase and thus inhibits the convertion of testosterone to its active metabolite dihydrotestosterone which acts mainly in the male urogenital tract.

Uses:

1. **Benign prostatic hypertrophy:** Fenasteride reduces the prostate size.
2. **Baldness in men:** Finasteride is tried either alone or with minoxidil.

Male Contraceptives

The requirement of a safe and effective chemical contraceptive in men has not been fulfilled largely because it is difficult to totally suppress spermatogenesis. Various compounds including testosterone with progestin, estrogens with progestins, anti-androgens like cyproterone acetate have been tried, but are neither reliable nor safe.

GnRH agonists and antagonists along with testosterone inhibit gonadotropin secretion and are being studied.

Gossypol, a cotton seed derivative has shown to produce oligozoospermia and impair sperm motility in Chinese studies. This effect is reversible in a few months. Hypokalemia is the major adverse effect.

Drugs Used in Sexual Impotence

Sexual impotence is the inability of a man to have satisfactory sexual intercourse due to inability to have and maintain an erection. Very often it is psychological while in some cases there could be an organic cause.

Several drugs have been tried including testosterone, yohimbine, papaverine and antidepressants. The recent introduction—Sildenafil (Viagra) has been a success in a large percentage of them.

Sildenafil

Sildenafil inhibits the enzyme phosphodiesterase in the penis and thus prolongs the life of cyclic GMP. This causes relaxation of smooth muscle in the corpus cavernosum and vasodilation—both resulting in cavernosal engorgement and penile erection.

Sildenafil is given orally (50–100 mg) 1 hour before sexual activity in patients with erectile dysfunction. Peak blood levels require 1–2 hr. VIAGRA, PENAGRA, EDEGRA 25, 50, 100 mg tab.

Sildenafil has also been found to be beneficial in several conditions in cardiology like pulmonary arterial hypertension, systemic hypertension and ischemic heart diseases. It is also useful in cystic fibrosis and benign prostatic hyperplasia.

Adverse effects and precautions: Due to vasodilation—headache, dizziness and nasal stuffiness can occur. Sildenafil potentiates the hypotensive action of nitrates and is contraindicated in patients on nitrates and in patients with coronary artery disease. Elderly men above 60 years need less dose (25 mg). Patients with liver disease, kidney disease, bleeding disorders and elderly people are at a higher risk of toxicity. Several deaths have been reported in such patients.

Vardenafil has properties similar to sildenafil. Dose 5–10 mg. **Tadalafil** is more potent and longer acting than sildenafil.

Other drugs used in male sexual dysfunction are alprostadil a prostaglandin E analog and papaverine with phentolamine (an α blocker) injected directly into the cavernosa.

ESTROGENS, PROGESTINS AND HORMONAL CONTRACEPTIVES

Physiologic Consideration

At puberty, the ovary begins its cyclic function called menstrual cycle which stretches over 30–40 years characterized by regular episodes of uterine bleeding.

The hypothalamus releases the GnRH in pulses which stimulates the release of FSH and LH from the anterior pituitary. At the beginning of each cycle, a number of follicles in the ovary begin to enlarge in response to FSH. After 5-6 days, one of the follicles begins to develop more rapidly. The granulosa cells of this follicle multiply and under the influence of LH, synthesize estrogens. This estrogen inhibits FSH release, resulting in regression of the smaller follicles. Just before the midcycle, the estrogen secretion reaches a peak, stimulating a brief surge in FSH and LH levels which results in **ovulation** by around the 14th day of the cycle (Fig. 10.4).

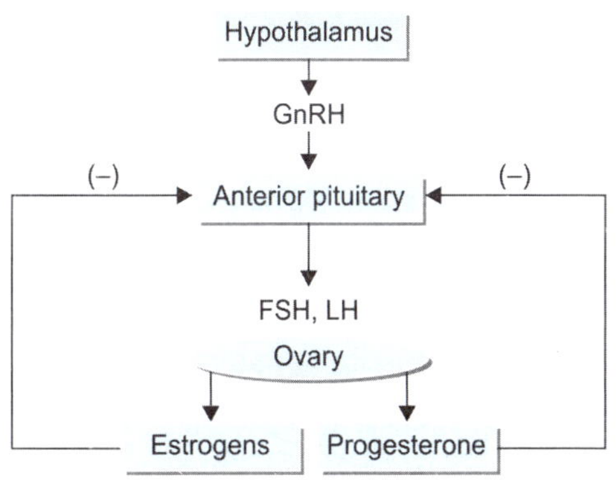

Fig. 10.4: Regulation of secretion of gonadal hormones.

Estrogens

The estrogens are produced by the ovaries, placenta and in small amounts by the adrenals and testes.

The major estrogens are:

- **Natural estrogens:**
  Estradiol, estrone, estriol.
- **Synthetic estrogens:**
  Ethinyl estradiol, stilboestrol, mestranol.

Estradiol is converted to estrone and estriol by the liver and other tissues.

Estrogens act on estrogen receptors ER-α and ER-β.

Actions: Estrogens are required for:

- The normal maturation of the female reproductive tract.
- Development of secondary sexual characters in the female.
- Stimulation of preovulatory endometrium.
- Metabolic effects—estrogens inhibit the resorption of bone and maintain the bone mass. They promote the fusion of epiphyses.
- Estrogens are important for the maintenance of normal structure of the skin and blood vessels in women.
- Estrogens decrease plasma LDL cholesterol and raise HDL cholesterol and triglycerides.
- Effect on blood coagulation—estrogens increase the coagulability of the blood.

Adverse effects:

Nausea, breast tenderness, migraine headaches, hyperpigmentation, hypertension and cholestasis may be seen. In men gynecomastia and feminization can occur.

Cancers: Increased incidence of endometrial and breast cancers are reported on long-term estrogen therapy. Therefore it should be combined with a progesterone.

Teratogenicity: When given to a pregnant lady, estrogens may cause the following teratogenic effects:

- In female child—increased risk of vaginal and cervical cancers.
- In male child—genital abnormalities.

Uses

1. **Replacement therapy:** In primary hypogonadism—an estrogen started at 11–13 years of age stimulates the development of secondary sexual characters and menstruation.

2. **Postmenopausal syndrome - Hormone replacement therapy (HRT):** Due to decreased estrogen production at menopause, hot flushes, anxiety, fatigue, sweating, muscle and joints pain are common. Other longer-lasting changes including osteoporosis, genital atrophy, skin changes, increased risk of cardiovascular disease and psychological disturbances may be seen. Estrogens given in low doses is highly effective in reversing most of the changes.
3. **Senile vaginitis** is common in elderly women due to lack of estrogen. Estrogen cream is used topically.
4. **Osteoporosis:** In postmenopausal osteoporosis, estrogens restore calcium balance and need to be given for a long time.
5. **Hormonal contraceptives:** Estrogens are used, along with progestins.
6. **Dysmenorrhea:** Estrogens combined with progestins suppress ovulation and such anovulatory cycles are painless.
7. **Dysfunctional uterine bleeding:** Estrogens are used along with progesterone.
8. **Carcinoma prostate** is an androgen dependent tumor. Estrogens antagonize the action of androgens, suppress androgen production and are useful for palliative therapy.
9. **Acne:** Estrogens oppose the action of androgens which cause acne. However estrogens should be avoided as safer topical drugs are available.

Contraindications: Estrogen dependent tumors, liver disease, thromboembolic disorders.

Selective Estrogen Receptor Modulators (SERMs) and Antiestrogens

Tamoxifen, raloxifene, ormeloxifene and toremifene are all termed selective estrogen receptor modulators (SERMs). SERMs bind to estrogen receptors and act as agonists, antagonists or partial agonists depending on the tissue:

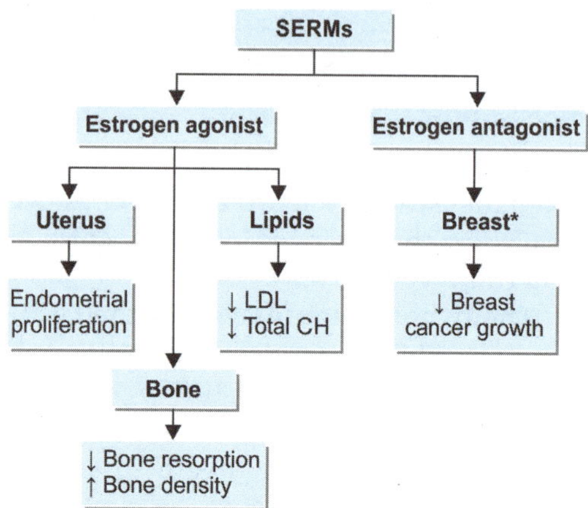

* Tamoxifen has prominent effects on breast tissue.
(CH: cholesterol)

SERMs have tissue-selective estrogenic activities, i.e.:

- They have agonistic effects on bone, lipid metabolism, brain and liver.
- Antagonists at breast, pituitary and endometrium.
- Partial agonists at genitourinary epithelium, bone remodeling and cholesterol metabolism.

Tamoxifen is given orally. Side effects include hot flushes, nausea, vomiting, vaginal bleeding and skin rashes.

Tamoxifen is used in advanced breast cancer in postmenopausal women with estrogen receptor-positive tumors.

Raloxifene: A nonsteriodal SERM—acts as an estrogen receptor agonist in the bone. In women with postmenopausal osteoporosis raloxifene prevents bone resorption. It reduces bone loss and may even help to gain bone mass. Raloxifene also lowers LDL. It acts as an estrogen antagonist in the breast due to which it reduces the incidence of breast cancer. Raloxifene does not stimulate the uterine endometrial proliferation.

Adverse effects include hot flushes, leg cramps and an increased risk of deep-vein thrombosis and pulmonary embolism.

Raloxifene is used in the prevention of postmenopausal osteoporosis.

Clomiphene citrate binds to the estrogen receptors and acts as a competitive inhibitor of endogenous estrogens. Clomiphene opposes the negative feedback of endogenous estrogens on the hypothalamopituitary axis resulting in increased gonadotropin secretion and thereby induces ovulation.

Side effects include ovarian hyperstimulation resulting in multiple pregnancy, ovarian cysts, hot flushes, headache and skin rashes.

Uses

1. **Infertility:** Clomiphene citrate is used to induce ovulation in infertility due to ovarian disorders.
2. ***In vitro* fertilization:** Clomiphene induced ovulation is also useful in *in vitro* fertilization.

Selective Estrogen Receptor Down Regulators

Fulvestrant is an estrogen receptor antagonist—it binds and blocks them. It is an antagonist at all tissues with estrogen receptors. The estrogen receptors all degraded and down regulated because of which it is called a SERD. It is used in breast cancer resistant to tamoxifen.

Progestins

Progesterone is the natural progestin synthesized in the ovary and placenta. It is also synthesized by the testis and adrenals where it acts as a precursor of various steroid hormones (see under corticosteroids).

Progestins	
1. Natural	Progesterone
2. Synthetic	Medroxyprogesterone acetate Allylestrenol Megestrol Norethisterone acetate Lynestrenol Levonorgestrel
3. Newer progestins	Norgestimate Desogestrel Gestodene

Actions

- **Uterus:** The secretory changes in the uterine endometrium are due to progesterone. In pregnancy, decidual changes in the endometrium take place under the influence of progesterone which is very important for the maintenance of pregnancy (*Progestin* = favors pregnancy).
- **Cervix:** The watery secretion of the cervix is changed to a thick scanty secretion by progesterone.
- **Vagina:** Vaginal epithelium changes to that seen in pregnancy by the influence of progesterone.
- **Breast:** Along with estrogen, progesterone is responsible for the development of the secretory apparatus in the breast and prepares the gland for lactation.
- **Body temperature:** Increase in the body temperature by 1°C that is seen during luteal phase which begins at ovulation is due to progesterone.

Adverse effects: Headache, breast engorgement, rise in body temperature, edema, acne and mood swings may be seen. Progesterone is teratogenic.

Uses

1. **Contraception** (*See* page 230).
2. **Hormone replacement therapy (HRT):** Progestins are combined with estrogens in HRT of postmenopausal women. Estrogen administration increases the risk of endometrial cancer—supplementing it with progestin counters this risk.
3. **Ovarian suppression:** Progestins are used to suppress ovulation in dysmenorrhea, endometriosis, dysfunctional uterine bleeding (DUB) and premenstrual syndrome.
4. **Threatened or habitual abortion:** Efficacy in such patients is not proved.
5. **Endometrial carcinoma:** Progestins are used as a palliative measure in cases with metastasis.

6. **Postponement of menstruation:** Progesterone given in the second half of the menstrual cycle prolongs the luteal phase thereby postponing the menstrual cycle. Norethisterone 5 mg (oral) started by day 16–20. Higher doses are needed if started later in the cycle.

Antiprogestins

Mifepristone binds to the progesterone receptor and blocks the actions of progesterone. When given in early pregnancy—abortion occurs.

Mechanism: Mifepristone blocks the progesterone receptors in the uterus and thereby causes decidual breakdown; blastocyst gets detached, HCG and progesterone secretions fall. This in turn increases prostaglandin levels and stimulates uterine contractions. It also softens the cervix and facilitates expulsion of the blastocyst.

If given during the follicular phase—it prevents the mid-cycle surge of gonadotropins and delays ovulation.

Mifepristone also binds to glucocorticoid receptors.

Uses

1. **Termination of pregnancy:** Early pregnancy up to 9 weeks can be terminated with a single oral dose—600 mg of mifepristone followed 48 hours later by a prostaglandin to increase uterine contractions and facilitate expulsion of the blastocyst.
   Adverse effects include heavy bleeding, nausea and abdominal pain.
2. **Postcoital contraception:** Mifepristone prevents implantation when given within 72 hours after coitus (a single dose of 600 mg).
3. **Monthly contraception:** When mifepristone is used regularly in late luteal phase—200 mg for 2 days after mid-cycle—it acts as a contraceptive. A single dose of 600 mg mifepristone taken on 27th day of the cycle every month acts as a contraceptive. This should however **not be used for long periods as a regular method** of contraception.
4. **Uterine fibroids:** Low dose mifepristone for 3 months reduces the size of the fibroid. This can be used to minimize blood loss when surgery has to be postponed for some reason.
5. **Ectopic pregnancy:** Mifepristone is injected into the unruptured sac of ectopic pregnancy to discourage the growth.
6. **Cervical ripening:** Given orally 1 day prior to labor mifepristone facilitates cervical ripening and softening of the cervix.
7. **Cushing's syndrome:** Due to its antiglucocorticoid effects, mifepristone is useful in Cushing's syndrome.

Hormonal Contraceptives

Millions of women around the world use hormonal contraceptives making them one of the most widely prescribed drugs. When properly used, they are the most effective spacing methods of contraception. Hormonal contraceptives have greatly contributed to the control of population throughout the world.

Hormonal contraceptives may be classified as in Flowchart 10.1.

Combined hormonal contraceptives contains low doses of an estrogen and a progestin. They are highly efficacious (success rate 98%). Newer progestins cause least side effects (Table 10.8).

Oral Pills

Monophasic: The pill is started on the fifth day of the menstrual cycle, taken daily for 21 days followed by a gap of 7 days during which bleeding occurs. This is monophasic regimen.

Biphasic: Estrogens for 10 days followed by a progestin for the next 11 days. Because of the risk of endometrial cancer, biphasic pills are not preferred.

Flowchart 10.1: Hormonal contraceptives.

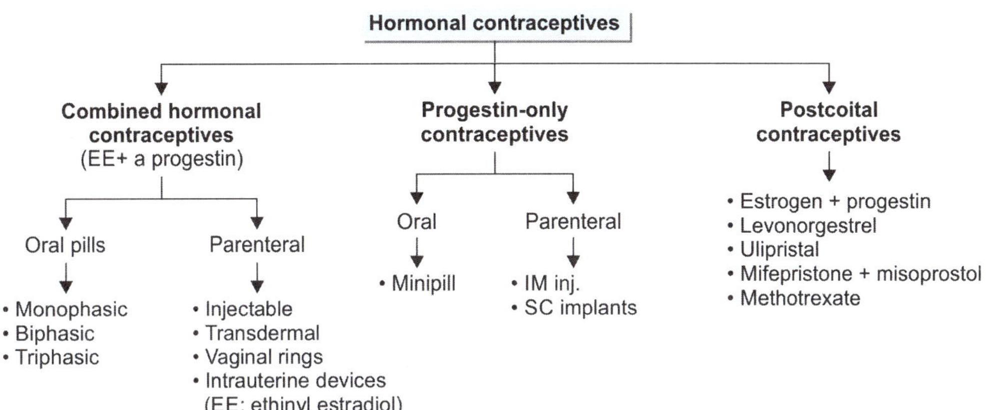

Table 10.8: Hormonal contraceptive preparations.

Regimen	*Estrogen*	*Progestin*	*Trade name*
Monophasic	Ethinyl estradiol 50 µg Ethinyl estradiol 30 µg	Norgestrel 0.5 mg Levonorgestrel 0.15 mg	Ovral-G Ovral-L
Biphasic	Ethinyl estradiol 35 µg	Norethindrone 0.5 mg (10 days) 1 mg (11 days)	—
Triphasic	6 days ethinyl estradiol 30 µg Next 5 days ethinyl estradiol 40 µg Next 10 days ethinyl estradiol 30 µg	Levonorgestrel 50 µg Levonorgestrel 75 µg Levonorgestrel 125 mg	Triquilar
Mini-pill	Nil	Norgestrel 75 µg	Ovrette
Postcoital pill	1. Levonorgestrel (1.5 mg single dose within 72 hours) Or 2. Combined pill (2 stat and 2 after 12 hours) Or 3. Mifepristone 600 mg (within 72 hours) followed 48 hours later by misoprostol 400 mg Or 4. Methotrexate 50 mg/m^2 Or 5. Diethyl stilboestrol (25 mg/day for 5 days)	—	iPILL OVRAL

Stat—at once

Triphasic: Low doses of an estrogen with a progestin → very effective with least side effects.

Use of oral pills—if a woman misses a pill, she should take two pills the next day and continue the course. If more than two pills are missed, then that course should be withdrawn, should follow an alternative method of contraception for that particular cycle and restart the course on the fifth day of the next menstrual cycle.

If the woman has conceived, pregnancy should be terminated as these hormones are teratogenic. However, recent studies have shown that in such **low doses**, the hormones are **not** teratogenic.

Parenteral Combined Contraceptives

Combined injectable contraceptives: An estrogen with a progestogen is injected at monthly intervals. They are highly effective with side effects similar to progesterone-only implants. They are better tolerated but further reports of long-term effects on reversal of ovulation are yet to be available.

Transdermal contraceptives: A transdermal patch containing a progestin and ethinylestradiol is applied once a week for 3 weeks and the next week withdrawal bleeding follows. It has the advantage of better compliance.

Vaginal rings: Containing levonorgestrel are placed in the vagina for 3 weeks of the cycle and then removed for 1 week. The hormone is absorbed gradually through the vaginal mucosa. The advantage is the need for a low dose of the hormone because the first-pass metabolism is avoided.

Mini-pill: A low dose progestin is taken daily. Different regimens are available to avoid adverse effects of estrogen, but the efficacy is lower, menstrual cycles may be irregular and is therefore not preferred.

Postcoital contraceptives: The following may be used for postcoital contraception:

1. Combination of low doses of **estrogen and progestins**—two tablets containing ethinylestradiol (100 mg) and a progestin levonorgestrel 0.5 mg are given as soon as possible (within 72 hours of coitus two tablets of OVRAL G). They can cause nausea and vomiting and have an efficacy of 90–98%. The dose is repeated after 12 hours. It is called **Yuzpe method.**
2. **Levonorgestrel** alone is also effective and commonly used (iPILL—1.5 mg single dose within 72 hours after coitus).
3. **Ulipristal** 30 mg orally within 5 days of coitus is effective.
4. **Mifepristone** 600 mg prevents implantation when given within 72 hours after coitus, followed 48 hours later by 400 mg misoprostol to improve success rate.
5. Insertion of an **intrauterine device** (IUD) like copper-T within 5 days of coitus can prevent implantation and thereby prevent pregnancy.
6. High dose of an **estrogen** (stilbestrol—25 mg daily for 5 days) was used earlier but this may cause severe nausea and vomiting and hence generally not preferred. If the pills are expelled in vomiting, they need to be repeated.
7. **Methotrexate** (50 mg/m^2) given orally or IM effectively induces abortion in the first trimester. Being a folic acid antagonist and also because its active metabolite gets concentrated in the placenta, methotrexate acts as an abortifacient. Misoprostol (Prostaglandin PGE1) is added to promote uterine motility.

Postcoital pills act by preventing implantation. The earlier they are started the better is their efficacy.

If postcoital pills fail, pregnancy should be terminated by other methods because oral contraceptives are likely to be teratogenic.

Post-coital contraception should be used as an emergency method in situations following rape or contraceptive failure.

Mechanism of action of hormonal contraceptives: The combined pill blocks the release of gonadotropins (FSH & LH) from the pituitary and thereby inhibits ovulation.

Progestins make the cervical mucus thick and scanty and thereby inhibit sperm penetration. They also inhibit tubal motility and delay ovum and sperm transport.

Adverse effects:

- Milder effects: Headache, nausea, vomiting, breast tenderness, amenorrhea and irregular menstrual cycles may be commonly seen. Weight gain, acne, mood swings and hirsutism may occur.
- More severe side effects include—cardiovascular effects—in women >35 years there is an increased risk of MI and venous thromboembolism.

Cancers: OCs may increase the incidence of cervical, breast and other cancers—but is controversial.

Cholestatic jaundice and gallstones: Incidence may be higher.

Contraindications to combined pill

- Thromboembolic and cerebrovascular disease
- Breast cancers
- Liver disease
- OCs should be used with caution in diabetes, hypertension, convulsive disorders, edema and CCF.

Benefits of combined pills

- Effective and convenient method of contraception.
- Reduced risk of ovarian and endometrial cancers.
- Reduced incidence of pelvic inflammatory disease and ectopic pregnancy.
- Menstrual benefits—loss menstrual blood less, less iron-deficiency; premenstrual tension and dysmenorrhea are less intense.

Centchroman or ormeloxifene has anti-estrogenic and antiprogestogenic activity and may act by preventing implantation. Dosage (Saheli, Centron) 30 mg twice a week for 3 months followed by once a week till contraception is desired.

Success rate claimed is 97-99% and is devoid of the side effects of hormonal contraceptives. It is well tolerated.

Centchroman may cause prolongation of menstrual cycles in 10% of women. It may cause ovarian enlargement and should be avoided in polycystic ovaries. It should also be avoided in renal and hepatic dysfunction, tuberculosis and in lactating mothers.

11

CHAPTER

Geriatric Pharmacology

Chapter Highlights

- Pharmacokinetic Changes
- Pharmacodynamic Changes
- Adverse Reactions in the Elderly
- Criteria for Safe Prescribing in the Elderly
- Dementia
- Drugs used in Alzheimer's Disease

INTRODUCTION

People above the age of '65' years are called the 'elderly'. Though the age considered is 65 years, it is just arbitrary and infact, by 5th decade many of the age related problems start. In women, it could be even earlier because, the onset of menopause itself may mark the beginning of such health problems.

The population of the elderly is constantly increasing and could result in a major change in the population structure. The increase in life expectancy consequent to better health services and growth of medical science have contributed to a rise in the number of the elderly. The population of the elderly is expanding. The population above 85 years of age will also grow bigger. Because women live longer than men, women form a larger percentage of the elderly. There are also associated social problems - a large number of women are widowed and this would add to their health problems. Loneliness, quite often financial problems, physiological changes including hormonal changes, all contribute to increasing number of problems in the elderly.

Elderly people take more drugs than younger. They tend to suffer from multiple diseases and would require multiple drugs with the risk of drug interactions.

In general, elderly are two to three times more likely to experience an adverse drug reaction. Elderly are more prone to adverse reactions for the following reasons:

1. The pattern of drug use in the elderly—it is estimated that >80 percent of people above 65 years suffer from one or more chronic diseases and consume 40 percent of all drugs. Thus elderly tend to have multiple diseases requiring multiple drugs.
2. Altered response to drugs in the elderly.

Some age-related physiological changes which could influence pharmacokinetics	
Pharmacokinetic changes	***Potential effect***
↓ Blood supply to oral mucosa	↓ Absorption by sublingual route
Delayed gastric emptying	Impaired absorption
↓ Splanchnic blood flow	↓ Presystemic elimination
↓ Lean body mass, body water	↓ Distribution volume
↓ Serum albumin	↑ Free drug concentration
↓ Mixed function oxidases	↓ Hepatic metabolism
↓ GFR, tubular function	↓ Renal clearance

3. Different doctors may be treating them and one may not know the other doctor's prescription, leading to risk of toxicity.
4. Older patients often have visual and auditory impairment which could lead to errors in drug intake.
5. **Dementia:** Many of the elderly patients may have dementia because of which they may make mistakes in drug intake like taking wrong drug or not remembering to take the drug.
6. Elderly may have financial constraints. They may take only some of the medication or even a smaller dose of drugs without knowing their importance.
7. Elderly are generally physically weaker section. They are also psychologically and emotionally helpless and down. These make them more susceptible for adverse effects.
8. Problems of drug education and compliance.
9. **Polypharmacy** is use of multiple drugs. Excessive and unnecessary use of multiple drugs is common in the elderly. It is predicted that by the year 2030, elderly will account for 21% of the population and consume 40% of all drugs. This indicates that elderly receive disproportionately more drugs than other age groups. This is understandable because elderly suffer from more diseases. Use of over-the-counter drugs is also high in the elderly. Polypharmacy adds to the problems. Each drug may result in some adverse effect and more drugs are given to treat these adverse drug reactions, e.g., antacids are given to treat gastritis induced by NSAIDs. Use of multiple drugs can also result in drug interactions. Polypharmacy would result in decreased compliance and increased financial burden to the patient. Elderly may also seek help from multiple doctors resulting in polypharmacy. Polypharmacy can be prevented by periodically checking the list of drugs received by the patients.
10. **Age-related changes:** There could be certain pharmacokinetic and pharmacodynamic changes in the elderly which make them more susceptible to adverse drug effects.

PHARMACOKINETIC CHANGES

Drug Absorption

Absorption is the process by which a drug passes from the GI tract to the bloodstream. Several functional changes could be seen in old age like a decrease in gastric acid production, blood flow to the gut, gastrointestinal motility and mucosal absorbing area. There is also an alteration in the gastric pH which may affect ionization and solubility of the drugs. However these changes may not have significant effects on the absorption of drugs. This could be because some of the changes counter each other. For example, factors that decrease absorption, like, decreased blood flow, may be opposed by decreased GI motility which allow drugs to remain longer in the gut. Some drugs have increased bioavailability in the elderly. A decrease in first pass metabolism may increase the bioavailability of drugs like propranolol, levodopa, nifedipine and morphine. Absorption of drugs by sublingual route may be reduced due to decrease in the blood supply to the oral mucosa. Absorption of drugs may be slower and somewhat less complete in the elderly. There are several age related changes in the gut that could influence absorption of drugs.

Distribution

Changes in the body composition due to older age can modify drug distribution. Changes such as decrease in total body water, body weight, lean body mass and plasma protein concentration and increase in percentage of body fat are common in the elderly. Depending on the properties of the drug, these changes can influence the drug distribution:

- Drugs that are extensively bound to plasma proteins will now have more free fraction to act and can produce a greater response (because of decreased plasma proteins).
- Water soluble drugs like morphine will have a higher concentration in the body because they are distributed in a smaller volume of body water.
- Lipid-soluble drugs have a larger volume of distribution, they are distributed in a larger volume of fat and therefore have a longer half-life. Increased body fat acts as a reservoir for such lipid-soluble drugs and can also result in problems related to drug storage—there could be accumulation of the drugs in the fatty tissue and thereby prolonged action. All these changes could put the elderly at a higher risk of toxicity from drugs. Hence, these problems should be anticipated and necessary dosage adjustments should be done.

Metabolism

The aim of drug metabolism is to inactivate the drugs and make them water soluble so that they can be easily excreted by the kidneys. Since liver is the primary site for drug metabolism, age related changes in liver function can affect the process of biotransformation. In the elderly, the drug metabolizing capacity of the liver decreases because of the decrease in the liver size, amount of blood flow and hepatic enzyme activity. Many drugs are metabolized more slowly and drugs would remain active for longer periods of time compared to young adults. Moreover, the oxidative pathways are inhibited. Hence drugs metabolized by oxidation like piroxicam, diazepam, ibuprofen and phenytoin have a longer half-life in the geriatric age group.

Excretion

The kidneys are the primary organs of drug excretion from the body. The renal function is depressed in the elderly because of a decline in renal blood flow, renal mass and function of renal tubules. As a result there is a decrease in GFR, tubular secretion and a consequent reduction in excretion of drugs. Studies have shown drug excretion to be reduced by 35–50 percent due to decrease in GFR. Thus age-related changes in the renal function can result in a significant reduction in drug excretion leading to accumulation of drugs and their metabolites in the body. The half-lives of the drugs get longer, and their clearance diminishes. Thus reduced renal function should be taken into account whenever drugs are prescribed in the elderly.

The overall effects of the pharmacokinetic changes associated with aging are that drugs remain active in the body for longer periods thereby prolonging their effects as well as adverse effects. For example, half-life of certain drugs like diazepam may be increased by as much as four times in the elderly. However, the extent of age-related pharmacokinetic changes vary from person-to-person. Thus drug dosages should be adjusted and adverse drug reactions minimized after considering all the above factors.

PHARMACODYNAMIC CHANGES

Age related alterations in the physiological functions can influence the systemic response to various drugs. Factors like decreased function of the smooth muscles of the viscera, decreased baroreceptor sensitivity, impaired postural control, altered thermoregulatory responses and a reduced cognitive function can all influence the response to a drug.

The receptor function may also be blunted, i.e., the affinity and binding of the drug to the receptor and the cellular functions may be altered in some tissues due to aging.

However, the extent of variations depends on the extent of changes in the physiological functions.

Other factors that influence response in the elderly include presence of multiple diseases, poor diet and poor general health.

ADVERSE REACTIONS IN THE ELDERLY

As discussed earlier, elderly are more prone to adverse effects. The adverse effects which are more common in the elderly and need special caution include—postural hypotension, dizziness, sedation, urinary retention, constipation, depression, dehydration, confusion, extrapyramidal symptoms, fatigue and weakness.

Postural hypotension: It is a fall in blood pressure by > 20 mm Hg upon assumption of an erect posture. Such hypotension causes dizziness and syncope because of reduced blood supply to the brain. This could result in falls and fractures, cerebral and cardiac infarcts. The older subjects have comparatively less physical activity and lower cardiovascular function—all these factors can increase the chances of postural hypotension in the elderly. Any additional impairment of these mechanisms by drugs would make them even more susceptible to postural hypotension. Physiotherapists should be aware of it because some of the procedures can result in episodes of postural hypotension and its complications.

Dizziness: Drug induced dizziness is common in the elderly. Drugs that produce sedation, altered vestibular function, antihypertensives and even some analgesics can cause dizziness. Orthostatic hypotension also results in dizziness. Some elderly who already have dizziness are all the more susceptible to drug induced dizziness. Apart from being troublesome to the patient as such, dizziness also increases the risk of falling due to imbalance. Hence it is necessary to be watchful in the elderly for this adverse effect.

Sedation and confusion: Several drugs produce sedation and confusion as side effects. Elderly people may also be on hypnotics as many of them may have insomnia. Such sedation may often result in confusion and disorientation.

Fatigue and weakness: Most geriatric subjects have a weaker muscle mass and many are already debilitated. Drugs that produce muscle weakness like skeletal muscle relaxants, drugs like β blockers which reduce heart rate and cardiac output; diuretics causing dehydration, decreased cardiac output and hyponaturemia and oral antidiabetics producing hypoglycemia can all result in worsening of fatigue and weakness.

Depression: Several drugs can cause depression as an adverse effect. Elderly are as such likely to be depressed due to problems of old age and social problems. They are more susceptible to drug induced depression. Symptoms of depression include sadness, lack of initiative and interest in the surroundings. These may interfere in their ability to assess them.

Dehydration: It is a common problem in the elderly. They are more susceptible to this particular side effect due to age-related physiological changes like decrease in lean body mass, increase in fat, and reduced capacity of the kidney to concentrate urine. Symptoms of dehydration include altered sensorium, dizziness, lethargy, confusion and weakness which are all vague and may be misinterpreted for other geriatric problems. Dehydration may also be due to drugs like diuretics, digoxin, vasodilators and laxatives. Dehydration would result in volume depletion, which in turn may reduce cardiac output. It also causes weakness and fatigue.

CRITERIA FOR SAFE PRESCRIBING IN THE ELDERLY

Guidelines are available for safe prescribing in the elderly, *viz.* Beer's criteria, START and STOPP criteria.

Beer's criteria: These serve as guidelines for good prescription practice in the elderly, particularly when multiple drugs are used. They help to avoid drug interactions and adverse drug reactions.

START: Screening Tool to Alert doctor to the Right Treatment.

STOPP: Screening Tool in Older persons for Potentially inappropriate Prescriptions. The START/STOPP criteria may also be used to guide clinicians in appropriate and safe use of drugs in the elderly.

DEMENTIA

Dementia is a degenerative disorder caused by gradual death of neurons in the cerebral cortex. It is characterized by impairment in memory, reasoning and behavior. Dementia could be due to Alzheimer's disease, vascular dementia due to decrease of blood flow to the brain and multi-infarct dementia due to multiple minor strokes. Incidence increases with age and is as high as 30–50% in elderly above 85 years of age.

DRUGS USED IN ALZHEIMER'S DISEASE

Alzheimer's disease (AD) is a neurodegenerative disorder, characterized by progressive impairment of memory and cognitive functions. Other symptoms like depression, anxiety and disturbed sleep may also be seen. Pathological features include atrophy of the cerebral cortex and loss of neurons—mainly cholinergic neurons with multiple senile (amyloid) plaques and neurofibrillary tangles in the brain. Since there is loss of cholinergic neurons, drugs that enhance cholinergic function have been tried. Many other drugs have also been used to improve cognitive functions with variable results as follows:

Cholinesterase inhibitors: Tacrine, rivastigmine, donepezil, galantamine

Nootropic agents (cognition enhancers): Piracetam, aniracetam

NMDA receptor antagonist: Memantine

Others: Piribedil, ginkgo biloba

Tacrine is a centrally acting cholinesterase inhibitor. It enhances cholinergic transmission in the brain. However, it is short acting and also causes various side effects including nausea, vomiting, abdominal cramps, diarrhea and hepatotoxicity. The newer agents ***rivastigmine, donepezil*** and ***galantamine*** are better tolerated with fewer side effects. They are selective central anticholinesterases—hence do not cause the GI side effects which are due to peripheral cholinergic activity. They increase acetylcholine levels in the surviving neurons and have produced good response—cognitive function improves and the symptom score shows benefit. They are not hepatotoxic and are longer acting. All are started at low doses which are gradually increased.

Donepezil has the advantage of longer action and once a day administration.

Dose

Rivastigmine 1.5–6 mg BD

Donepezil: 5 mg HS. **Galantamine:** 4 mg BD.

Nootropic agents have not shown consistent results in Alzheimer's disease.

Memantine is an N-methyl-D-aspartate (NMDA) receptor antagonist found to be useful in patients with moderate to severe AD. The benefit is thought to be due to blockade of glutamate-induced excitotoxicity.

Memantine is well tolerated as the adverse effects are mild and reversible—may cause dizziness and headache. It is used in moderate to severe AD. Started with 5 mg OD and increased to 10 mg BD.

Nonsteroidal anti-inflammatory drugs (NSAIDs): Small doses of aspirin (and other NSAIDs) have been shown to delay the onset of AD. However, further studies are needed to prove their benefit.

12

CHAPTER

Chemotherapy

INTRODUCTION

Chemotherapy can be defined as the use of chemicals in infectious diseases to destroy microorganisms without damaging the host tissues. **Antibiotics** are substances produced by microorganisms which suppress the growth of or destroy other microorganisms.

Pasteur and Joubert were the first to identify that microorganisms could destroy *other* microorganisms. Paul Ehrlich 'The father of Modern Chemotherapy' coined the term 'chemotherapy'. He showed that certain dyes can destroy microbes and demonstrated that methylene blue can be used in malaria. He also synthesized some arsenical compounds for the treatment of syphilis and sleeping sickness. Domagk in 1936 demonstrated that prontosil, a sulfonamide dye is effective in some infections. Sir Alexander fleming discovered penicillin in 1928. It was produced for clinical use in 1941 and this marked the beginning of the 'golden era' of antibiotics. In the last 60 years, several powerful antibiotics and their semi-synthetic derivatives have been produced.

Many infectious diseases which were earlier incurable can now be completely cured with just a few doses of antimicrobial drugs. Thus the development of antimicrobial drugs is one of the important advances of modern medicine. Infact antimicrobials are one of the most commonly prescribed drugs and are often the most over-used and misused drugs.

Classification

Based on their mechanisms of action, antimicrobials are classified (Fig. 12.1) as drugs that:

1. **Inhibit cell wall synthesis:** Penicillins, cephalosporins, vancomycin, bacitracin, cycloserine.
2. **Damage cell membrane:** Causing leakage of cell contents—Polymyxins, amphotericin B, nystatin.
3. **Bind to ribosomes and inhibit protein synthesis:** Chloramphenicol, tetracyclines, erythromycin, aminoglycosides, clindamycin.
4. **Inhibit DNA gyrase:** Fluoroquinolones like ciprofloxacin, norfloxacin.
5. **Inhibit DNA function** (↓DNA dependant RNA polymerase)—Rifampicin.

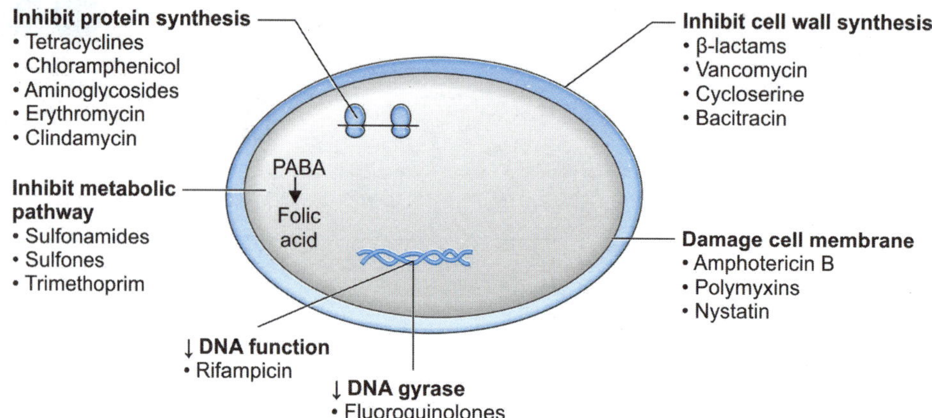

Fig. 12.1: Classification of antimicrobials based on their mechanisms of action.

6. **Interfere with metabolic steps:** Sulfonamides, sulfones, trimethoprim, pyrimethamine (antimetabolite action).

Antimicrobials may also be classified as:

1. **Bacteriostatic drugs:** Suppress the growth of bacteria. For example, tetracyclines, sulfonamides.
2. **Bactericidal drugs:** Kill or destroy the bacteria. For example, Penicillins, aminoglycosides.

Antibiotics may also be grouped based on their antibacterial spectrum of activity as:

1. **Narrow-spectrum antibiotics:** For example, penicillin, aminoglycosides.
2. **Broad-spectrum antibiotics**: For example, tetracyclines, chloramphenicol.

Resistance to Antimicrobial Agents

Resistance is the unresponsiveness of a microorganism to the antimicrobial agent. The resistance may be natural or acquired.

Natural resistance: When resistance is natural, the organisms never respond to the antimicrobial—may be due to the absence of the particular enzyme or target site affected by the drug, e.g., gram-negative bacilli are not sensitive to PnG. But this type of resistance is clinically not a problem as alternate drugs are available.

Acquired resistance: Here, the microbes which were previously sensitive to the antimicrobial agents become resistant to it. Clinically this poses a problem.

Bacteria acquire resistance by a change in their DNA. Such DNA changes may occur by: (i) Mutation or (ii) Transfer of genes.

Mutation is a genetic change that occurs spontaneously. In any population of bacteria, a few resistant mutants may be present. When the sensitive organisms are destroyed by the antibiotic, the resistant mutants freely multiply.

Transfer of genetic material: Many bacteria contain genetic material called **plasmids** in the cytoplasm which carry genes coding for resistance. These plasmids are transferred to other bacteria and spread resistance (Fig. 12.2).

This spread may take place by:

1. **Transduction:** Plasmid DNA is transferred through bacteriophage, i.e., virus which infects bacteria.

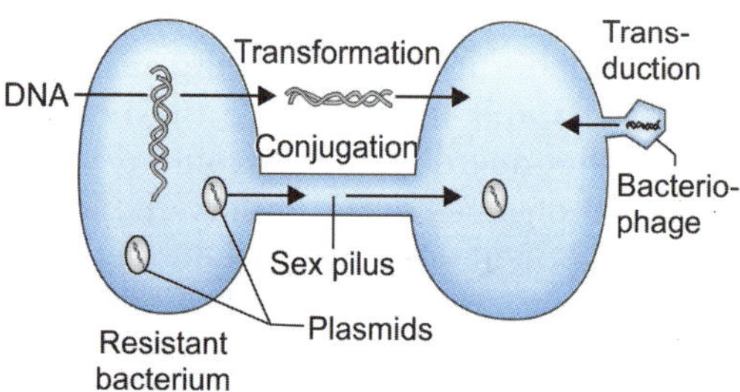

Fig. 12.2: Mechanisms of transfer of resistance.

2. **Transformation:** Resistant bacteria may release genetic material into the medium which is taken up by other bacteria.
3. **Conjugation:** This is the most important mode of spread of resistance. The plasmid is transferred from cell to cell by direct contact through a sex pilus or bridge and the process is known as conjugation.

   The resistance acquired by the bacteria may result in the following:
   - Production of enzymes that inactivate the drug, e.g., β-lactamase by staphylococci; aminoglycoside inactivating enzymes by *E. coli.*
   - Decreased accumulation of the drug in the bacterium, e.g., resistance to tetracyclines by gram-positive and gram-negative bacteria.
   - Altered target for the drug—the binding site may be altered, e.g., binding sites for aminoglycosides on the ribosomes may be altered.
   - Altered metabolic pathway—bacteria may produce folic acid by an alternate pathway.

Cross resistance is the resistance seen among chemically related drugs. When a microorganism develops resistance to one drug, it is also resistant to other drugs of the same group, even when not exposed to it, e.g., resistance to one tetracycline means resistance to all other tetracyclines.

Prevention of Resistance to Antimicrobials

Development of resistance to drugs can be avoided to some extent by the following measures:

- Antibiotics should be used only when necessary.
- Selection of the correct antibiotic is absolutely important.
- Correct dose and duration of treatment should be followed.
- Combination of drugs should be used as in tuberculosis to delay the development of resistance.

Antimicrobial Stewardship Program

Antimicrobial stewardship is a program to promote appropriate use of antimicrobials by the prescriber, to reduce their overuse and prevent resistance. The program is meant to control and supervise the use of antibiotics in order to decrease the emergence and spread of infections due to multidrug-resistant organisms.

Combination of Antimicrobials

A combination of antimicrobial agents is indicated in certain specific situations. The combination serves one of the following purposes:

1. **To obtain synergism:** Combination of antibiotics is recommended in conditions like:
   - **Bacterial endocarditis:** Penicillin + streptomycin is synergistic.
   - **Amoxicillin + clavulanic acid:** β-lactamase producing organisms like *H. influenzae.*
2. **Treatment of mixed infections:** In mixed infections with aerobic and anaerobic organisms, two or more antibiotics may be used.
3. **Initial treatment of severe infections:** Drugs covering both gram-positive and gram-negative pathogens may be used initially till the culture report is available, e.g., penicillin + aminoglycoside.
4. **To prevent the emergence of resistance:** In the treatment of tuberculosis and leprosy, combination of drugs is used to prevent development of resistance.
5. **To reduce the adverse effects:** The doses needed may be lower when a combination is used. This may reduce the incidence and severity of adverse effects, e.g., Amphotericin B + flucytosine in cryptococcal meningitis.

Disadvantages of Antimicrobial Combination

- Risk of toxicity from each agent
  Vancomycin + aminoglycoside → more severe renal toxicity.
- **Growth of resistant strains:** The few resistant mutants that remain may multiply unchecked.
- Emergence of organisms resistant to multiple drugs.
- Increased cost of therapy.

Chemoprophylaxis

Chemoprophylaxis is the use of antimicrobial agents to prevent infection. This is recommended in the following situations:

1. **To protect healthy persons**
   - Penicillin G is given for prevention of gonorrhea or syphilis in patients after contact with infected persons.
   - Malaria, leprosy, tuberculosis.
2. **To prevent infection in high risk patients**
   - In neutropenic patients—penicillin or fluoroquinolones or cotrimoxazole may reduce the incidence of bacterial infection.
   - In patients with valvular heart diseases even minor procedures like dental extraction, tonsillectomy or endoscopies may result in bacterial endocarditis (damage to mucosa results in bacteremia). Penicillin is used for prophylaxis.
3. **Surgical prophylaxis:** Certain guidelines are to be followed:
   - The drug should be started before surgery and should not be continued beyond 24 hours (risk of resistance) after surgery.
   - A single dose of 1 g IV cefazolin injection is the most commonly used.
4. **In close contacts:** Chemoprophylaxis is recommended particularly in children when infectious (open) cases of leprosy or tuberculosis are in close contact.

Superinfection

Superinfection/suprainfection is the appearance of a new infection resulting from the use of antimicrobials. Antibacterials alter the normal microbial flora of the intestinal, respiratory and genitourinary tracts. The normal flora help in host defence mechanisms by producing antibacterial substances called bacteriocins and by competing for nutrients. When the normal flora are destroyed by antibacterials, there can be dangerous infections due to various organisms especially the normal commensals. The broader the antibacterial spectrum of a drug, the more are the chances of superinfection, as the alteration of the normal flora is greater (Table 12.1).

Candida, Staphylococci, E. coli, Pseudomonas and *Clostridium difficile* commonly cause superinfection.

Table 12.1: Common microorganisms causing superinfection.

Microorganisms	*Manifestations*	*Treatment*
Candida albicans	Oral thrush, diarrhea, vaginitis	Clotrimazole
Staphylococci	Enteritis	Cloxacillin
Clostridium difficile	Pseudomembranous colitis	Metronidazole, vancomycin
E. coli	UTI	Norfloxacin
Pseudomonas	UTI	Carbenicillin, ticarcillin

Misuse of Antibiotics

Antibiotics are one of the most overused or misused drugs. Faulty practices like the use of antibacterials in viral infections, using too low doses or unnecessary prolonged treatment, using antibiotics in all fever cases—are all irrational and can do more harm than any benefit.

Probiotics are products containing viable non-pathogenic microorganisms administered orally to alter the intestinal microflora. *Lactobacillus, Streptococcus* *salivarius* and some enterococci are tried as probiotics in diarrhea, ulcerative colitis and irritable bowel syndrome.

Prebiotics are non-digestible substances which stimulate the growth of intestinal flora and thereby prevent the colonization by pathogenic bacteria, e.g., lactulose, inulin.

SULFONAMIDES

Sulfonamides were the first effective antibacterial agents to be used systemically in man. They contain a sulfonamide group.

Classification

- **Short-acting:** Sulfisoxazole, sulfadiazine.
- **Intermediate-acting:** Sulfamethoxazole.
- **Long-acting:** Sulfamethoxypyridazine, sulfadoxine.
- **Poorly absorbed:** Sulfasalazine.
- **Topical:** Sulfacetamide, mefenide, silver sulfadiazine.

Antibacterial spectrum: Sulfonamides inhibit gram-positive and some gram-negative bacteria, nocardia, chlamydiae and some protozoa.

Mechanism of action: Bacteria synthesize their own folic acid from p-amino benzoic acid (PABA) with the help of the enzyme folic acid synthetase (Fig. 12.3). Sulfonamides are structurally similar to PABA and competitively inhibit the enzyme folic acid synthetase. This results in folic acid deficiency and injury to the bacterial cell.

Sulfonamides are **bacteriostatic.**

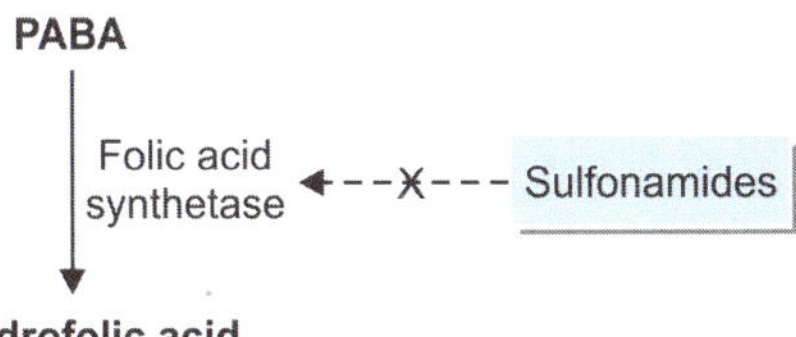

Fig. 12.3: Inhibition of folic acid synthesis by sulfonamides.

Presence of pus, blood and tissue breakdown products make sulfonamides ineffective as these are rich in PABA.

Resistance: Bacteria acquire resistance to sulfonamides by:

- Mutations—resulting in overproduction of PABA.
- Using alternate metabolic pathway for folic acid synthesis.
- Low permeability to sulfonamides.

Pharmacokinetics: Sulfonamides are well-absorbed, extensively bound to plasma proteins and are well distributed to all tissues. They are metabolized in the liver by acetylation.

Adverse Effects

- Renal irritation, hematuria, albuminuria and crystalluria—due to precipitation of the drug in acidic urine. This can be avoided by intake of large volumes of fluids and by alkalinizing the urine.
- **Allergic reactions** like rashes, fever, Stevens-Johnson syndrome and rarely exfoliative dermatitis.
- Anorexia, nausea and abdominal pain.
- Hemolytic anemia in patients with G6PD deficiency.
- **Kernicterus**—sulfonamides displace bilirubin from binding sites which crosses BBB and may cause kernicterus in the newborn. Hence contraindicated in pregnancy and in infants.

Uses: Because of the development of resistance and availability of better antimicrobials, sulfonamides are not commonly used now except in a few cases (Table 12.2).

1. **Urinary tract infections:** Sulfonamides may be used in areas where resistance is not high.
2. **Nocardiosis:** High doses of sulfonamides can be used.
3. **Toxoplasmosis:** Sulfonamides with pyrimethamine is the treatment of choice.
4. **Trachoma and inclusion conjunctivitis:** Tetracylines are the drugs of choice, sulfonamides are used as alternatives.
5. **Lymphogranuloma venereum and chancroid:** Sulfonamides are used as alternatives to tetracyclines.

Table 12.2: Choice of antibiotics recommended in the treatment of some common infections.

Microorganisms	*Clinical diagnosis*	*Drug of first choice*	*Alternate drugs*
Gram-positive organisms			
Group A *Streptococcus*	Pharyngitis, otitis media, sinusitis, cellulitis, erysipelas, impetigo, bacteremia dento-alveolar abscess	Penicillin or amoxicillin	Erythromycin, a first generation cephalosporin
Group B *Streptococcus*	Bacteremia, endocarditis meningitis	Ampicillin or penicillin + an aminoglycoside	A first generation cephalosporin
Staphylococcus aureus	Furuncle, cellulitis, bacteremia, osteomyelitis, pneumonia		
• Methicillin sensitive		Cloxacillin or dicloxacillin	A first generation cephalosporin or vancomycin
• Methicillin resistant		Vancomycin	Ciprofloxacin + rifampicin
Pneumococcus	Pneumonia, sinusitis, otitis, endocarditis, meningitis	Penicillin, amoxicillin	A first generation cephalosporin
Penicillin resistant	—	Ceftriaxone, cefotaxime vancomycin	Clindamycin cotrimoxazole
Enterococcus	Endocarditis	Penicillin G + gentamicin	Vancomycin + gentamicin
Gonococcus	Gonorrhea, pelvic inflammatory disease	Ceftriaxone	Ampicillin, amoxicillin doxycycline, erythromycin
Meningococcus	Meningitis Carrier state	Ceftriaxone, cefotaxime rifampicin	Penicillin G, chloramphenicol minocycline
Corynebacterium diphtheriae	Diphtheria	Erythromycin	A first generation cephalosporin, clindamycin
Clostridium tetani	Tetanus	Penicillin G	Clindamycin, doxycycline
Clostridium difficile	Pseudomembranous colitis	Metronidazole	Vancomycin
Clostridium perfringens	Gas gangrene	Penicillin G	Ceftizoxime, cefoxitine chloramphenicol doxycycline
Bacillus anthracis	Malignant pustule, pneumonia	Penicillin G	Erythromycin, doxycycline, a first generation cephalosporin
Gram-negative organisms			
Escherichia coli	Urinary tract infection	Norfloxacin, ciprofloxacin, cotrimoxazole	Ampicillin + gentamicin; Amoxicillin + clavulinic acid; Aztreonam
Proteus mirabilis	Urinary tract infection Bacteremia and other infections	Ampicillin or amoxicillin	Ciprofloxacin A cephalosporin, gentamicin
Pseudomonas aeruginosa	Urinary tract infection	Amoxicillin Ciprofloxacin	Gentamicin A cephalosporin, imipenem
Klebsiella pneumoniae	Urinary tract infection Pneumonia	A cephalosporin A cephalosporin + gentamicin	Mezlocillin, an aminoglycoside mezlocillin, aztreonam Amoxicillin + clavulinic acid

Contd...

Contd...

Microorganisms	*Clinical diagnosis*	*Drug of first choice*	*Alternate drugs*
Salmonella	Typhoid fever, bacteremia	Ciprofloxacin, ceftriaxone	Chloramphenicol, ampicillin, cotrimoxazole
Shigella	Gastroenteritis	Ciprofloxacin or norfloxacin	Cotrimoxazole, ampicillin
Hemophilus influenzae	Sinusitis Pneumonia Otitis media Meningitis	Amoxicillin + clavulinic acid Cotrimoxazole Ceftriaxone	Amoxicillin, ciprofloxacin Azithromycin A cephalosporin Chloramphenicol Ampicillin + sulbactam
Hemophilus ducreyi	Chancroid	Ceftriaxone Cotrimoxazole	Ciprofloxacin, erythromycin doxycycline
Brucella	Brucellosis	Doxycycline + rifampicin	Cotrimoxazole, gentamicin
Yersenia pestis	Plague	A tetracycline + streptomycin	Doxycycline, chloramphenicol ciprofloxacin
Vibrio cholerae	Cholera	Doxycycline Ciprofloxacin	Cotrimoxazole Chloramphenicol
Campylobacter jejuni	Enteritis	Ciprofloxacin	Erythromycin
Treponema pallidum	Syphilis	Penicillin G	Ceftriaxone, doxycycline
Leptospira	Weil's disease, meningitis	Penicillin G	Doxycycline
Other agents			
Mycoplasma pneumoniae	Atypical pneumonia	Erythromycin Doxycycline	Azithromycin
Rickettsia	Typhus fever, Q fever Rocky mountain, spotted fever	Doxycycline	Chloramphenicol
Chlamydia trachomatis	Lymphogranuloma venereum, trachoma Inclusion conjunctivitis, urethritis	Doxycycline	Erythromycin, azithromycin
Chlamydia psittaci	Psittacosis	Doxycycline	Chloramphenicol
Chlamydia pneumoniae	Pneumonia	Doxycycline	Erythromycin, azithromycin
Pneumocystis carinii	Pneumonia	Cotrimoxazole	Trimethoprim + dapsone

6. **Malaria:** Sulfadoxine is used with pyrimethamine in chloroquine resistant malaria.
7. **Prophylactic use:** In patients allergic to penicillins, sulfonamides may be used for prophylaxis of streptococcal pharyngitis in rheumatic fever.
8. **Topical:** Sulfacetamide eyedrops are used in bacterial conjunctivitis; mafenide and silver sulfadiazine are used in burns to prevent infection.
9. **Ulcerative colitis:** Sulfasalazine is useful in ulcerative colitis and rheumatoid arthritis.

COTRIMOXAZOLE

The combination of **trimethoprim and sulfamethoxazole** is cotrimoxazole. Trimethoprim is effective against several gram-positive and gram-negative organisms - but when used as a single drug, resistance develops rapidly.

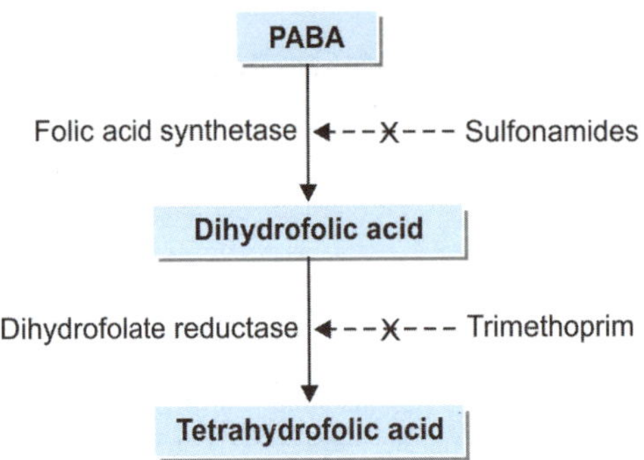

Fig. 12.4: Sequential blockage in folic acid synthesis.

Mechanism of action: Sulfonamides inhibit the conversion of PABA to dihydrofolic acid (DHF) and trimethoprim inhibits dihydrofolate reductase (DHFR) and thus prevents the reduction of DHF to tetrahydrofolic acid (THF). The two drugs thus block sequential steps in folic acid synthesis and the combination is bactericidal (Fig. 12.4).

The ratio of 'trimethoprim: sulfamethoxazole' used is 1:5 to attain the right plasma concentration. Among sulfonamides, sulfamethoxazole is chosen since its pharmacokinetic properties closely match with that of trimethoprim.

Antibacterial spectrum: Cotrimoxazole is effective against several gram-positive and gram-negative organisms like *Staphylococcus aureus,* streptococci, meningococci, *C. diphtheriae, E. coli, Proteus, H. influenzae, Salmonella* and *Shigella.* Cotrimoxazole also has good efficacy in *Pneumocystis jiroveci* infections.

Resistance: Development of resistance to the combination is slower when compared to either drugs given alone. Bacteria may acquire resistance by mutation or by acquisition of a plasmid coding for an altered DHFR.

Adverse Effects

- Nausea, vomiting, headache, glossitis, stomatitis and allergic skin rashes are relatively common.
- In patients with folate deficiency, cotrimoxazole may precipitate megaloblastic anemia.
- Hematological reactions like anemia and granulocytopenia are rare.
- AIDS patients are more likely to develop adverse effects to cotrimoxazole.

Preparations

Trimethoprim	Sulfamethoxazole (Septran, Ciplin)
80 mg	400 mg
160 mg	800 mg—double strength (DS).

Uses

1. **Urinary tract infection:** Uncomplicated acute UTI is treated for 7-10 days with cotrimoxazole.
   Chronic and recurrent UTI—small doses are given for prophylaxis.
   Bacterial prostatitis—Trimethoprim attains high concentration in prostatic fluid.
2. **Respiratory tract infections:** Upper and lower respiratory infections including bronchitis, sinusitis and otitis media respond.
3. **Bacterial gastroenteritis** due to *Shigella* and *E. coli* respond to cotrimoxazole.
4. **Typhoid:** Cotrimoxazole is used as an alternative to fluoroquinolones.
5. ***Pneumocystis jiroveci* infection:** Cotrimoxazole is used for prophylaxis and treatment (high doses) of *Pneumocystis* pneumonia in neutropenic and AIDS patients. It also protects against infection with other gram-negative bacteria.
6. **Chancroid:** Cotrimoxazole is the drug of choice.
7. **Melioidosis:** Caused by *B. pseudomallei* may be treated with cotrimoxazole but severe infection requires combination of antibiotics.
8. **Toxoplasmosis:** As an alternative to pyrimethamine-sulfadoxine.
9. **Intravenous cotrimoxazole:** Generally cotrimoxazole is used orally. In serious infections as in **typhoid, Pneumocystis**

pneumonia and UTI, cotrimoxazole can be given intravenously.

QUINOLONES

The quinolones are a group of synthetic antimicrobial agents. Nalidixic acid is the older agent in the group.

Nalidixic acid: Nalidixic acid is bactericidal against various gram-positive organisms like *E. coli, Shigella, Proteus* and *Klebsiella*. It is excreted too rapidly to have systemic effects but attains high concentration in the urine. Mechanism of action is similar to fluoroquinolones.

Allergic reactions including hemolytic anemia and CNS effects like headache, myalgia and drowsiness may be encountered.

Uses: Nalidixic acid is used in uncomplicated UTI and diarrhea due to *E. coli, Shigella* and *Proteus*.

Fluoroquinolones

The quinolones were fluorinated to get fluoroquinolones with the below advantages:

- Wider spectrum of activity,
- Fewer side effects,
- Lesser chances of resistance development,
- Better tissue penetration when compared to quinolones.

The fluoroquinolones (FQs) include:

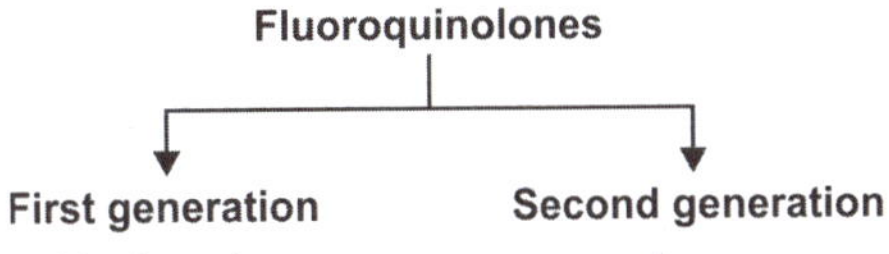

1. Respiratory fluoroquinolones
2. Withdrawn in many countries

Mechanism of action: Fluoroquinolones are bactericidal. They inhibit the bacterial enzyme DNA gyrase which is required for DNA replication and transcription.

Resistance: Resistance is due to mutations in the DNA gyrase enzyme or a change in the permeability of the organism. Several strains of *E. coli, Staphylococci, Pseudomonas* and *Serratia* have now developed resistance.

Antibacterial spectrum: Gram-negative organisms like *gonococci, meningococci, H. influenzae, E. coli, Salmonella, Shigella, enterobacteria; H. pylori,* gram-positive organisms like staphylococci; others like *Chlamydiae, Mycoplasma, Myobacterium* are also sensitive. Some of the newer agents are effective against some anaerobic organisms.

Pharmacokinetics: On oral administration, fluoroquinolones are well-absorbed and widely distributed. Food and antacids interfere with absorption; these are excreted by kidneys.

Adverse reactions: Fluoroquinolones are well-tolerated. Nausea, vomiting, abdominal discomfort, diarrhea and rashes may be seen. Tendinitis with associated risk of tendon rupture has been reported. Fluoroquinolones damage the growing cartilage resulting in arthropathy and are therefore contraindicated up to 18 years of age.

Uses (Table 12.3)

1. **Urinary tract infections:** Very effective in UTI even when caused by multidrug resistant bacteria—norfloxacin is generally used.
2. **Typhoid:** Ciprofloxacin is the drug of choice (500 mg BD—10 days)—also eradicates carrier state.
3. **Diarrhea** due to *Shigella, E. coli* and *Campylobacter* respond.
4. **Gonorrhea:** Single dose 250 mg ciprofloxacin is curative.
5. **Chancroid:** As an alternative to cotrimoxazole.
6. **Respiratory tract infection**—due to *H. influenzae, Legionella and Mycoplasma* can be treated with fluoroquinolones.
7. **Bone, joint, soft tissue and intra-abdominal infections:** Osteomyelitis and joint infections require prolonged treatment. Soft tissue infections due to sensitive bacteria can be treated with fluoroquinolones.

Table 12.3: Dose of some fluoroquinolones.

Drug	*Dose (oral)*
Norfloxacin (NORFLOX)	400 mg BD
Ciprofloxacin (CIPLOX)	250–750 mg BD
Pefloxacin (PEFLOX)	400 mg BD
Ofloxacin (TARIVID)	200–400 mg OD
Lomefloxacin (LOMEF)	400 mg OD
Sparfloxacin (SPARLOX)	200–400 mg OD

8. **Tuberculosis:** Ciprofloxacin is one of the drugs in multidrug regimens used for resistant tuberculosis. It is also useful in atypical mycobacterial infections.
9. **Bacterial prostatitis and cervicitis**—FQs are useful.
10. **Eye infections:** Ciprofloxacin and ofloxacin may be used topically in the treatment of eye infections.
11. **Anthrax**—also responds to fluoroquinolones.
12. **Neutropenic patients**—fluoroquinolones are used in neutropenic patients to prevent infections.
13. **Gram-negative septicemia**—FQs may be combined with a III generation cephalosporin/aminoglycoside in the treatment of gram-negative septicemia.
14. **Meningococcal carrier state**—FQs eradicate carrier state.

Mnemonic for Uses

FQs **GET RID** of **Bacillus SANCTUM**
G—Gonorrhea
E—Eye infection
T—Typhoid
R—Respiratory tract infections
I—Intra-abdominal infections
D—Diarrhea
of
B—Bacterial prostatitis/cervicitis
S—Septicemia
A—Anthrax
N—Neutropenia patients
C—Chancroid
T—Tuberculosis
U—UTI
M—Meningococcal carrier state

BETA-LACTAM ANTIBIOTICS

The β-lactam antibiotics have a β-lactam ring. Penicillins, cephalosporins, monobactams and carbapenems are β-lactams.

Penicillins

Sir Alexander Fleming discovered penicillin in 1928. Penicillins are one of the most important groups of antibiotics. Penicillin is now obtained from the fungus *Penicillium chrysogenum*.

Mechanism of action: β-lactam antibiotics act by inhibiting cell wall synthesis in the bacteria. The rigid cell wall of the bacteria protects it from lysis. Peptidoglycan, is an important component which gives strength to the cell wall. β-lactam antibiotics inhibit the synthesis of this peptidoglycan, resulting in the formation of cell wall deficient bacteria. These undergo lysis. Thus, penicillins are bactericidal.

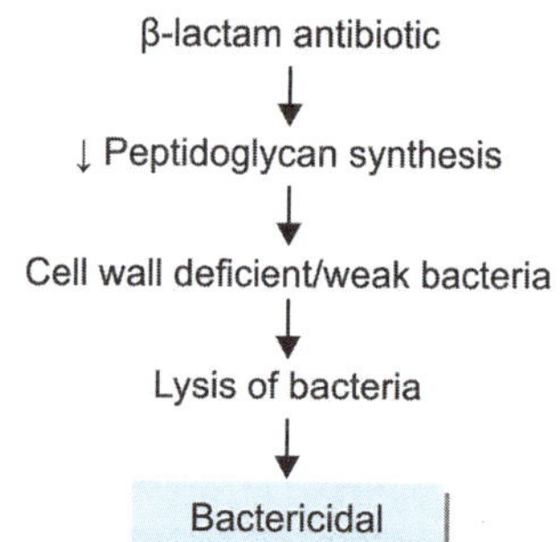

Classification of Penicillins

A. ***Natural:***
   - Penicillin G
   - Repository penicillins
     - Procaine penicillin
     - Benzathine penicillin

B. ***Semisynthetic:***
   1. **Acid resistant:** Penicillin V
   2. **Penicillinase resistant:** Methicillin, oxacillin, cloxacillin, nafcillin
   3. **Aminopenicillins:** Ampicillin, bacampicillin, pivampicillin, talampicillin, amoxicillin

4. **Antipseudomonal penicillins:**
   - **Carboxypenicillins:** Carbenicillin, ticarcillin
   - **Ureidopenicillins:** Azlocillin, mezlocillin, piperacillin.

Natural Penicillins

Penicillin G (Benzyl Penicillin)

Antibacterial Spectrum: Penicillin G (PnG) has a narrow antibacterial spectrum and is effective against gram-positive cocci and bacilli and a few gram-negative cocci. Thus streptococci, pneumococci, gonococci, meningococci, *B. anthracis, C. diphtheriae*, clostridia, listeria and spirochetes are highly sensitive.

Resistance: Many organisms like staphylococci produce an enzyme called penicillinase which is a beta-lactamase—which opens the β-lactam ring and inactivates penicillins.

Pharmacokinetics: PnG is destroyed by gastric juice; food interferes with its absorption —hence it is to be given 2 hours after food. It has a short t½ of 30 minutes. Though it does not readily cross the blood-brain barrier (BBB), in presence of inflammation, therapeutic concentration is attained in the cerebrospinal fluid (CSF). It is excreted by the kidneys. Probenecid blocks the renal tubular secretion of penicillin and thereby prolongs its duration of action.

Preparations

For preparations and doses (*See* Table 12.4).

Adverse Effects

Hypersensitivity: PnG is the most common cause of drug allergy. It can cause skin rashes, urticaria, fever, bronchospasm, serum sickness and rarely exfoliative dermatitis and anaphylaxis. Though all forms of penicillins can cause allergy, anaphylaxis is more common with parenteral than oral preparations. The highest incidence is with procaine penicillin where allergy is most often due to the procaine component. There is cross-sensitivity among different penicillins. Topical penicillins are highly sensitizing and their use is banned.

Table 12.4: Doses and route of administration of penicillins.

Drugs	*Doses*	*Routes*
Natural Penicillins		
Sodium penicillin G (Crystalline penicillin)	0.5–5 MU 4–6 hr	IM/IV
Procaine penicillin G	0.5–1 MU 12–24 hr	IM
Benzathine penicillin G	1.2–2.4 MU every 3–4 weeks	Deep IM
Semisynthetic Penicillins		
Penicillin	250–500 mg QID	Oral
Cloxacillin	250–500 mg QID	Oral
Dicloxacillin	250–500 mg QID	Oral
Nafcillin	1–2 g 4–6 hr	IV
Ampicillin	250 mg or 1 g QID	Oral IM/IV
Ampicillin + sulbactum	1 g Ampi + 0.5 g sulb 6–8 hr	IV
Amoxicillin	250–500 mg TID	Oral
Amoxicillin + clavulanic acid	250 mg Amox + 125 mg Clav TID	Oral
Piperacillin	3–4 g 4–6 hr	IV
Ticarcillin	3 g 4–6 hr	IV

History of allergy to penicillins should be taken before prescribing. A **scratch test** or intradermal sensitivity test with 2–10 units should be done. Even if this is negative, it does not completely rule out allergy. Penicillin should be given cautiously and a syringe loaded with adrenaline to treat anaphylaxis should be kept ready.

Other Adverse Effects

Local: Pain at the site of injection, thrombophlebitis on IV injection.

CNS: Large doses of PnG may produce confusion, muscle twitchings, convulsions and coma.

Suprainfections: These are rare due to its narrow spectrum of activity.

Jarisch-Herxheimer reaction: When penicillin is injected in a patient with syphilis, there is sudden destruction of spirochetes and release of its products. This triggers a reaction with fever, myalgia, shivering, exacerbation of syphilitic lesions and vascular collapse.

Uses

Penicillin G is the antibiotic of choice for several infections unless the patient is allergic to it.

1. **Pneumococcal infections:** For infections due to penicillin-sensitive pneumococci, like pneumonia, meningitis and osteomyelitis, PnG is the ***drug of choice***.
2. **Streptococcal infections:** Pharyngitis, sinusitis, pneumonia, meningitis and endocarditis are all treated with penicillin. Infective endocarditis due to *Strep. viridans* is treated with high dose PnG ± an aminoglycoside.
3. **Meningococcal infections:** PnG is the drug of choice for all meningococcal infections.
4. **Staphylococcal infections:** Since most staphylococci produce penicillinase, a penicillinase resistant penicillin should be used.
5. **Syphilis:** It is treated with procaine penicillin for 10 days or with benzathine penicillin.
6. **Diphtheria:** Antitoxin is the only effective treatment. PnG eliminates carrier state.
7. **Anaerobic infections:** Pulmonary, periodontal and brain abscesses due to anaerobes respond to PnG.
8. **Actinomycosis:** PnG is the drug of choice for all forms of actinomycosis.
9. **Tetanus and gas gangrene:** Antitoxin is the treatment for tetanus—but PnG kills the bacteria.

   Gas gangrene—PnG is the **drug of choice**.
10. **Other infections:** PnG is the **agent of choice** for infections like anthrax, trench mouth and listeria infections.
11. **Prophylactic uses:**
    - **Rheumatic fever:** Benzathine penicillin 1.2 MU every month prevents colonization by streptococci and thereby decreases the recurrences of rheumatic fever. It is to be continued for several years.
    - **Gonorrhea and syphilis:** Sexual contacts are effectively protected against these diseases when treated with penicillin within 12 hours of exposure.
    - **Valvular heart diseases:** 25 percent cases of bacterial endocarditis are seen following dental extractions. Such patients undergoing dental extractions, endoscopies and other minor surgical procedures that may cause bacteremia should be given penicillin prophylaxis.

Mnemonic

PADMA STOPS Syphilis

P—Pneumococcal
A—Anaerobic
D—Diphtheria
M—Meningococcal
A—Actinomycosis
S—Staphylococcal
T—Tetanus
O—Other infections
P—Prophylactic
S— Streptococcal
S— Syphilis

Disadvantages of Natural Penicillins

- Narrow-spectrum of activity
- Not effective orally—acid labile
- Susceptible to penicillinase
- Risk of hypersensitivity

Semisynthetic penicillins were obtained in an effort to overcome these disadvantages.

Semisynthetic Penicillins

1. **Acid resistant penicillins:** ***Penicillin V*** (phenoxymethyl penicillin) is acid stable and can be given orally. It is used only in mild streptococcal pharyngitis, sinusitis and trench mouth.
2. **Penicillinase resistant penicillins** like methicillin and cloxacillin are resistant to hydrolysis by penicillinase produced by

bacteria. However, against other microorganisms—they are less effective than PnG.

Methicillin is destroyed by gastric juice—hence given parenterally. Cloxacillin is given orally.

Uses: Penicillinase resistant penicillins are the drugs of choice for infections with penicillinase producing staphylococci. Methicillin resistant strains have now emerged and are treated with vancomycin.

3. **Aminopenicillins:** Aminopenicillins are ***Extended Spectrum Penicillins*** have a wider antibacterial spectrum including many gram-negative bacilli. They are orally effective but are sensitive to beta-lactamases.

Antibacterial spectrum: Both gram-positive and gram-negative organisms including streptococci, meningococci, pneumococci, *H. influenzae, E. coli, Proteus, Salmonella, Shigella* and *Klebsiella* are sensitive. Many strains are now resistant.

Ampicillin is well-absorbed orally; food interferes with absorption. It is excreted mainly through kidneys.

Adverse Effects

Diarrhea due to irritation of the gut by the unabsorbed drug is the most common adverse effect with ampicillin. **Skin rashes** are also fairly frequent.

Uses

1. **Respiratory tract infections** like bronchitis, sinusitis and otitis media respond to ampicillin.
2. **Urinary tract infections:** Though ampicillin was the drug of choice earlier, many organisms have now become resistant.
3. **Meningitis:** Ampicillin is given with a cephalosporin.
4. **Typhoid:** Ampicillin is an alternative to ciprofloxacin.
5. **Septicemia due to gram-negative organisms:** Ampicillin may be used with an aminoglycoside.
6. **Bacillary dysentry due to shigella** - some strains respond but many are now resistant to ampicillin.

Bacampicillin: It is an ester of ampicillin. It is a prodrug that is better absorbed (hence diarrhea is less common) and longer-acting than ampicillin.

Amoxicillin is used in similar infections as ampicillin like respiratory infections, *Salmonella gastroenteritis* and urinary tract infection. Amoxicillin is a component of the various regimens to eradicate *H. pylori.* Amoxicillin is preferred over ampicillin because of below advantages:

- Amoxicillin is better absorbed orally.
- Food does not interfere with its absorption.
- Diarrhea is rare.
- Given thrice daily.

Antipseudomonal Penicillins

Carboxypenicillins

Carbenicillin is effective in *Pseudomonas aeruginosa* and *Proteus* infections. It is given parenterally while carbenicillin indanyl is effective orally. Both are susceptible to penicillinase.

Adverse effects: Carbenicillin is used as a sodium salt and in higher doses this excess sodium may cause edema and CCF; may also cause bleeding due to abnormal platelet aggregation.

Ureidopenicillins: Ureidopenicillins have a wider antibacterial spectrum than ticarcillin and are effective against a variety of gram-negative organisms including *Pseudomonas* and *Klebsiella.*

Beta-lactamase inhibitors: β-lactamases are enzymes produced by bacteria that open up the β-lactam ring and inactivate the β-lactam antibiotics. β-lactamase inhibitors bind to and inactivate β-lactamases preventing the destruction of the β-lactam antibiotics.

They broaden the antibacterial spectrum of penicillins so that they can be used against penicillinase producing staphylococci, gonococci, *E. coli, H. influenzae* and others. The antibacterial spectrum depends on the penicillin used.

Clavulanic acid, sulbactam, tazobactam and avibactam are β-lactamase inhibitors available for use and newer ones are **vaborbactam and relebactam.**

Clavulanic acid/sulbactam/tazobactam

↓

Inhibit bacterial β-lactamases

↓

Prevent degradation of β-lactam antibiotics

↓

Broaden antibacterial spectrum

Clavulanic acid is combined with amoxicillin for both oral and parenteral administration. It extends the antibacterial spectrum of amoxicillin. The combination is used for mixed nosocomial infections.

Sulbactam is combined with ampicillin. It is given parenterally for mixed pelvic and other infections. **Tazobactam** is combined with piperacillin.

They are available in fixed dose combinations.

Cephalosporins

Cephalosporins are semisynthetic antibiotics with a beta-lactam ring related to penicillins. They are derived from cephalosporin-C and have a wider spectrum of activity than penicillins (Table 12.5).

Table 12.5: Preparations, doses and routes of administration of some cephalosporins.

Drugs	*Dose*	*Routes*
Cephalothin (KAFLIN)	1–2 g q 6 hr	IV
Cefazolin (ALCIZON)	0.5–1 g q 6 hr	IM/IV
Cephalexin (SPORIDEX)	0.25–1 g QID	Oral
Cefadroxil (DROXYL)	0.5–1 g BID	Oral
Cefamandole (KEFADOL)	0.5–2 g q 4–8 hr	IM/IV
Cefuroxine (SUPACEF)	0.75–1.5 g q 8 hr	IM/IV
Cefuroxime axetil (CEFTUM)	0.25–0.5 g BD	Oral
Cefachlor (KEFLOR)	0.25–0.5 g q 8 hr	Oral
Cefotaxime (OMNATAX)	1–2 g q 8 hr	IM/IV
Ceftriaxone (OFRAMAX)	1–2 g q 12–24 hr	IM/IV
Cefoperazone (CEFOBID)	1–2 g q 8–12 hr	IM/IV
Cefixime (CEFSPAN)	0.2–0.4 g q 12 hr	Oral
Cefpirome (CEFROM)	1–2 g q 12 hr	IV

Mechanism of Action

Cephalosporins inhibit the bacterial cell wall synthesis similar to penicillins. They are bactericidal.

Classification

Cephalosporins are classified into five generations.

	Parenteral	*Oral*
First generation	Cephalothin Cefazolin	Cephalexin Cefadroxil
Second generation	Cefamandole Cefuroxime Cefoxitin Cefotetan	Cefachlor Cefuroxime axetil
Third generation	Cefotaxime Ceftrioxone Cefoperazone Ceftizoxime Ceftazidime	Cefixime Cefpodoxime proxetil Ceftibuten
Fourth generation	Cefepime Cefpirome	
Fifth generation	Ceftaroline Ceftobiprole	

Resistance

As in the case of penicillins, beta-lactamases determine resistance to cephalosporins.

First Generation Cephalosporins

First generation cephalosporins are very effective against gram-positive organisms. Cephalothin is resistant to penicillinase, hence can be used in staphylococcal infections. Cefazolin has a longer t½ and its tissue penetrability is good—therefore used for surgical prophylaxis. Cephalexin is used orally for minor infections like abscesses or cellulitis.

Second Generation Cephalosporins

Second generation cephalosporins are more active against some gram-negative organisms compared to first generation ones. *H. influenzae, E. coli, Proteus and Klebsiella* are inhibited. Cefuroxime is resistant to β-lactamases; attains good CSF concentration and is useful in meningitis.

Cefoxitin and cefotitan are effective against *Bacteroides fragilis* and are used in mixed infections like in intra-abdominal infections.

Third Generation Cephalosporins

Third generation cephalosporins are highly resistant to β-lactamases; have good activity against gram-negative organisms. Many cross BBB and are useful in meningitis. Ceftrioxone has a long t½ and can be given once daily. It is excreted mainly through biliary tract and no dosage adjustment is needed in renal failure.

Ceftazidime is effective against *Pseudomonas aeruginosa*. Third generation cephalosporins can be life-saving in serious gram-negative infections including aminoglycoside resistant ones.

Fourth Generation Cephalosporins

Cefepime and cefpirome have activity similar to III generation ones except that they are more resistant to β-lactamases and are effective against organisms resistant to other cephalosporins. Cefepime attains very good CSF levels.

Fourth generation cephalosporins are used in **serious gram-negative infections** including septicemia, nosocomial infections and in immuno-compromised patients.

Fifth Generation Cephalosporins

Fifth generation cephalosporins including ceftaroline and ceftobiprole are antiMRSA cephalosporins. Both are effective against MRSA and penicillin resistant *Streptococcus pneumoniae*. They inhibit PBP which is specific to MRSA. They are approved for use in skin and skin structure infections and community acquired pneumonia. Ceftarolin dose: 600 mg slow IV over 1 hour 12th hourly. Ceftobiprole is also effective against *Pseudomonas*.

Adverse Reactions to Cephalosporins

Cephalosporins are generally well-tolerated.

1. **Hypersensitivity reactions:** Like skin rashes, fever, serum sickness and rarely anaphylaxis are seen. Twenty percent of patients allergic to penicillin show cross-reactivity to cephalosporins. There are no reliable skin tests for testing allergy.
2. **Nephrotoxicity:** Mild nephrotoxicity is noted with some cephalosporins. Combination with other nephrotoxic drugs should be avoided.
3. **Diarrhea** can result from some of the cephalosporins.
4. **Bleeding** is due to hypoprothrombinemia which is more common in malnourished patients.
5. **Low** WBC count may be seen though rarely.
6. **Pain** at the injection site may occur.
7. **Disulfiram-like reaction** with alcohol is reported with some cephalosporins.

Uses of Cephalosporins

1. **Gram-negative infections:** Urinary, respiratory and soft tissue infections due to gram-negative organisms respond.
2. **Surgical prophylaxis:** Cefazolin is preferred.
3. **Gonorrhea:** Ceftriaxone (single dose 250 mg) is the drug of choice.
4. **Meningitis:** Due to *H. influenzae, N. meningitidis and S. Pneumoniae*—3rd generation agents are used.
5. **Mixed aerobic-anaerobic infections:** Common following pelvic surgeries—a 3rd generation agent is used.
6. **Typhoid:** As an alternative to ciprofloxacin.
7. **Nosocomial infections** can be treated with 3rd generation cephalosporins.

Carbapenems

Carbapenems contain a β-lactam ring fused with a five-membered penem ring. Carbapenems include **imipenem, meropenem, ertapenem, faropenem and doripenem**.

Antibacterial spectrum: Carbapenems have a wide antibacterial spectrum and inhibit various gram-positive, gram-negative organisms and anaerobes including streptococci, staphylococci, enterococci, *Listeria, Enterobacteriaceae, Pseudomonas* and *B. fragilis*.

Mechanism of action: Carbapenems inhibit bacterial cell wall synthesis similar to penicillins.

Imipenem is not absorbed orally and is administered intravenously (250–500 mg every 6–8 hours); it has good tissue penetrability. Imipenem is inactivated quickly by an enzyme in the renal tubules. Hence it is always combined with **cilastatin** which inhibits the renal enzyme and prolongs the plasma half-life of imipenem.

Adverse effects to imipenem include nausea, vomiting and diarrhea. Allergic reactions are seen especially in patients allergic to other β-lactam antibiotics. High doses can occasionally cause seizures.

Uses: Imipenem-cilastatin is used in UTI, respiratory, skin, bone, soft tissue, intra-abdominal and gynecological infections due to susceptible microorganisms. It is particularly useful in nosocomial infections resistant to other antibiotics. It is used in pseudomonas infection (along with an aminoglycoside).

Meropenem has the following advantages over imipenem.

- It is not destroyed by renal dipeptidase and therefore does not require to be combined with cilastatin.
- Risk of seizures is less than with imipenem.

Indications are similar to imipenem.

Ertapenem is similar to meropenem except that it is not useful against *P. aeruginosa*. It is longer acting and given once daily.

Monobactams

Monobactams are monocyclic beta lactams, i.e., they contain a single ring—the beta-lactam ring.

Aztreonam is the monobactam available. It is active against gram-negative bacilli including *Pseudomonas aerugenosa* but is *not* effective against gram-positive organisms and anaerobes. Aztreonam acts by inhibiting cell wall synthesis like penicillins. It is given parenterally.

Aztreonam can be used in patients allergic to penicillins as there is no cross allergenicity with other β-lactams . The only reported adverse effects are occasional skin rashes. Aztreonam is used in *Pseudomonas* infections especially nosocomial and in other gram-negative infections.

AMINOGLYCOSIDES

Aminoglycosides are antibiotics with amino sugars in glycosidic linkages. They are derived from the soil actinomycetes.

Aminoglycosides include:

- Streptomycin
- Kanamycin
- Tobramycin
- Neomycin
- Gentamicin
- Netilmicin
- Amikacin

Common Properties of Aminoglycosides (AG)

1. Aminoglycosides are not absorbed orally and are therefore given parenterally
2. They remain extracellularly and penetration into CSF is very poor.
3. They are all bactericidal.
4. They act by inhibiting bacterial protein synthesis.
5. They are mainly effective against gram-negative organisms.
6. They produce ototoxicity and nephrotoxicity as adverse effects.
7. They are excreted unchanged by the kidneys.

Antibacterial spectrum: Aminoglycosides have a narrow-spectrum and are effective mainly against aerobic gram-negative bacilli like *E. coli, Proteus, Pseudomonas, Brucella, Salmonella, Shigella* and *Klebsiella.*

Mechanism of action: Aminoglycosides bind to 30S ribosomes and inhibit bacterial protein synthesis. They are *bactericidal.* Aminoglycosides have a postantibiotic effect, i.e., the antibacterial activity remains for a long time even after the drug in excreted.

Resistance to aminoglycosides is acquired by:

- Aminoglycoside inactivating enzymes.
- Low affinity of ribosomes—acquired by mutation.
- Decrease in permeability to the antibiotic.

There is partial cross-resistance among various aminoglycosides.

Adverse Effects

1. **Ototoxicity:** This is the most important toxicity. Both vestibular and auditory dysfunction can occur depending on the dose and duration. The aminoglycosides get concentrated in the inner ear and damage both cochlear hair cells and vestibular sensory cells. As the cochlear cells cannot regenerate, there is progressive, **permanent deafness**. Elderly people are more susceptible. Stopping the drug can prevent further damage. Vestibular dysfunction results in headache, nausea, vomiting, dizziness, vertigo, nystagmus and ataxia. Recovery is slow over 1–2 years.
2. **Nephrotoxicity:** Aminoglycosides attain high concentration in the kidney and cause damage to the renal tubules. These effects are reversible.
3. **Neuromuscular blockade:** Aminoglycosides have curare-like effects and block neuromuscular transmission.

Precautions in Using Aminoglycosides

1. Avoid use of other ototoxic drugs like loop diuretics with aminoglycosides.
2. Avoid use of other nephrotoxic drugs like amphotericin B and cisplatin with aminoglycosides.
3. To be avoided with other skeletal muscle relaxants.
4. To be used cautiously in elderly, in renal dysfunction and in combination with skeletal muscle relaxants.
5. Contraindicated in pregnancy.
6. Do not mix aminoglycosides with any other drug in the same syringe.
7. Determination of plasma levels of aminoglycosides may be needed in severe infections and in patients with renal dysfunction.

Streptomycin obtained from *Streptomyces griseus* is mainly effective against aerobic gram-negative bacilli. When used alone, bacteria, especially the tubercle bacillus rapidly develops resistance to it. Streptomycin is the least nephrotoxic among aminoglycosides.

Uses

1. **Tuberculosis** (*See* page 264).
2. **Subacute bacterial endocarditis (SBE):** Combination of streptomycin and penicillin is synergistic in this condition.
3. **Plague, tularemia and brucellosis:** Streptomycin is given with a tetracycline.

Gentamicin obtained from *Micromonospora purpurea* is more potent and has a broader spectrum of action compared to streptomycin. Development of resistance has limited its use.

Uses

- **UTI:** Gentamicin is effective in uncomplicated UTI as it is released for a long time from the renal cortex.
- **Pneumonia** due to gram-negative organisms may be treated with gentamicin + penicillin.
- **Osteomyelitis, peritonitis, septicemia** caused by gram-negative organisms respond to gentamicin.
- **Meningitis due to gram-negative bacilli:** Gentamicin is used with a III generation cephalosporin.
- **Bacterial endocarditis:** Gentamicin may be used in place of streptomycin.

- **Topical:** Gentamicin cream is used topically in burns and other infected wounds. Gentamicin eyedrops is used in bacterial conjunctivitis.

Tobramycin has better activity against *Pseudomonas* and is used with an anti-pseudomonal penicillin in such infections.

Kanamycin—due to its toxicity, its use is limited to multi-drug resistant tuberculosis.

Amikacin

Amikacin has widest antibacterial spectrum among the aminoglycosides. It is resistant to aminoglycoside inactivating enzymes.

Uses

- Nosocomial infections due to gram-negative organisms.
- **Tuberculosis:** Amikacin is useful in multidrug resistant tuberculosis in combination with other drugs.
- It is also used in infections due to *atypical mycobacteria* in patients with AIDS.

Netilmicin like amikacin, netilmicin is resistant to aminoglycoside inactivating enzymes. It is used in serious infections due to gram-negative bacilli.

Sisomicin has actions, toxicity and uses similar to gentamicin.

Neomycin has a wide antibacterial spectrum. As it is highly ototoxic, it is not given systemically. It is used topically as ointment, cream and powder.

Adverse effects: Neomycin can cause skin rashes on topical use. Oral use can cause diarrhea, steatorrhea and malabsorption due to damage to the intestinal villi. Superinfection with *Candida* can also occur.

Uses

- **Topical:** Neomycin is used topically in skin infections, burns, ulcers and wounds; eye and ear infections.
- **Orally:** Neomycin is not absorbed when given orally. But it is used to prepare the bowel for surgery, i.e., for preoperative gut sterilization.
- **Hepatic coma:** Normally ammonia produced by colonic bacteria is absorbed and converted to urea by the liver. But in severe hepatic failure, liver is unable to handle this ammonia and blood ammonia levels rise resulting in encephalopathy. Neomycin inhibits intestinal flora and decreases ammonia production.

BROAD-SPECTRUM ANTIBIOTICS

Tetracyclines

Tetracyclines are antibiotics with four cyclic rings (hence the name) obtained from the soil actinomycetes. In addition to gram-positive and gram-negative bacteria, tetracyclines also inhibit the growth of other microorganisms like Rickettsiae, Chlamydiae, *Mycoplasma* and some protozoa. Therefore, they are called **broad-spectrum antibiotics.** The tetracyclines include:

Tetracyclines	*Semisynthetic derivatives*
Chlortetracycline Tetracycline Oxytetracycline	Demeclocycline Methacycline Doxycycline Minocycline
Newer tetracycline	Tigecycline

Antibacterial Spectrum

Antibacterial spectrum is broad including gram-positive and gram-negative organisms like *Streptococci, Staphylococci, Gonococci, Meningococci, H. influenza, Brucella, V. cholerae, Campylobacter, Y. pestis* and many anaerobes. They also inhibit rickettsiae, chlamydiae, *Mycoplasma, Actinomyces, E. histolytica* and *Plasmodia.* Many organisms have now become resistant.

Mechanism of Action

Tetracyclines are bacteriostatic. They bind to 30S ribosomes and inhibit protein synthesis.

Pharmacokinetics

Older tetracyclines are incompletely absorbed from the gut; food interferes with their absorption. Doxycycline and minocycline are 100 percent absorbed and food does not affect the absorption of these two agents. Tetracyclines chelate calcium and other metals which reduce their absorption. Hence tetracyclines should not be given with **milk, iron preparations and antacids**.

Tetracyclines except doxycycline and minocycline are excreted through kidneys. Doxycycline and minocycline are excreted through gut and are therefore safe in patients with renal insufficiency.

Adverse Effects

1. **GIT:** Gastrointestinal irritation, nausea, vomiting and diarrhea—tetracyclines are to be given with food to minimize these effects.
2. **Hepatotoxicity** may result in jaundice. Acute hepatic necrosis may occur in pregnant women but is rare.
3. **Renal toxicity:** Renal failure may be aggravated. Outdated tetracyclines cause a syndrome like Fanconi's syndrome with vomiting, polyuria, proteinuria, glycosuria and acidosis due to metabolites of the outdated tetracyclines.
4. **Phototoxicity:** Skin reactions and dermatitis on exposure to sun are more likely with doxycycline and demeclocycline.
5. **Effect on teeth and bones:** Tetracyclines chelate calcium. The calcium-tetracycline-orthophasphate complexes get deposited in the developing teeth and bones. The deformities depend on the time of tetracycline administration. Brownish discoloration and pigmentation of the teeth occur. The growth of skeleton is also depressed when given up to 8 years of age. Hence tetracyclines are teratogenic.
6. **Suprainfections:** Since the intestinal flora are extensively suppressed by tetracyclines, these are the most common antibiotics to cause suprainfections.
7. **Hypersensitivity reactions** are not very common.

Uses

A. **Tetracyclines are the drugs of choice in:**
   1. **Rickettsial infections:** All rickettsial infections respond to tetracyclines.
   2. **Chlamydial infections:**
      - *Lymphogranuloma venereum*
      - Trachoma—both topical and oral administration.
      - Inclusion conjunctivitis.
      - *Chlamydia pneumoniae* - causes pneumonia.

      Tetracyclines are effective in all the above chlamydial infections.
   3. **Atypical pneumonia:** Due to *Mycoplasma pneumoniae.*
   4. **Cholera:** Tetracyclines reduce the duration of illness and are of adjuvant value.
   5. **Brucellosis:** Doxycycline 200 mg + Rifampicin 600 mg daily for 6 weeks is the treatment of choice.
   6. **Plague:** Tetracyclines may be combined with an aminoglycoside.

B. **Tetracyclines are useful in other conditions like:**
   7. **Traveller's diarrhea:** Doxycycline reduces the incidence of traveller's diarrhea.
   8. **Sexually transmitted diseases** like syphilis, gonorrhea and chancroid also respond to tetracyclines—but are not preferred.
   9. **Acne:** The propioni bacteria in the sebaceous follicles metabolize lipids into irritating free fatty acids which trigger the development of acne. Tetracyclines inhibit these bacteria. Low doses are given for a long time (250 mg BD for 4 weeks).
   10. **Protozoal infections:**
       - **Amebiasis:** Tetracyclines are useful in chronic intestinal amebiasis.
       - **Malaria:** Doxycycline is given with quinine in multi-drug resistant malaria.

11. **Other infections:** Treatment of tularemia, lyme disease, relapsing fever and leptospirosis.
12. **Topical use:** Tetracycline eye drops are used for eye infections.

Contraindications

Tetracyclines are contraindicated in pregnancy, lactation and in children up to 8 years of age.

Dosage of some tetracyclines	
Tetracyclines	*Doses*
Chlortetracycline	250–500 mg Qid
Tetracycline	250–500 mg Qid
Doxycycline	200 mg initially then 100 mg OD
Minocycline	200 mg initially then 100 mg OD

Doxycycline and minocycline are semisynthetic tetracyclines.

- Given orally they are nearly 100% absorbed.
- Food does not interfere with their absorption.
- Have long t½—can be given once daily.
- Excreted through gut hence can be given in renal impairment.
- Minocycline causes vestibular toxicity - causes vertigo, ataxia, dizziness, nausea and vomiting.

Tigecycline

Tigecycline is a derivative of minocycline. It has a broad antibacterial spectrum including many resistant strains of staphylococci, streptococci, multidrug resistant enterococci, many gram-positive and gram-negative aerobes and anaerobes that are resistant to tetracyclines.

Tigecycline is given iv—initial dose of 100 mg followed by 50 mg twice daily. It has a long t½ of 36 hours. Penetrability into cells and tissues is good. It is excreted through the gut and therefore does not require dose reduction in renal dysfunction. Tigecycline can cause nausea and vomiting apart from other adverse effects of tetracyclines. Tigecycline is used in life-threatening infections due to drug resistant microorganisms and nosocomial pathogens including skin and skin structure infections and intra-abdominal infections.

Chloramphenicol

Chloramphenicol is a broad-spectrum antibiotic first obtained from *Streptomyces venezuelae* in 1947.

Mechanism of action: Chloramphenicol is bacteriostatic but to some organisms it is bactericidal. It binds to 50S ribosomal subunit and inhibits protein synthesis.

Antibacterial spectrum: It has a broad-spectrum and includes gram-negative organisms, some gram-positive organisms, anaerobic bacteria, Rickettsiae, Chlamydiae and *Mycoplasma*. Thus *H. influenzae, Salmonella, Shigella, Bordatella, Brucella,* gonococci, meningococci, streptococci, staphylococci, *Clostridium, E. coli* and *Klebsiella*—are inhibited apart from Rickettsiae, Chlamydiae and *Mycoplasma.*

Pharmacokinetics: Chloramphenicol is rapidly absorbed from the gut; penetration into tissues is excellent; attains high concentration in CSF. It is metabolized in the liver by conjugation.

Adverse Reactions

1. **Gastrointestinal disturbances:** Nausea, vomiting, diarrhea.
2. **Bone marrow depression:** Chloramphenicol may cause bone marrow depression by an idiosyncratic response—resulting in aplastic anemia which may be fatal. It may be due to a toxic metabolite.
3. **Gray baby syndrome:** Newborn babies given high doses of chloramphenicol may develop vomiting, refusal of feeds, hypotonia, hypothermia, abdominal distension and ashen gray cyanosis—described as 'gray baby syndrome'. It may be fatal. Because the newborn cannot

metabolize and excrete chloramphenicol adequately (liver and kidneys are not fully developed), toxicity results.
4. **Hypersensitivity reactions** like rashes and fever are uncommon.
5. **Superinfection** can occur because it is a broad spectrum antibiotic.

Drug Interactions

Chloramphenicol inhibits hepatic microsomal enzymes and thereby prolongs the duration of action of drugs metabolized by this system. This may result in toxicity of some drugs like phenytoin, tolbutamide and dicumarol.

Uses

Because of the risk of bone marrow toxicity and availability of safer drugs, chloramphenicol is not generally preferred. The indications are:

1. **Typhoid fever:** Very effective in typhoid.
2. **Bacterial meningitis:** Chloramphenicol is an alternative to penicillin.
3. **Anaerobic infections:** Chloramphenicol + penicillin + an aminoglycoside can be used in severe anaerobic infections as an alternative to metronidazole and clindamycin.
4. **Rickettsial infections:** As an alternative when tetracyclines are contraindicated.
5. **Eye infections:** Chloramphenicol is used as eye drops because of the good penetration into aqueous humor.

MACROLIDES AND OTHER ANTIBACTERIAL AGENTS

Macrolides are antibiotics with a macrocyclic lactone ring.

Macrolides include: Erythromycin, roxithromycin, azithromycin, clarithromycin. Their doses are given in Table 12.6.

Erythromycin

Erythromycin is obtained from *Streptomyces erythreus.*

Antibacterial spectrum: Erythromycin has a narrow spectrum and is effective against aerobic gram-positive bacteria and a few gram-negative organisms; some atypical mycobacteria are sensitive.

Mechanism of action: Erythromycin is bacteriostatic at low and bactericidal at high concentrations. It binds to 50S ribosomes and inhibits bacterial protein synthesis.

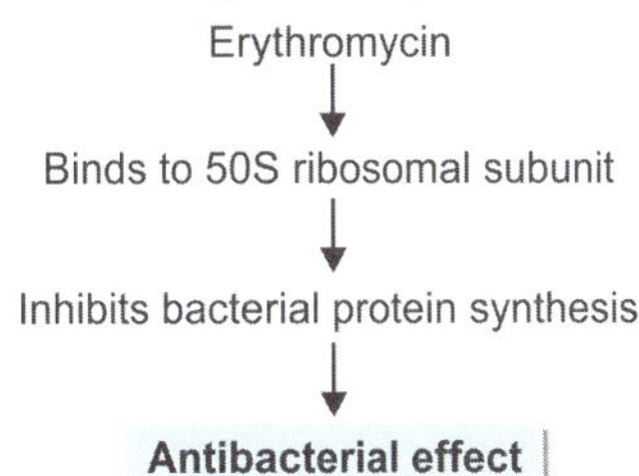

Resistance: Resistance to macrolides is acquired through plasmids.

Pharmacokinetics: Erythromycin is destroyed by gastric acid and is therefore given as enteric coated tablets. It is mainly excreted through bile; dose adjustment is not needed in renal failure.

Adverse Effects

1. **Hepatitis with cholestatic jaundice**—starts after 2–3 weeks of treatment and is more common with the estolate salt. The symptoms—nausea, vomiting and abdominal cramps are similar to acute cholecystitis and may be wrongly treated. These are followed by jaundice and fever. It may be an allergic response to the estolate salt. The patient recovers on stopping the drug.
2. Epigastric distress, nausea, vomiting and diarrhea are often reported.
3. Allergic reactions including fever and skin rashes can occur.
4. Cardiac arrhythmias are reported in patients with cardiac diseases or those who are on other drugs that cause arrhythmias.
5. Erythromycin can also cause reversible hearing impairment in some patients.

Drug interactions: Erythromycin inhibits the hepatic metabolism of many drugs like carbamazepine, valproate, and warfarin resulting in toxicity due to these drugs.

Table 12.6: Dose of macrolide antibiotics.

Drug	*Dose (oral)*
Erythromycin stearate (Erythrocin)	250–500 mg q6 hr
Erythromycin estolate (Althrocin)	250–500 mg q6 hr
Roxithromycin (Roxid)	150 mg q12 hr (to be taken 30 minutes before food)
Clarithromycin (Claribid)	250–500 mg q12 hr
Azithromycin (Azithral)	Ist day 500 mg OD 250 mg OD for next 3–4 days

Uses

Erythromycin can be used as an alternative to penicillin in patients allergic to penicillin.

1. **Atypical pneumonia due to *Mycoplasma pneumoniae*:** Erythromycin is the **drug of choice.**
2. **Legionnaire's pneumonia:** It is treated with erythromycin.
3. **Whooping cough (pertussis):** Erythromycin is the drug of choice for treatment and prophylaxis.
4. **Diphtheria:** Erythromycin is very effective in acute stage though antitoxin is life saving. Erythromycin also eradicates carrier state.
5. **Tetanus:** Erythromycin eradicates carrier state.
6. **Streptococcal infections:** Pharyngitis and tonsillitis respond to erythromycin.
7. **Staphylococcal infections:** Minor infections may be treated. But now resistant strains are common.
8. **Syphilis and gonorrhea:** Erythromycin is used as an alternative.
9. **Campylobacter gastroenteritis and anthrax:** Erythromycin is used as an alternative
10. **Topical:** Erythromycin ointment is used for skin infections, boils and acne.
11. **Anthrax**—erythromycin is an alternative to penicillin.
12. **Prophylaxis**—erythromycin may be used as an alternative to penicillin in valvular heart disease patients undergoing dental and other minor procedures.
13. **Other uses:** Erythromycin can be used in post operative gastroparesis because it stimulates gut motility (motilin receptor agonist)

Roxithromycin is longer-acting, acid stable, more potent, better absorbed and has better tissue penetrability compared to erythromycin. It does not inhibit the metabolism of other drugs—hence drug interactions are avoided. It should be taken 30 minutes before food because food can reduce its absorption.

Roxithromycin can be used as an alternative to erythromycin.

Clarithromycin compared to erythromycin, clarithromycin is longer-acting, acid stable and better absorbed; it is more effective against atypical mycobacteria, *H. pylori* and some protozoa.

Clarithromycin is used:

- As a component of triple regimen for *H. pylori* infections in peptic ulcer patients.
- Atypical mycobacterial infections.

Though clarithromycin is effective in other indications of erythromycin, its higher cost makes it less preferable.

Azithromycin is a derivative of erythromycin with activity similar to clarithromycin.

Advantages

- It is acid stable
- Rapidly absorbed
- Has better tissue penetrability
- Longer acting - once daily dose
- Given as a single loading dose of 500 mg once daily followed by 250 mg for the next 4 days.
- Better tolerated than erythromycin
- Free of drug interactions as azithromycin does not suppress hepatic metabolism of other drugs.

Uses: Azithromycin is used in the prophylaxis and treatment of atypical mycobacterial infections in AIDS patients. Like erythromycin it can also be used in respiratory, genital and skin infections and in pneumonias.

Ketolides

Ketolides are modified macrolides that are similar to newer macrolides except that they are effective against macrolide-resistant pneumococci.

Telithromycin is a ketolide. It is used in mild to moderate community acquired bacterial pneumonia, streptococcal pharyngitis and sinusitis.

Miscellaneous Antibiotics

1. Lincosamides

Clindamycin is a congener of lincomycin. It binds to 50S ribosomal subunit and suppresses protein synthesis. Streptococci, staphylococci, pneumococci and many anaerobes are inhibited by clindamycin. Clindamycin is well-absorbed on oral administration. It attains good concentration in the bone and many other tissues.

Adverse effects include diarrhea due to pseudomembranous colitis, skin rashes and neuromuscular blockade. Intravenous use can cause thrombophlebitis.

1. **Anaerobic infections:** Abdominal, pelvic, bone and joints infections due to anaerobes are treated with clindamycin. It may be combined with an aminoglycoside or a cephalosporin.
2. **Streptococcal and staphylococcal infections:** Clindamycin is effective in skin and soft tissue infections due to *Streptococcus* and *Staphylococcus* including MRSA infections.
3. ***P. jiroveci* infection:** Clindamycin is also useful in *Pneumocystis jiroveci* pneumonia and toxoplasmosis in AIDS patients.
4. ***Toxoplasma gondii:*** Clindamycin and pyrimethamine combination is used.

2. Glycopeptides

Glycopeptides include vancomycin and teicoplanin.

Vancomycin produced by *Streptococcus orientalis* is active against gram-positive bacteria particularly staphylococci including those resistant to methicillin. It acts by inhibiting cell wall synthesis and is bactericidal. Vancomycin is not absorbed orally—given IV. It is widely distributed and excreted through kidneys.

Adverse effects are skin rashes, pain at the site of injection, thrombophlebitis, ototoxicity and nephrotoxicity. **Redman's syndrome**—rapid IV injection can cause fever, chills, urticaria and flushing.

Uses

1. **Pseudomembranous colitis:** Oral vancomycin is used.
2. **Methicillin resistant staphylococcal infection:** Vancomycin is given IV for serious infections like osteomyelitis, endocarditis and soft-tissue abscesses.
3. **Enterococcal endocarditis**—as an alternative to penicillin.
4. **Penicillin resistant pneumococcal infections**—vancomycin is recommended with a cephalosporin.

Teicoplanin has mechanism of action and antibacterial spectrum similar to vancomycin, but teicoplanin can be safely given intramuscularly. It is also less toxic. Occasionally causes allergic reactions. It is used in osteomyelitis and endocarditis due to methicillin resistant staphylococci and enterococci. Dose: 200-400 mg/day

Telavancin a derivative of vancomycin and **dalbavancin** a derivative of teicoplanin are newer glycopeptides which are longer acting.

Ramoplanin, an analog of teicoplanin, is highly active against enterococci and *C. difficile*. It is given orally (but is not absorbed) to clear the gut of enterococci and to treat pseudomembranous colitis due to *C. difficile*. It is well tolerated.

3. Polypeptide Antibiotics

Polymyxin and Colistin

Polymyxin obtained from *Bacillus polymyxa* and colistin from *Bacillus colistinus* are effective against gram-negative bacteria.

Mechanism of action: Polymyxin and colistin alter the permeability of the cell membrane resulting in leakage of the cell contents. They are bactericidal.

Polypeptide antibiotics are not absorbed orally; applied topically, they may rarely cause skin rashes.

Systemically (parenteral) given colistin causes **nephrotoxicity**, muscle weakness, paresthesias, vertigo and dysarthria.

Uses

- Used topically for skin infections, ear and eye infections.
- Oral colistin is used in children for diarrhea due to gram-negative bacilli.
- Colistin is also used systemically in severe infections but is toxic.

4. Other Antimicrobial Drugs

A. Metronidazole

Metronidazole has good activity against anerobic bacteria. It is a powerful amebicide - effective against amebiasis. Apart from this it also inhibits *Trichomonas vaginalis, Giardia lamblia* and *Balantidium coli.*

Mechanism of action: In the microorganisms, metronidazole is reduced to a derivative which is toxic to the DNA.

Metronidazole is well-absorbed and reaches adequate concentrations in the CSF.

Adverse effects: Gastrointestinal effects like nausea, anorexia, abdominal pain and metallic taste in the mouth are the most frequent. Headache, stomatitis, dizziness, insomnia, skin rashes and rarely peripheral neuropathy can occur. High doses can cause convulsions.

Metronidazole has a disulfiram like effect; on alcohol intake, antabuse like reaction can follow.

Uses

1. **Anaerobic infections:** Metronidazole is the drug of choice for anaerobic infections. It is given intravenously for serious anaerobic infections. It is also useful for surgical prophylaxis of abdominal and pelvic infections.
2. **Amebiasis:** Metronidazole is the drug of choice in all forms of amebiasis in the dose of 400–800 mg TDS for 7–10 days. However, it does not eradicate the cysts.
3. **Trichomonas vaginitis:** Metronidazole 200 TDS for 7 days is the drug of choice.
4. **Giardiasis:** Metronidazole given 200 mg TDS for 7 days is the treatment of choice.
5. ***H. pylori* infections** seen in peptic ulcer patients can be treated with a combination of metronidazole, clarithromycin and omeprazole/ranitidine.
6. **Pseudomembranous colitis due to *Clostridium difficile:*** Responds to metronidazole.
7. **Acute ulcerative gingivitis:** As an alternative to penicillin G.
8. **Dracunculosis:** Metronidazole facilitates extraction of the guinea worm.

B. Bacitracin

Bacitracin produced by *Bacillus subtilis* is effective against gram-positive bacteria. It inhibits the cell wall synthesis and is bactericidal. It is too toxic to be given systemically and is therefore used only for topical application—in skin infections, surgical wounds, ulcers and ocular infections (neosporin powder is bacitracin + neomycin).

C. Sodium fusidate (fusidic acid)

Sodium fusidate is effective against gram-positive organisms particularly staphylococci. It is bactericidal. It is mainly used topically as a 2% ointment (Fucidin). It may be given orally for resistant staphylococcal infections.

D. Mupirocin

Mupirocin is bactericidal against gram-positive and some gram-negative organisms.

It is used as an ointment for skin infections particularly due to staphylococci and streptococci.

5. Newer Agents

A. Streptogramins

A combination of **quinupristin** and **dalfopristin** in the ratio 30:70 is bactericidal against gram-positive cocci including methicillin-resistant staphylococci. Streptogramins bind to 50S ribosomal subunit and inhibit protein synthesis. Streptogramins are given intravenously; they are rapidly metabolized and excreted largely through feces. Hence adjustment of dose is not required in renal insufficiency.

Adverse effects include myalgia and pain at the site of injection. The combination is used in the treatment of serious infections due to streptococci and methicillin-resistant staphylococci.

B. Linezolid

Linezolid is an oxazolidinone effective against gram-positive bacteria including methicillin resistant staphylococci and gram-positive anaerobic organisms. It acts by inhibiting protein synthesis on binding to 50S ribosomes. Linezolid binds to the 23S ribosomal RNA of the 50S subunit and prevents initiation of protein synthesis—the first step in protein synthesis.

An advantage with linezolid is that it is completely (100%) absorbed; food does not interfere with its absorption and can be given oral or IV. It is widely distributed and has a half life of 4–6 hours. In patients undergoing hemodialysis, linezolid should be given after dialysis because it can be excreted through dialysis. **Dose:** 600 mg BD.

Tadazolid is similar to linezolid.

C. Daptomycin

Daptomycin is a lipopeptide obtained from *Streptomyces roseosporus*. Though the exact mechanism of action is not known, daptomycin appears to have a unique mechanism of action. It binds to the cell membrane and depolarizes it. This leads to outward movement of potassium ions resulting in rapid cell death. Daptomycin is thus **bactericidal**. It is synergistic with gentamicin.

Antibacterial spectrum: It is effective against aerobic gram-positive microorganisms including methicillin and vancomycin resistant staphylococci and also against anaerobes.

Daptomycin can cause **myopathy**. It should not be used to prevent pneumonia because surfactant in the lungs antagonizes the effects of daptomycin.

Uses:

- Complicated skin and soft tissue infections.
- As an alternative to vancomycin.

D. Fidaxomicin

Fidaxomicin is effective against gram-positive bacteria. Given orally, it is poorly absorbed and may be used in the treatment of colitis due to *Cl. difficile*.

CHEMOTHERAPY OF URINARY TRACT INFECTIONS

Infection of the urinary tract is quite common and may be acute or chronic. *Urinary antiseptics* are drugs which exert antibacterial activity only in the urinary tract (and no systemic activity). They include nitrofurantoin and methenamine mandelate.

Nitrofurantoin is effective against many gram-positive and gram-negative bacteria. It attains high concentration in urine and is used in acute UTI, long-term suppression of chronic UTI and for prophylaxis of UTI.

Methenamine mandelate: A salt of mandelic acid and methenamine, releases formaldehyde in acidic urine below pH 5.5. Formaldehyde is bactericidal and resistance does not develop to it. It is used orally in chronic UTI that is resistant to other drugs.

Other drugs: Used in UTI are sulfonamides, cotrimoxazole, nalidixic acid, fluoroquinolones, ampicillin, cloxacillin, carbenicillin, aminoglycosides, tetracyclines and cephalosporins.

Urinary analgesic: Phenazopyridine has analgesic actions on the urinary tract and relieves burning symptoms of dysuria and urgency.

CHEMOTHERAPY OF TUBERCULOSIS

Tuberculosis is a chronic granulomatous disease caused by *Mycobacterium tuberculosis*. In developing countries, it is a major public health problem; 5 lakh people die in India every year due to this disease. After the spread of AIDS, the problem has become more complex, as tuberculosis and *Mycobacterium avium* complex (MAC) infections are more common and rapidly progress in patients with AIDS.

The government of India has initiated NTEP or National Tb Elimination Program with the aim to eliminate Tb by 2025.

Drugs used in Tuberculosis (*See* Flowchart 12.1) may be classified as:.

First-line Drugs

Isoniazid (INH) is the most effective and cheapest primary antitubercular drug. It is tuberculocidal for rapidly multiplying bacilli but static for resting bacilli. INH destroys: (i) intracellular bacilli as it penetrates into the cells, i.e., tubercle bacilli in the macrophages, and (ii) bacilli multiplying in the walls of the cavities. Thus it is effective against both intra- and extracellular organisms (Table 12.7). If used alone, mycobacteria develop resistance to it. Hence it should be used in combination with other drugs.

Mechanism of action: INH inhibits the synthesis of mycolic acids which is an important component of the mycobacterial cell wall.

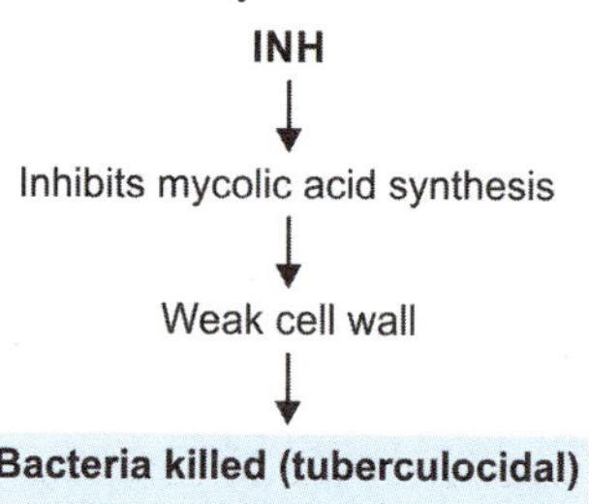

Adverse effects: Peripheral neuritis (which is due to interference with utilization and increased excretion of pyridoxine) can be avoided by giving prophylactic pyridoxine with INH. Hepatitis is another major adverse effect, more common in alcoholics. It can cause CNS toxicity including psychosis and seizures but are rare. Other minor effects like anorexia, GI discomfort and allergic reactions can occur.

Rifampicin is obtained from *Streptomyces mediterranei*. It is bactericidal to *M. tuberculosis, M. leprae* and atypical mycobacteria. It also inhibits most gram-positive and gram-negative bacteria like *Staph. aureus, N. meningitidis, E. coli, Proteus* and *Pseudomonas*.

Flowchart 12.1: Classification of drugs used in tuberculosis.

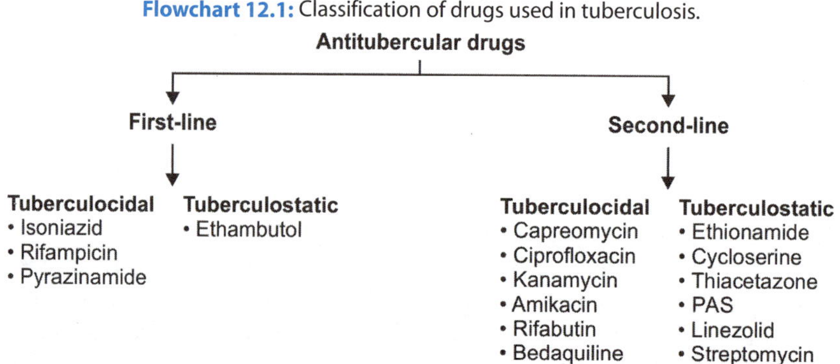

Table 12.7: Antitubercular actions and characteristic adverse effects of some antitubercular drugs.

Drug	*Antitubercular action*	*Serious toxicity*
Isoniazid	Tuberculocidal; acts on intra and extracellular organisms	Peripheral neuritis, seizures, psychosis
Rifampicin	Tuberculocidal; Acts on intra and extracellular organisms, persisters and drug resistant organisms	Hepatotoxicity, flu-like syndrome, nephritis; urine and secretions are colored orange-red
Pyrazinamide	Tuberculocidal; kills intracellular organisms; more active in acidic pH	Hepatotoxicity, arthralgia, hyperuricemia
Ethambutol	Tuberculostatic; inhibits tubercle bacilli in the walls of cavities	Optic neuritis with ↓ visual acuity and red-green color blindness
Bedaquiline	Tuberculocidal; inhibits mycobacterial ATP synthase and energy generation	Hepatotoxicity, QTc prolongation, arthralgia
Streptomycin	Tuberculocidal; acts on extracellular organisms	Ototoxicity, nephrotoxicity

Antitubercular action: Rifampicin is highly effective, tuberculocidal and is the only drug that acts on **persisters**; acts on both intra- and extracellular organisms and is effective against tubercle bacilli resistant to other drugs it is called a **sterilizing agent**. If used alone resistance develops.

Mechanism of action: Rifampicin binds to DNA dependent RNA polymerase and inhibits RNA synthesis in bacteria. It is bactericidal.

Pharmacokinetics: Rifampicin is well-absorbed and has **good tissue penetrability**—reaches caseous material, cavities and CSF. It is a microsomal enzyme inducer.

Adverse effects: Rifampicin is well-tolerated. Skin rashes, diarrhea, nephritis and hepatotoxicity can occur. In intermittent dosing regimen, a flu-like syndrome can occur.

The urine and other secretions turn orange yellow color.

Uses

1. Tuberculosis and atypical mycobacterial infections.
2. Leprosy (*See* page 267).
3. Prophylaxis of *H. influenzae* meningitis in close contacts.
4. Resistant staphylococcal infections—as an alternative.
5. Brucellosis—Rifampicin + doxycycline—drug of choice.
6. To eradicate meningococcal carrier state.

Pyrazinamide is tuberculocidal, and is more active in acidic pH. Mechanism of action is not known. It is effective against intracellular bacilli. If used alone resistance develops. It is well-absorbed and reaches good concentration in the CSF. Hepatotoxicity is the most common adverse effect. Hyperuricemia (due to ↓ excretion of uric acid), arthralgia, anorexia, vomiting and rashes are the adverse effects.

Ethambutol is tuberculostatic and acts on fast multiplying bacilli in the cavities. It is also effective against atypical mycobacteria. It inhibits the incorporation of mycolic acids into the mycobacterial cell wall.

Optic neuritis resulting in decreased visual acuity and inability to differentiate red from green is an important adverse effect which needs stopping of the drug. Other adverse effects include nausea, anorexia, headache, fever and allergic reactions.

Second-line Drugs

Second-line drugs are generally less effective and more toxic than first line drugs. They are used only if organisms are resistant to first-line drugs.

Bedaquiline, a newly introduced antibacterial, binds to and inhibits mycobacterial ATP synthase and thereby interferes with the generation of energy.

It is tuberculocidal. Co-administration of other microsomal enzyme inducers, such as rifampicin and also enzyme inhibitors should be avoided.

Adverse effects: Hepatotoxicity, nausea, arthralgia, headache and QTc prolongation are reported.

Bedaquiline is used in the treatment of MDR tuberculosis along with other drugs.

Delamanid: Delamanid a nitroimidazole acts by inhibiting the synthesis of mycolic acid in the mycobacterial call wall. It should be taken with food because food increases absorption.

Delamanid is approved for treatment of MDR-TB.

Thiacetazone is tuberculostatic with low efficacy; it delays the development of resistance to other drugs and its low cost makes it a suitable drug in combination regimens. Hepatotoxicity, dermatitis, allergic reactions and GI side effects may occur.

Ethionamide: This tuberculostatic drug is effective against both intra and extracellular organisms. It is also effective in atypical mycobacteria.

Anorexia, nausea, vomiting and metallic taste in the mouth are the most common adverse effects. It can also cause hepatitis, skin rashes and peripheral neuritis (needs prophylactic pyridoxine).

Ethionamide is a secondary agent used only when primary drugs are ineffective.

Para-aminosalicylic acid (PAS) related to sulfonamides is tuberculostatic. Gastrointestinal effects like nausea, anorexia, epigastric pain and diarrhea make it a poorly tolerated drug. Allergic reactions and hepatitis are also seen. It is rarely used.

Streptomycin is tuberculocidal, acts only against extracellular organisms due to poor penetrating power. It has to be given IM. When used alone resistance develops. Because of these disadvantages and its toxicity (oto and nephrotoxicity), streptomycin is not preferred now.

Amikacin, kanamycin and capreomycin are second line drugs that need parenteral administration. They are oto and nephrotoxic and are used only in resistant cases. Amikacin is also effective against atypical mycobacteria.

Cycloserine is an antibiotic that inhibits cell wall synthesis, is tuberculostatic and is also effective against some gram-positive organisms. It causes CNS toxicity including psychosis. It is used only in resistant tuberculosis.

Fluoroquinolones: Ciprofloxacin, ofloxacin and sparfloxacin inhibit tubercle bacilli and atypical mycobacteria. They are useful in multidrug resistant tuberculosis in combination with other drugs.

Linezolid is effective in tuberculosis along with second-line drugs. Its penetrability into cells is good and is lethal to intracellular bacilli. It can be used in a single daily dose of 600 mg along with second-line drugs only in the treatment of MDR tuberculosis.

Treatment of Tuberculosis

Tuberculosis is one of the most difficult infections to cure. The need for long-term treatment, drug toxicity, cost of treatment and poor patient compliance have all made the problem more complex. AIDS patients have more severe disease due to depressed immunity. However, with the availability of effective drugs, most patients can now be treated as outpatients (Tables 12.8 and 12.9).

A combination of drugs is used in tuberculosis to:

- Delay the development of resistance.
- Reduce toxicity.
- Shorten the course of treatment.

Treatment is given in 2 phases—initial intensive phase followed by continuation phase.

Resistant tuberculosis should be treated with 4–5 drugs, of which 3 are first line drugs and treatment is continued for at least 1 year after the sputum becomes negative.

Table 12.8: Treatment categories of tuberculosis as per WHO recommendation.

Type of patient	Regimen	
	Intensive phase (IP)	*Continuation phase (CP)*
New/Previously treated*	8 weeks 2HRZE (56 doses)	16 weeks 4HRE (112 doses)

*Should be evaluated for DRTB. H: INH; R: Rifampicin; Z: Pyrazinamide; E: Ethambutol

Table 12.9: NTEP recommendation of Fixed Dose Combination (FDC) for tuberculosis.

Weight	Number of tablets	
	Intensive phase 4 FDC	*Continuation phase 3 FDC*
25–34	2	2
35–49	3	3
50–64	4	4
65–74	5	5
≥75 kg	6	6

4 FDC-HRZE; 3 FDC-HRE

Chemoprophylaxis is given with INH for 6–12 months only in:

- Close contacts of open cases especially children.
- Patients with old inactive disease who have not been adequately treated.

Drugs for *Mycobacterium avium* complex (MAC): Infection with MAC is more common in HIV patients. The drugs effective are rifabutin, clarithromycin, azithromycin, fluoroquinolones, ethambutol, clofazimine, amikacin and ethionamide. Clarithromycin + ethambutol is the preferred regimen for MAC infection and needs lifelong treatment. Rifabutin is used for prophylaxis.

CHEMOTHERAPY OF LEPROSY

Leprosy caused by *Mycobacterium leprae* is a chronic infectious disease affecting skin, mucous membranes and nerves. Hansen discovered lepra bacillus in 1873.

In India leprosy was a major public health problem affecting millions of people but now its largely controlled.

Drugs used in leprosy:

- Sulfones: Dapsone.
- Rifampicin.
- Clofazimine.
- Ethionamide.

Dapsone is diaminodiphenylsulfone (DDS) and is related to sulfonamides.

Mechanism of action: Like sulfonamides, it inhibits the incorporation of PABA into folic acid.

Actions: Dapsone is leprostatic. Though it inhibits the growth of many other bacteria, the dose needed is high and is therefore not used. The lepra bacillus develops resistance to dapsone on prolonged use.

Dapsone is completely absorbed on oral administration and reaches high concentrations in skin. It is metabolized in the liver and excreted in bile.

Adverse effects: Dapsone is well-tolerated—anorexia, nausea and vomiting are common and allergic reactions can occur. Hemolytic anemia is dose dependent and needs iron supplementation. Hepatitis and agranulocytosis can occur. Patients with lepromatous leprosy may develop lepra reactions.

Uses

- **Leprosy:** Dapsone is the primary drug in leprosy used for both treatment and chemoprophylaxis.
- ***P. jiroveci:*** Dapsone is used along with trimethoprim as an alternative in *P jiroveci* infections in patients with AIDS—both for the prevention and treatment.
- **Dermatitis herpetiformis** a chronic blistering skin disease seen in patients with celiac disease can be treated with dapsone.

Rifampicin is rapidly bactericidal to *M. leprae* and is highly effective. It can be conveniently given once monthly. Used in combination with dapsone, it shortens the duration of treatment. Given alone—resistance develops.

Clofazimine a dye, has weak bactericidal actions against *M. leprae.* It also has anti-inflammatory properties which is useful in suppressing lepra reactions. It is used orally in multidrug regimens.

Clofazimine causes reddish-black discoloration of the skin specially on the exposed parts which remains for several months. It can also cause dryness of skin, itching and phototoxicity.

Treatment of Leprosy

For the sake of treatment, leprosy is divided into paucibacillary (non-infectious) and multibacillary (infectious) leprosy.

WHO has recommended a combination of drugs in leprosy to:

- Eliminate persisters.
- Prevent drug resistance.
- Reduce the duration of therapy.

Multidrug Regimen

Drugs	*Multibacillary leprosy (for 12 months)*	*Paucibacillary leprosy (for 6 months)*
Rifampicin	600 mg once a month supervized	600 mg once a month supervized
Dapsone	100 mg daily self-administered	100 mg daily self-administered
Clofazimine	300 mg once monthly supervized 50 mg daily self-administered	— —
All drugs are given orally		

Lepra reactions are the acute exacerbations that occur in leprosy. They are triggered by acute infections, stress, anxiety and treatment with dapsone.

Type I reactions seen in tuberculoid leprosy is a delayed hypersensitivity reaction to the antigens of *M. leprae*. Skin ulcerations occur and existing lesions become red. It is treated with aspirin in mild and corticosteroids or clofazimine in severe cases.

Type II reactions are seen in lepromatous leprosy (known as *erythema nodosum leprosum* (ENL). New lesions appear and the existing lesions become worse. Fever, lymphadenitis and neuralgia may occur. It is a hypersensitivity reaction to the antigens of *M. leprae.* Type II reactions can be treated with **aspirin** or **clofazimine** which are effective due to their anti-inflammatory properties. **Chloroquine, corticosteroids** or **thalidomide** are also effective. **Dapsone** should be continued throughout.

ANTIFUNGAL DRUGS

Fungal infections may be systemic or superficial. There has been an increase in the incidence and severity of fungal infections in the recent years. Several unusual and drug-resistant organisms have emerged. These may be due to the use of broad spectrum antibiotics, anticancer drugs and HIV infection. Antifungal drugs may be classified into (Fig. 12.5):

Classifications

1. **Drugs acting on cell membrane**
   a. **Antifungal antibiotics:** Amphotericin B, nystatin, hamycin, natamycin.
   b. **Azoles:**
      - *Imidazoles:* Clotrimazole, econazole, miconazole, ketoconazole, butoconazole, oxiconazole, sulconazole, isoconazole.
      - *Triazoles:* Fluconazole, itraconazole, terconazole, voriconazole, posaconazole, ravuconazole, isavuconazole.
   c. **Others:** Terbinafine, naftifine
2. **Drugs acting of cell wall**
   - Pneumocandins—caspofungin, micafungin, anidulafungin

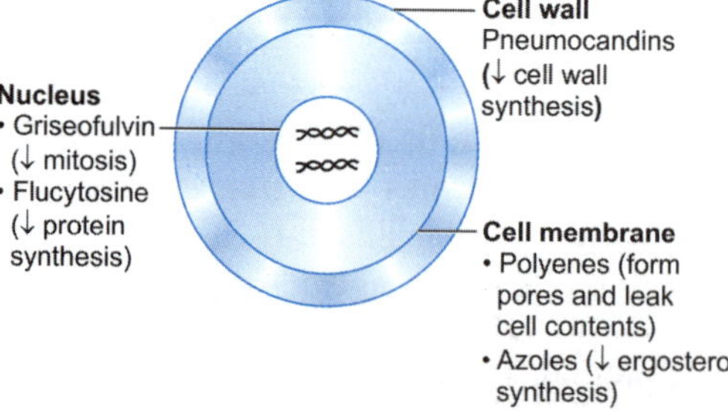

Fig. 12.5: Sites of action of antifungal drugs.

3. **Drugs acting on nucleus:** Griseofulvin, flucytosine
4. **Other topical agents:** Tolnaftate, undecylenic acid, benzoic acid, salicylic acid, selenium sulfide, ciclopirox olamine.

Antifungal Antibiotics

Amphotericin B obtained from *Streptomyces nodosus* is a polyene antibiotic containing many double bonds.

Antifungal spectrum: Amphotericin B has a wide antifungal spectrum. It inhibits the growth of *Candida albicans, Histoplasma capsulatum, Cryptococcus neoformans, Coccidioides, Aspergillus* and *Blastomyces dermatitidis.* It is fungistatic at low and fungicidal at high concentrations. It is also effective agonist leishmania.

Mechanism of action: Amphotericin B binds to ergosterol present in fungal cell membrane and forms pores in the cell membrane. Through these pores, cell contents leak out resulting in cell death.

Pharmacokinetics: Amphotericin B is not absorbed orally and hence given IV. It has a long t½ of 15 days.

Adverse effects: Fever, chills, muscle spasms, vomiting, headache and **hypotension** can be encountered on IV infusion. **Renal impairment**, neurotoxicity and anemia due to bone marrow depression can also occur. Other nephrotic drugs should not be given with it.

Uses

1. Amphotericin B is the drug of choice for all life-threatening mycotic infections.
2. Used topically in candidiasis. In infection of the bladder (cystitis) due to candida, amphotericin is used to irrigate the bladder.
3. Given orally in fungal infections of the gut for local action.
4. **Leishmaniasis:** In kala-azar and mucocutaneous leishmaniasis, amphotericin is used as an alternative.

Nystatin obtained from *Streptomyces noursei* has actions similar to amphotericin B. Because it is too toxic for systemic use, it is used topically for local candidial infections like oral thrush and vaginal candidiasis.

Hamycin is similar to nystatin. It is used topically for cutaneous candidiasis and otomycosis.

Azoles

Imidazoles and triazoles: The older antifungals need to be given intravenously and are quite toxic. Azoles are newer antifungals that are effective orally and are less toxic.

Azoles include imidazoles and triazoles. The triazoles have more selective antifungal action and are longer acting.

Antifungal spectrum: Azoles have a broad spectrum antifungal activity. They inhibit *dermatophytes, candida, cryptococcus neoformans* and other *deep mycoses.*

Mechanism of action: Azoles inhibit the synthesis of ergosterol, an important component of the fungal cell membrane.

Ketoconazole (KTZ) is the first oral azole to be available. It is well-absorbed from the gut. Food and low gastric pH increase absorption. In large doses it inhibits the biosynthesis of adrenal and gonadal steroids in humans—resulting in gynecomastia, infertility and menstrual irregularities.

Adverse reactions include gastric irritation, headache, allergic reactions, gynecomastia, decreased sexual desire (libido) infertility and rarely hepatotoxicity.

Drug interactions: Rifampicin and phenytoin induce KTZ metabolism and decrease its efficacy.

Uses: Mucocutaneous candidiasis and dermatophytosis can be treated with ketoconazole. It is also useful in Cushing's syndrome.

Fluconazole is well-absorbed orally and attains good CSF concentration.

Adverse effects are mild gastrointestinal disturbances, headache and rashes. Since it has very little effect on hepatic microsomal enzymes, drug interactions are less common.

Uses:

1. Fluconazole is used in cryptococcal meningitis after initial treatment with amphotericin B.
2. Drug of choice in coccidial meningitis.
3. Systemic candidiasis and other systemic fungal infections.
4. Also effective in tinea infections and mucocutaneous candidiasis.
5. Leishmaniasis—used as an alternative.

Itraconazole is the most potent azole. Given orally, its absorption is increased by food and gastric acid. Its effect on hepatic microsomal enzymes is less; does not affect steroid synthesis. Thus, it is preferred over ketoconazole. Itraconazole is the drug of choice in most systemic mycoses (without meningitis).

It is also useful in dermatophytosis, candidiasis, and onychomycosis.

Clotrimazole and miconazole are used topically in dermatophytic infections (ringworm) and mucocutaneous candidiasis. Clotrimazole troche is available for oral thrush. Miconazole has better efficacy. Both can cause mild irritation at the site of application.

Others

Econazole, terconazole, tioconazole, butoconazole, oxiconazole and **sulconazole** are all azoles available for topical use as creams and lotions for use in dermatophytoses and mucocutaneous candidiasis.

Voriconazole, posaconazole and ravuconazole are broad spectrum antifungals.

Voriconazole and posaconazole are effective in invasive aspergillosis. Posaconazole and Ravuconazole are also effective for the prophlaxis of fungal infection in bone marrow transplantation.

Terbinafine is a synthetic antifungal that is effective against dermatophytes and *Candida*. It is orally effective and is fungicidal. It gets concentrated in the keratin like griseofulvin. It inhibits an enzyme needed for biosynthesis of ergosterol by fungi.

Adverse effects are rare—gastrointestinal disturbances, rashes and headache. Terbinafine is used in dermatophytosis, pityriasis, onychomycosis and candidiasis. Sebifin—250 mg tab, 1 percent cream.

Drugs Acting on Cell Wall

Pneumocandins or **echinocandins** inhibit the formation of the fungal cell wall. They inhibit the synthesis of an important component of the fungal cell wall—a glucose polymer, as a result of which the fungal cell lysis occurs.

Echinocandins include caspofungin, micafungin and amorolfine. Caspofungin has activity in candidiasis, aspergillosis and in *Pneumocystis jiroveci* infections. Micafungin is effective against candida and aspergillosis while amorolfine is useful in fungal infections of the nail.

Drugs Acting on Nucleus

Griseofulvin is derived from *Penicillium griseofulvum*. It is effective in superficial dermatophytosis (caused by *Trichophyton, Microsporum* and *Epidermophyton*). Griseofulvin is the antifungal given orally for superficial dermatophytes. It gets deposited in the newly forming skin, binds to keratin and protects the skin from getting newly infected.

Griseofulvin binds to protein in the nucleus and inhibits multiplication in the fungus.

Adverse effects include allergic reactions, hepatitis and neurotoxicity.

Flucytosine is effective against *Cryptococcus neoformans* and some strains of *Candida*. It is taken up by the fungal cells and converted to 5-fluorouracil which inhibits DNA synthesis.

Bone marrow depression and gastrointestinal disturbances are the most common adverse effects. It is used with amphotericin B (used alone, resistance develops rapidly) in cryptococcal meningitis and systemic candidiasis.

Other Topical Antifungal Agents

Apart from nystatin, clotrimazole, miconazole and terbinafine, some drugs like salicyclic acid, benzoic acid, tolnaftate, cyclopirox olamine are used topically for dermatophytosis and pityriasis versicolor.

Selenium sulfide is useful in tinea versicolor caused by *Malassezia furfur,* and also in dandruff. Selsun is 2.5% suspension of selenium sulfide in a shampoo base. It is irritant to the eyes and the odor is unpleasant.

ANTIVIRAL DRUGS

Viruses are intracellular parasites and depend on the host cells for their food, growth and multiplication. The virus attaches itself to the host cell membrane, penetrates it and DNA/RNA is released in the host cell. The viral components are assembled and the mature viral particle is then released from the host cell. Chemotherapy can interfere with any of these steps. But drugs that interfere with viral replication may also interfere with host cell function.

Classification

1. **Antiherpes virus agents:** Acyclovir, ganciclovir, idoxuridine, trifluridine, foscarnet.
2. **Anti-influenza virus agents:** Amantadine, rimantadine.
3. **Antihepatitis agents:** Adefovir, tenofovir, lamivudine
4. **Others:** Ribavirin, interferons, oseltamivir, zanamivir.
5. **Antiretroviral agents:**
   - **Nucleoside reverse transcriptase inhibitors (NRTIs)—**
     Zidovudine, lamivudine, abacavir, tenofovir.
   - **Nonnucleoside reverse transcriptase inhibitors—**
     Nevirapine, efavirenz, delavirdine, etravirine, rilpivirine
   - **Protease inhibitors—**
     Saquinavir, indinavir, ritonavir, nelfinavir, amprenavir, lopinavir, atazanavir, darunavir
   - **Entry inhibitors—**
     Enfuvirtide, maraviroc
   - **Integrase Strand Transfer Inhibitors (INSTIs)—**
     Raltegravir, elvitegravir, dolutegravir

Antiherpes Virus Agents

Acyclovir is effective against herpes simplex virus (HSV) type 1 and type 2, varicella zoster virus (VZV) and Epstein-Barr virus (EBV).

Mechanism of action: Acyclovir inhibits viral DNA synthesis by inhibiting viral DNA polymerases and causing DNA chain termination as in Figure 12.6.

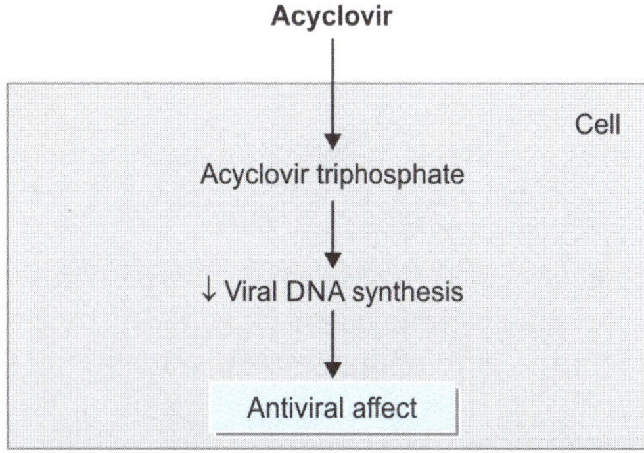

Fig. 12.6: Mechanism of action of acyclovir.

Adverse effects: Acyclovir is well-tolerated; nausea, diarrhea, headache and rashes may occur occasionally. Topical acyclovir can cause burning and irritation. Given IV, it may cause renal and neurotoxicity but are uncommon.

Uses (Table 12.10)

1. **HSV infections:** Infection with HSV-1 causes diseases of the mouth, face, skin, esophagus or brain. HSV-2 usually causes

Table 12.10: Indications of some commonly used antiviral drugs.

Drugs	*Routes*	*Indications*
Acyclovir	Topical Oral IV	Herpes genitalis, HSV eye infections Herpes genitalis/mucocutaneous HSV chickenpox HSV encephalitis, severe herpes genitalis, chickenpox/herpes zoster in immunocompromised patients
Idoxuridine Trifluridine	Topical	HSV keratitis
Ganciclovir	IV/oral	CMV infections
Foscarnet	IV	CMV retinitis, acyclovir resistant HSV infections
Amantadine Rimantadine	Oral	Influenza A
Ribavirin	Aerosol oral/IV	RSV bronchiolitis, severe influenza and measles
Interferon α	IV	Chronic hepatitis B and C, genital warts, Kaposi's sarcoma

infections of the genitals, rectum, skin, hands or meninges. Acyclovir is effective in infection by both HSV-1 and HSV-2.

2. **Herpes zoster:** Acyclovir shortens the duration of illness.
3. **Chickenpox:** In adults and in immunodeficient patients, acyclovir reduces duration and severity of illness. In children, routine use is not recommended.

Valacyclovir is a prodrug of acyclovir. Famciclovir is a prodrug of penciclovir—used in HSV and VZV infections.

Ganciclovir is effective against herpes viruses especially cytomegalovirus (CMV). Toxicity includes myelosuppression and gonadal toxicity. It is used in immunocompromised patients with CMV retinitis.

Idoxuridine is effective in DNA viruses. It acts by inhibiting viral DNA synthesis. Idoxuridin is used topically in HSV keratitis (it is too toxic for systemic use). Eyelid edema, itching and allergic reactions may occur.

Trifluridine is used topically in HSV eye infections.

Foscarnet is given intravenously to treat CMV retinitis as an alternative to ganciclovir.

Anti-influenza Virus Agents

Amantadine and rimantadine inhibit the replication of influenza A viruses. Generally well-tolerated, nausea, vomiting, diarrhea, dizziness, insomnia and ankle edema are reported. Rimantadine is longer-acting and has fewer adverse effects.

Uses

- Treatment of influenza A during an epidemic—reduces duration and severity—dose: 200 mg/day for 5 days.
- Prophylaxis of influenza A during an epidemic especially in high-risk patients. Also for seasonal prophylaxis in high-risk patients.
- Parkinsonism—amantadine enhances the release of dopamine and is beneficial in parkinsonism.

Oseltamivir and Zanamivir

Oseltamivir and zanamivir gained wide popularity in the recent **H1N1** pandemic that spread across different countries including India. They inhibit viral replication by **inhibiting the neuraminidase** activity which is essential for the release of daughter virions. Oseltamivir and zanamivir are effective against both influenza A including H1N1 infections and influenza B. To be effective, these drugs should be administered within a few hours after the onset of symptoms (within 36–48 hour). They reduce both the duration and severity of illness.

Oseltamivir is given orally. It is a prodrug, well absorbed from the gut and activated in the liver by esterases. Oseltamivir is well tolerated—can cause nausea, vomiting, headache, diarrhea and abdominal discomfort. It should not be given in children <1 year of age. Oseltamivir can casue nausea and vomiting while zanamivir is given by inhalation which can occasionaly cause respiratory distress.

Uses: Oseltamivir and zanamivir are used in the prevention and treatment of influenza including H1N1 flu (swine flu).

Dose: Oseltamivir 75 mg BD for 5 days. TAMIFLU 75 mg tab. Zanamivir 10 mg inhalation twice daily for 5 days RELENZA inhaler.

Antihepatitis Agents

Adefovir is converted to adefovir diphosphate which inhibits viral DNA polymerase. Entecavir is effective in chronic HBV infection. It is used orally in chronic HBV infection. **Lamivudine**, a nucleoside analog is also useful against HBV. **Tenofovir** an adenosine analog used in AIDS is found to be effective in chronic hepatitis in lamivudine resistant strains.

Interferons (IFN) are cytokines produced by host cells in response to viral infections.

They also have immunomodulating and antiproliferative properties. There are three types—α, β and γ interferons in man. They inhibit the multiplication of many DNA and RNA viruses. Interferons are given parenterally (SC/IM).

Uses

1. **Chronic hepatitis B:** Interferons administered for 4-6 months for an overall improvement.
2. **Chronic hepatitis C infection:** Interferons + ribavirin → response is better and longer lasting.
3. Kaposi's sarcoma in AIDS patients.
4. **Genital warts** caused by papilloma—interferons are injected into the lesion.
5. Some leukemias and lymphomas, mutiple myeloma and CML
6. **Multiple sclerosis:** Interferon β reduces severity.
7. **Rhinovirus cold:** Interferon α is given intranasally for prophylaxis.

Antihepatitis C Agents

Hepatitis C can vary in severity from mild infection of few weeks to serious lifelong disease. Hepatitis C related liver diseases include cirrhosis and liver cancer. Drugs used to treat HCV infection include:

- Interferons, Ribavirin, Sofosbuvir
- Protease inhibitors—boceprevir, simeprevir and telaprevir.

HCV is treated with a combination of interferon alpha and ribavirin or newer drugs.

Sofosbuvir—Inhibits RNA-dependent RNA polymerase. Sofosbuvir is used in combination with inteferons and ribavirin to attain high cure rates. It is given orally and is well-tolerated; fatigue and headache are reported.

Protease inhibitors—boceprevir, simeprevir and telaprevir inhibit HCV protease and are used in combination with IFNs and ribavirin.

Other Antiviral Agents

Ribavirin has broad-spectrum antiviral activity. It is effective against influenza A and B, respiratory syncytial virus (RSV) and many DNA and RNA viruses. It is used as an aerosol in RSV bronchiolitis in children. Also it can be used in severe influenza and measles in immunocompromised patients.

Interferons are cytokines produced by host cells in response to viral infections. There are three types α, β, γ interferons in man. They also have immunomodulating and antiproliferative properties. They inhibit the multiplication of many DNA and RNA viruses.

Adverse effects include myelosuppression, hypotension, arrhythmias, alopecia, headache and arthralgia. It can also cause neurotoxicity resulting in confusion, sedation and rarely seizures.

Uses

- Chronic hepatitis B and C.
- Kaposi's sarcoma in AIDS patients.
- Genital warts caused by Papilloma virus—interferons are injected into the lesion.
- Hairy cell leukemia.
- HSV, herpes zoster and CMV infections in immunocompromised patients.
- Rhinovirus cold—interferon α is given intranasally for prophylaxis.

Antiretroviral Agents

Nuclease reverse transcriptase (NRT) inhibitors.

Zidovudine (azidothymidine, AZT) is a thymidine analog, active against HIV infections and other retroviruses.

Mechanism of action: NRT inhibitors are converted to their triphosphate derivatives by cellular enzymes which inhibit reverse transcriptase.

Adverse effects: Bone marrow suppression, headache, nausea, vomiting and insomnia can occur. High doses cause myopathy and neurotoxicity.

Uses: AZT is used with other drugs in HIV infections.

Given during pregnancy and continued in newborns for 6 weeks, AZT reduces the risk of transmission to the baby. It is used in combination therapy regimen.

Emtricitabine, lamivudine, tenofovir and abacavir are used in combination regimens of Antiretroviral therapy (ART).

Non-nucleoside reverse transcriptase (NNRT) inhibitors like nevirapine, delavirdine, efavirenz and etravirine inactivate the enzyme reverse transcriptase. They are useful in HIV-1 infections.

Protease inhibitors like saquinavir indinavir, atazanavir and others bind to HIV protease and block viral maturation. They are well tolerated with mild adverse effects like gastrointestinal disturbances. They are used in combination with other drugs in HIV infections.

Entry Inhibitors

Enfuvirtide blocks the entry of the virus (HIV-1) into the cell. It is given as subcutaneous injection-causes local reactions. It can also cause allergic reactions.

Maraviroc selectively binds to a receptor that is necessary for the entry of the HIV-1 into the $CD4^+$ cells and blocks the entry of the virus into it. It is well-tolerated; adverse effects are upper respiratory infection, cough, myalgia, arthralgia, sleep disturbances and diarrhea.

Integrase Strand Transfer Inhibitors (INSTIs)

Integrase is a viral enzyme necessary for viral replication in both HIV-1 and HIV-2 viruses.

Raltegravir, elvitegravir and dolutegravir are INSTIs. They prevent viral replication by inhibiting the enzyme integrase. Dolutegravir (DTG) has the below advantages:

- Highly effective against HIV-1 and HIV-2
- Well tolerated
- Effective in HIV resistant to other drugs
- Convenient to use - once daily
- Drug interactions are low.

Uses

DTG is now the first-line drug along with abacavir and lamivudine in the treatment of HIV infection (Tables 12.11A and B).

Table 12.11A: Antiretroviral drug regimen (as per NACO Guidelines—2021).

Group	Regimen
Adults Adolescent Pregnant	TDF + 3TC + DTG/EFV
Children	ABC + 3TC + DTG
Neonates	AZT + 3TC + RAL

(AZT: azidothymidine (Zidovudine); 3TC: lamivudine; TDF: tenofovir)

Table 12.11B: Post-exposure prophylaxis as per NACO guidelines.

Group	Regimen
Adults and Adolescent	TDF + 3TC/FTC + DTG
Children	AZT + 3TC or ABC + 3TC or TDF + 3TC + DTG

(AZT: azidothymidine (Zidovudine); 3TC: lamivudine; TDF: tenofovir; FTC: emtricitabine)

ANTIPROTOZOAL DRUGS

Treatment of Malaria

Malaria is caused by protozoa of the genus *Plasmodium,* transmitted through the bite of a female Anopheles mosquito. It is a major public health problem in most of the developing countries including India.

Lifecycle of the malaria parasite: The bite of an infected female anopheles mosquito introduces the parasite into the bloodstream of man. These multiply in the liver cells and then in RBCs. Once they mature in RBCs, they rupture and cause the symptoms of malaria. The male and female sexual forms enter the mosquito when they suck the blood and undergo sexual cycle in the mosquito.

Antimalarial drugs can be classified as:

Classification	
Therapeutic	
1. ***Causal prophylactics*** (primary tissue schizonticides) (destroy parasite in liver cells and *prevent invasion of erythrocytes)*	Primaquine, pyrimethamine
2. ***Blood schizonticides*** (suppressives) *(destroy parasites in the RBCs and terminate clinical attacks of malaria)*	Chloroquine, quinine, mefloquine, halofantrine, pyrimethamine, chloroguanide, artemisinin
3. ***Tissue schizonticides (used to prevent relapse)*** (hypnozoitocidal drugs—*act on hypnozoites of P. vivax* and *P. ovale* that produce relapses)	Primaquine
4. ***Radical curatives*** *(Eradicate P. vivax and P. ovale)*	Blood schizonticides + hypnozoitocidal drugs
5. ***Gametocidal drugs*** *(destroy gametocytes and prevent transmission)*	Primaquine, chloroquine, quinine

Chloroquine is a synthetic 4-aminoquinoline. It is a highly effective blood schizontocide with activity against all 4 species of plasmodia. It also destroys gametocytes of *P. vivax, P. ovale* and *P. malaria* and completely cures falciparum malaria. Patients become afebrile in 24-48 hours.

Chloroquine is safe in pregnancy. It also has anti-inflammatory properties.

Mechanism of action is not clear. Chloroquine is a base. It concentrates in acidic food vacuoles of the parasite and causes accumulation of toxic haeme in the parasite leading to death of the parasite.

Adverse effects: Nausea, vomiting, pruritus, headache, visual disturbances, insomnia and skin rashes may occur. Prolonged treatment with high doses can cause irreversible retinopathy. High doses can also cause cardiomyopathy and psychiatric problems.

Uses (Table 12.12)

1. *Malaria*—Chloroquine is highly effective in the treatment of malaria due to sensitive strains of all 4 species (600 mg base stat, 300 mg after 6 hours and 300 mg for the next 2 days). It is also used for prophylaxis—300 mg/week (Flowchart 12.2).
2. Extraintestinal amoebiasis
3. Giardiasis
4. Rheumatoid arthritis
5. Photogenic reactions
6. Lepra reactions

(3–6: Chloroquine is effective in these because of its anti-inflammatory property)

Quinine is an alkaloid obtained from the bark of the cinchona tree. It destroys erythrocytic forms of the parasite similar to chloroquine and is useful as a suppressive. It is also gametocidal *(except for P. falciparum).*

Quinine also has mild **analgesic and antipyretic activity**; myocardiac depressant and local anesthetic properties. It is a **skeletal muscle relaxant**.

Adverse effects are high. Quinine is a gastric irritant and causes nausea, vomiting and epigastric pain. Cinchonism with ringing in the ears, headache, nausea, visual disturbances and vertigo may be encountered. In quinine poisoning, hypoglycemia, fever, delirium, confusion, hypotension, cardiac

Table 12.12: Preferred antitmalarials in the treatment and prophylaxis of malaria.	
Chloroquine-sensitive vivax malaria	
Treatment	Chloroquine (oral)—1 g day 1, 1g day 2, 0.5 g day 3 + primaquine 15 mg daily for 14 days
Chloroquine-sensitive falciparum malaria	
Treatment	Chloroquine (dose as above) + Primaquine 45 mg single dose
Prophylaxis	Chloroquine 2 tabs/week; start 1 week before and continue for 4 weeks after leaving the endemic area
Chloroquine-resistant and MDR falciparum malaria	
Treatment	Choices are: • Artemisinin-based combination therapy – Artesunate 100 mg BD oral (or 2.4 mg/kg/IV/IM) × 3 days with sulfadoxine/pyrimethamine (1500 mg–75 mg) single dose or Mefloquine 750 mg on day 2 and 500 mg on day 3 – Artemether 80 mg BD + lumefantrine 480 mg BD for 2 days • Quinine oral—600 mg TDS for 3 days followed by one of the following: – Doxycycline 100 mg BD for 7 days or – Clindamycin 600 mg BD for 7 days
Prophylaxis	• Mefloquine 250 mg weekly; start 1 week before and continue for 4 weeks after leaving the area or • Doxycycline 100 mg daily; start 2 days before and continue for 4 weeks after leaving the area

For all cases of *P. vivax* and *P. ovale,* Primaquine 15 mg/day should be given for 2 weeks.

arrhythmias and coma may develop. Death is due to respiratory arrest.

Uses: Quinine is used in the treatment of resistant falciparum malaria and cerebral malaria and for nocturnal muscle cramps.

Artemisinin

Obtained from the plant *Artemisia annua* has been used in chinese traditional medicine 'Quinghaosu' for almost 2000 years.

It is a potent, rapidly acting, blood schizontocide effective against all the 4 plasmodial species, including MDR *P. falciparum.* Mechanism of action is not known. It is useful in cerebral malaria.

Artemisinin + Heme
↓
Free radicals generated
↓
Damage parasite membrane
↓
Death of parasite

Artemisinin is the best tolerated antimalarial—mild GI symptoms, fever, itching and bradycardia are reported.

Uses: Drug of choice for MDR falciparum malaria. It is used in combination with other drugs (Table 12.12).

Mefloquine in a single dose is highly effective against erythrocytic forms of vivax and falciparum malaria—even the multidrug resistant (MDR) strains of *P. falciparum.* It is well-tolerated. Nausea, vomiting, dizziness, confusion, abdominal pain and bradycardia are common.

Mefloquine is indicated only in MDR strains of falciparum malaria.

Halofantrine is schizonticidal against erythrocytic forms of all *Plasmodium* species including MDR strains of *P. falciparum.*

It is used as an alternative in MDR strains of falciparum malaria. **Lumefantrine** is used along with artemisinin in falciparum malaria.

Primaquine

It is effective against liver forms (persistent tissue forms) of *P. vivax* and *P. ovale* and prevents relapse in these cases. It is also a causal prophylactic and gametocidal agent.

Flowchart 12.2: Revised guidelines by NVBDCP.

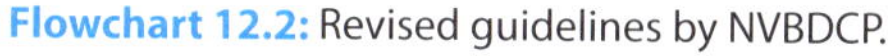

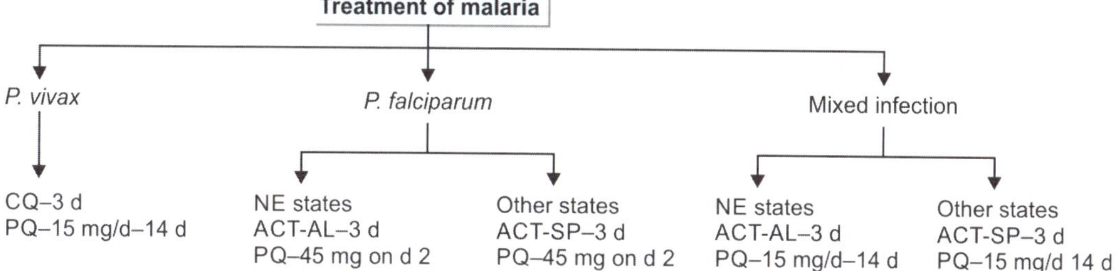

(CQ: Chloroquine; PQ: Primaquine; ACT-AL: Artesunate + lumefantrine; ACT–SP: Artesunate + sulfadoxine–pyrimethamine; NE: North-Eastern; NVBDCP: National Vector Borne Disease Control Programme)

Primaquine is used for *radical cure* along with a blood schizontocide in *P. vivax* and ovale and as a gametocidal agent in all strains including *P. falciparum* malaria.

Sulfadoxine-Pyrimethamine: Pyrimethamine is effective against the erythrocytic forms of all 4 species of plasmodia. When given with sulfadoxine (a sulfonamide), the combination is synergistic and the development of resistance is slower. They act by inhibiting folic acid synthesis.

Uses

1. **Malaria**
   - **Acute attacks:** Sulfadoxine + pyrimethamine combination is used with artemisinin.
   - **Prophylaxis:** 1-2 tablets once weekly for prophylaxis against MDR falciparum malaria—when a person is visiting an endemic area but not preferred now.
2. **Toxoplasmosis:** Sulfadoxine + pyrimethamine combination is the treatment of choice for toxoplasmosis.
3. ***Pneumocystis jiroveci*** infection responds to sulfadoxine + pyrimethamine

Proguanil (Chloroguanide) is a schizontocide with causal prophylactic activity against *P. falciparum.* It is used along with atovaquone for MDR falciparum malaria.

Atovaquone is effective against the erythrocytic forms of the plasmodia. When combined with proguanil, the activity is synergistic and development of resistance is less common. Proguanil potentiates the action of atovaquone.

Atovaquone is also effective against *T. gondii* and *Pneumocystis jiroveci* infections.

Adverse effects include vomiting, headache and abdominal pain. It is contraindicated in pregnancy.

Uses: Atovaquone + proguanil can be used in chloroquine resistant and multidrug resistant falciparum malaria.

Atovaquone may also be used in *Pneumocystis jiroveci* infection as an alternative to cotrimoxazole.

ANTIAMEBIC DRUGS

Amebiasis caused by the protozoan *Entamoeba histolytia* is a tropical disease common in developing countries. It spreads by fecal contamination of food and water. Though it primarily affects colon, other organs like liver, lungs and brain are the secondary sites. Acute amebiasis is characterized by bloody mucoid stools and abdominal pain. Chronic amebiasis manifests as anorexia, abdominal pain, intermittent diarrhea and constipation. Cyst passers are symptom free but they are carriers of infection.

Classification

- **Drugs effective in both intestinal and extraintestinal amebiasis:** Metronidazole, tinidazole, secnidazole, ornidazole.

- **Drugs effective only in intestinal amebiasis (luminal amebicides):** Diloxanide furoate, nitazoxamide, tetracyclines.
- **Drugs effective only in extraintestinal amebiasis:** Chloroquine.

Metronidazole a nitroimidazole, is a powerful amebicide. Apart from this it also inhibits *Trichomonas vaginalis, Giardia lamblia* and *Balantidium coli.* Anaerobic bacteria are also sensitive.

Mechanism of action: In the microorganisms including anaerobic bacteria and amoeba, metronidazole is reduced to a derivative which is toxic to the DNA.

Metronidazole pharmacology - *See* page 262.

Use in amoebiasis: Metronidazole is the drug of choice in all forms of amebiasis in the dose of 400–800 mg TDS for 7–10 days. But it does not eradicate the cyst.

Tinidazole is longer-acting and is better tolerated than metronidazole due to lesser side effects. It can be given 2 grams once daily for 3 days in amebiasis and as a single dose for other indications.

Secnidazole is longer-acting and can be given as a single 2 grams dose for most indications of metronidazole.

Diloxanide furoate is directly amebicidal. Flatulence, nausea and occasionally abdominal cramps and rashes can occur. It is used alone in asymptomatic cyst passers, mild intestinal amoebiasis and along with a nitroimidazole—for the cure of amebiasis, because diloxanide eradicates cysts.

Nitazoxanide is a derivative of niclosamide effective against *Entamoeba histolytica, Trichomonas vaginalis, Giardia* and also some intestinal helminths like *Ascaris* and *Hymenolepis nana*.

Nitazoxanide is used in giardia, diarrhea due to *Cryptosporidium, Cryptosporidium parvum, H. nana, Ascaris, Trichuris trichura* and *Enterobius vermicularis.*

It is well-tolerated as adverse effects are rare. It imparts a **greenish tint** to the urine; should be avoided in pregnancy.

Chloroquine attains high concentration in the liver, is directly toxic against trophozoites and is therefore useful in hepatic amebiasis. As chloroquine is completely absorbed from the small intestines, it is not effective against amebae in the colon. It is used as an alternative to metronidazole in hepatic amebiasis.

Tetracyclines: The older tetracyclines are not well-absorbed and large amounts reach the colon—hence these are useful in intestinal amoebiasis. They inhibit the intestinal flora and break the symbiosis between them and the amebae. Tetracyclines are used as adjuvants in chronic cases.

DRUGS USED IN LEISHMANIASIS

Leishmaniasis is caused by protozoa of the genus *Leishmania*—kala-azar or visceral leishmanias is caused by *Leishmania donavani*; oriental sore by *L. tropica* and mucocutaneous leishmaniasis by *L. braziliensis.* The infection is transmitted by the bite of the female sandfly phlebotomus. It is endemic in Bihar.

Drugs used in leishmaniasis include:

Sodium stibogluconate is an antimony compound which is effective in kala-azar and in mucocutaneous and cutaneous leishmaniasis.

Adverse effects include a metallic taste in the mouth, nausea, vomiting, diarrhea, headache, myalgia, arthralgia, pain at the injection site, bradycardia, skin rashes, hematuria and jaundice. Some cases of sudden death due to shock have occurred. ECG should be monitored as arrhythmias can occur during the later days of therapy.

Meglumine antimonate and **ethyl stibamine** can also be used in all forms of leishmaniasis.

Pentamidine is effective against *Leishmania donovani,* trypanosomes, *Pneumocystis carinii* and some fungi.

Adverse effects: Pentamidine liberates histamine which is responsible for vomiting, diarrhea, flushing, pruritis, rashes,

Table 12.13: Preferred drugs for helminthiasis infection.

Worms	Drugs of choice	Alternative drugs
• Roundworm *(Ascaris lumbricoides)*	Mebendazole/albendazole/pyrantel	Piperazine
• Hookworms *(Ancylostoma duodenale, Necator americanus)*	Mebendazole/albendazole	Pyrantel
• Pinworm *(Enterobius vermicularis)*	Mebendazole/albendazole/pyrantel	Piperazine
• Whipworm *(Trichuris trichura)*	Mebendazole	Albendazole
• Strongyloides stercoralis	Albendazole	Thiabendazole
• Guineaworm *(Dracunculous medinensis)*	Metronidazole	Mebendazole
• Tapeworms *(Taenia saginata, Taenia solium, H. nana, D. latum)*	Niclosamide/praziquantel	Albendazole
Neurocysticercosis	Albendazole	Praziquantel
• Hydatid disease *(E. granulosus, E. multilocularis)*	Albendazole	Mebendazole
• Filaria *(Wuchareria bancrofti, Brugia malayi)*	Diethylcarbamazine	—
• Schistosomes	Praziquantel	—

tachycardia and hypotension apart from pain at the injection site.

Pentamidine is useful in visceral *leishmaniasis, trypanosomiasis* and in *Pneumocystis jeroveci* infections.

Miltefosine is the first drug that could be used orally in leishmaniasis. It has a high efficacy against both visceral and cutaneous leishmaniasis.

It is effective also in leishmania resistant to stibogluconate. It is approved for use in India in visceral leishmaniasis—700 mg/kg/day for 4 weeks. Miltefosine is safe—vomiting and diarrhea are common while raised liver enzymes and creatinine are reversible. It is contraindicated in pregnancy.

Other Drugs

Amphotericin B, ketoconazole, allopurinol and **paramomycin** have been tried in leishmaniasis in the endemic areas where antimonials may be ineffective.

ANTHELMINTICS

Worm infestations are more common in the developing countries. It is seen in people with poor hygiene. Anthelmintics are deworming agents. A **vermicidal** kills while a **vermifuge** promotes expulsion of worms.

Mebendazole a broad-spectrum anthelmintic cures roundworm, hookworm, pinworm and strongyloides infestations. The eggs and larvae are also destroyed. It blocks the glucose uptake in the parasite. It is well-tolerated; nausea, abdominal pain and diarrhea are seen in heavy infestations.

Uses: Mebendazole is used in the treatment of roundworm, hookworm, pinworm, tapeworm, trichuriasis and hydatid disease (Table 12.13). It is of special value in multiple worm infestations.

Albendazole is similar to mebendazole, in actions but is *better tolerated* and is effective in a *single dose.* Adverse effects are similar to mebendazole but milder.

Uses

1. Albendazole is the drug of choice in **roundworm, hookworm, pinworm, trichuriasis** infestations in a single 400 mg dose. Dose to be repeated after 2 weeks in pinworm infestation to prevent reinfection from ova that have matured later.
2. **Trichinosis, tapeworms and strongyloidosis** require 3 days treatment.
3. **Neurocysticercosis:** Albendazole is the drug of choice.

4. **Hydatid disease:** Albendazole is the drug of choice; given for 4 weeks.
5. **Filariasis**—combination of albendazole (400 mg) with DEC (6 mg/kg) or ivermectin (0.3 mg/kg) given as a single dose is found to be effective in *W. bancrofti* in suppressing microfilariae for one year. This also prevents the spread of filariasis and may be given once a year for 5–6 years.

Pyrantel pamoate is effective against roundworm, hookworm and pinworms. It stimulates the nicotinic cholinergic receptor in the worm leading to persistant depolarization and spastic paralysis (depolarizing neuromuscular blocker). The paralyzed worms are expelled.

Uses: In the treatment of roundworm, hookworm and pinworm infestations.

Piperazine citrate is effective in roundworm and pinworm infestations. It competitively blocks the action of acetylcholine and thereby contractions in the worms. Flaccid paralysis results and the worms are expelled.

Levamisole is effective against roundworms and hookworms and can be used as an alternative drug in these infestations. It is well-tolerated and is effective in a single dose. It is also an immunomodulator.

Niclosamide is effective against most tapeworms. The segments of the dead tapeworms are partly digested and in case of *T. solium,* may result in visceral cysticercosis. A purgative may be given 2 hours after niclosamide to wash off the worms and avoid cysticercosis.

Uses: Niclosamide is the drug of choice in infestations by tapeworms like *T. solium, T. saginata, H. nana* and *D. latum.* It is also an alternative drug in intestinal fluke infestation.

Praziquantel is effective against schistosomes of all species, most other trematodes and cestodes including cysticercosis.

Adverse effects are mild and include GI disturbances, headache, dizziness, drowsiness, rashes and myalgia.

Uses

1. **Schistosomiasis:** Praziquantel is the drug of choice in all forms of schistosomiasis.
2. **Tapeworms:** Single dose (10 mg/kg) of praziquantel is effective in all tapeworm infestations. In *T. solium* it has the advantage that it kills the larvae and therefore visceral cysticercosis is avoided.
3. **Neurocysticercosis:** Praziquantel is an alternative to albendazole.

Diethylcarbamazine (DEC) is the drug of choice in filariasis. It immobilizes the microfilariae resulting in their displacement in the tissues.

Adverse effects are mild; anorexia, nausea, vomiting, dizziness and headache; an allergic reaction with itching, rashes and fever due to release of antigens from the dying worms may occur. Antihistamines are given with DEC to minimize these reactions. DEC can be given during pregnancy.

Uses

- **Filariasis:** DEC is the drug of choice (2 mg/kg TDS for 21 days). In 7 days patients are rendered non-infective to mosquitoes as microfilariae rapidly disappear. But adult worms may need repeated courses.
- **Tropical eosinophilia (2 mg/kg TDS for 7 days):** Symptoms rapidly disappear.

Ivermectin obtained from *Streptomyces avermitilis* is effective against many nematodes, arthropods and filariae that infect animals and human beings. It is microfilaricidal and also blocks the release of microfilariae from the uterus of adult worms. There is a rapid decrease in the microfilarial count in the skin and eyes.

Ivermectin is believed to act by paralyzing the worms by binding to GABA-gated chloride channels and increasing GABA activity.

Ivermectin is as effective as DEC against *W. bancrofti* and *B. malayi.* It is also effective against *Strongyloides stercoralis, Ascaris lumbricoides*, and cutaneous larva migrans, scabies (*Sarcoptes scabiei*) and lice.

Adverse effects: Ivermectin is well-tolerated. Apart from nausea and vomiting, allergic reactions can result due to hypersensitivity to the dying microfilarial proteins (Mazzotti reaction).

Ivermectin should not be used with other drugs that influence GABA activity (e.g. benzodiazepines, valproic acid), and in patients with meningitis and sleeping sickness as these conditions impair the blood brain barrier.

Uses

1. Ivermectin is the preferred drug in the treatment of **onchocerciasis**.
2. Ivermectin is also useful in the treatment of **lymphatic filariasis**. A single dose of 400 mg/kg ivermectin with 400 mg albendazole is given once a year for mass chemotherapy of lymphatic filariasis.
3. **Strongyloidiasis**—a single dose of 200 mg/kg is curative in **strongyloidiasis**. However the dose is to be repeated on the second day.
4. Ivermectin is also useful in **cutaneous larva migrans, ascariasis,** in **scabies** and **lice** infestations in a single dose of 200 mg/kg.
5. **COVID-19:** Ivermectin had shown efficacy against COVID-19 *in vitro* and therefore was used extensively for treatment and prophylaxis. However, its utility could not be established.

CANCER CHEMOTHERAPY

Cancer is one of the major causes of death. The treatment of cancers remains unsatisfactory due to certain characteristics of the cancer cells—like capacity for uncontrolled proliferation, invasiveness and metastasis. Moreover, the cancer cells are our own cells unlike microbes which means that, drugs which destroy these cells also can affect normal cells. The host defence mechanisms which help us in infections are not doing so in cancers because these cancer cells are also host cells. Moreover, the cancer cells can be in a resting phase during which they are not sensitive to anticancer drugs but can start multiplying later—resulting in recurrence. These features have made cancer chemotherapy more difficult.

Classification

1. **Alkylating agents and platinum analogs**	
Nitrogen mustards	Cyclophosphamide Ifosfamide Chlorambucil Melphalan
Alkyl sulfonate	Busulfan
Nitrosoureas	Carmustine Streptazocin
Triazine	Dacarbazine
Platinum analogs	Cisplatin Carboplatin
2. **Antimetabolites**	
Folate antagonist	Methotrexate
Purine analogs	6-Mercaptopurine
Pyrimidine analogs	5-Fluorouracil, Floxuridine, Cytarabine, Thioguanine, Pentastatin Fludarabin, Cladribin
3. **Antibiotics**	Actinomycin-D Daunorubicin Doxorubicin Bleomycin Mitomycin-C Mithramycin (Plicamycin)
4. **Topoisomerase II inhibitors** (Epipodophyllotoxins)	Etoposide teniposide
5. **Topoisomerase I inhibitors** Camptothecins	Topotecan Irinotecan

6. **Microtubule toxins**
   - ***Taxanes*** Paclitaxel, Docetaxel
   - ***Vinca alkaloids*** Vincristine, Vinblastine, Vinorelbine
7. **Hormones** Glucocorticoids, Androgens, Antiandrogens, Estrogens, Antiestrogens, Progestins
8. **Miscellaneous** Procarbazine, L-asparaginase, Interferon-α, Imatinib
9. **Biological Response Modifiers** Interferon alpha, amifostin, Interleukin 2, Hematopoietic growth factors

Common Adverse Effects to Anticancer Drugs

Since most anticancer drugs act on the rapidly multiplying cells, they are also toxic to the normal rapidly multiplying cells in the bone marrow, epithelial cells, lymphoid organs and gonads. Thus the common adverse effects are:

1. **Bone marrow depression** resulting in leukopenia, anemia, thrombocytopenia and in higher doses—aplastic anemia. In such patients, infections and bleeding are common.
2. **Other proliferating cells**
   GIT: Stomatitis and ulcers;
   alopecia (loss of hair),
   reduced spermatogenesis in men and amenorrhea in women (due to damage to the germinal epithelium).
3. **Immediate adverse effects:** Nausea and vomiting are very common with most cytotoxic drugs. Prior treatment with powerful antiemetics is required.
4. **Hyperuricemia:** Rapid tumor cell lysis can result in an increased plasma uric acid levels.
5. **Teratogenicity:** All cytotoxic drugs are teratogenic and are therefore contraindicated in pregnancy.
6. **Carcinogenicity:** Cytotoxic drugs themselves may cause secondary cancers, e.g., leukemias are common after treatment of Hodgkin's lymphoma.

Apart from the above, the adverse effects unique to some drugs are discussed under individual drugs (Table 12.14).

Alkylating Agents

Actions: Alkylating agents exert cytotoxic, immunosuppressant and radiomimetic effects (similar to radiotherapy).

Table 12.14: Specific adverse effects of some anticancer drugs.

Drugs	*Specific adverse effects*	*Other prominent adverse effects*
Cyclophosphamide	Cystitis	Bone marrow depression, alopecia, stomatitis, vomiting, amenorrhea, teratogenicity
Busulfan	Pulmonary fibrosis	Bone marrow depression, alopecia, stomatitis, vomiting, amenorrhea, teratogenicity
Cisplatin	Ototoxicity	Renal dysfunction
Bleomycin	Pulmonary fibrosis, edema of hands	Stomatitis, alopecia
Daunorubicin	Cardiotoxicity, red colored urine	Bone marrow depression, alopecia
Doxorubicin	Cardiotoxicity	Bone marrow depression, alopecia
Mithramycin (Plicamycin)	Hepatotoxicity	Thrombocytopenia
Vincristine	Neurotoxicity, peripheral neuritis	Muscle weakness, alopecia
Asparaginase	Pancreatitis, hepatotoxicity, mental depression	Allergic reactions
Mitotane	Dermatitis, mental depression	Diarrhea

Mechanism of action: These drugs form highly reactive derivatives which transfer alkyl groups to various cellular constituents and bind them with covalent bonds. Alkylation of DNA results in breakage of DNA strand.

Cyclophosphamide is converted to its active metabolite aldophosphamide in the body. It can be given orally. It causes cystitis (inflammation of the urinary bladder) due to a metabolite acrolein. This can be prevented by giving IV **Mesna**, irrigating the bladder with **acetylcysteine**, and by in take of large amounts of **fluids** orally. Mesna and acetylcystine contain sulfhydryl (SH) groups which bind the toxic metabolites and inactivate them.

Uses: Cyclophosphamide is used in Hodgkin's lymphoma, leukemias in children and as an immunosuppressive agent.

Cisplatin gets converted to its active form in the cell, inhibits DNA synthesis and causes cytotoxicity. It causes ototoxicity, nephrotoxicity, peripheral neuropathy, nausea, vomiting, anemia and anaphylactoid reactions. It is relatively less toxic to bone marrow. Cisplatin is used in ovarian and testicular tumors and cancers of the head and neck. Carboplatin is a less toxic derivative of cisplatin and is better tolerated than cisplatin.

Antimetabolites

Folate Antagonist

Methotrexate is a folic acid antagonist. It binds to dihydrofolate reductase (DHFR) and prevents the formation of tetrahydrofolate (THF). This THF is a coenzyme essential in several reactions in protein synthesis. The deficiency results in inhibition of protein synthesis. Thus rapidly multiplying cells are the most affected.

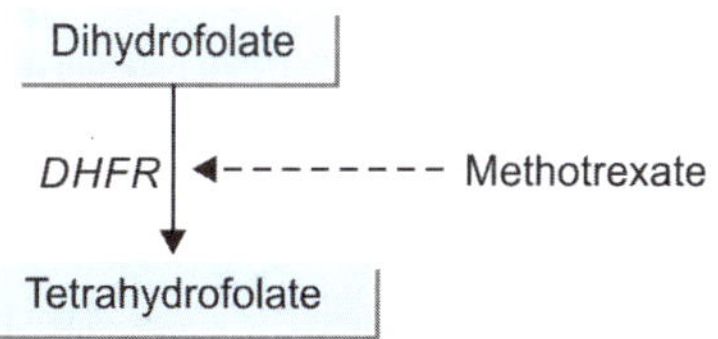

Actions: Cytotoxic actions—methotrexate mainly affects bone marrow, skin and gastrointestinal mucosa.

It also has immunosuppressant and anti-inflammatory properties.

Methotrexate toxicity can be largely prevented by administering folinic acid. This folinic acid gets converted to a form of THF that can be utilized by the cells.

Uses:

- Methotrexate is curative in chorio-carcinoma.
- It is useful in acute leukemias, breast cancer and soft tissue sarcomas.
- It is also used in rheumatoid arthritis and psoriasis.

Purine Analogs

6-Mercaptopurine (6-MP) is converted to a metabolite which inhibits purine synthesis.

Drug interaction: 6-MP is metabolized by xanthine oxidase. Allopurinol inhibits xanthine oxidase and thus prolongs the action of 6-MP.

Uses: 6-MP is used in acute leukemias in children, choriocarcinoma and some solid tumors.

Pyrimydine Analogs

5-Fluorouracil inhibits the synthesis of thymidylate and thereby inhibits DNA synthesis. It is used in carcinoma of the stomach, colon, rectum, breast and ovaries.

Cytosine arabinoside is the drug of choice in acute myeloid leukemia in adults.

Antibiotics

Actinomycin D acts by inhibiting DNA-dependent RNA synthesis. It is one of the most potent anticancer drugs and is used in Wilms' tumor, rhabdomyosarcoma, chorio-carcinoma and some soft tissue sarcomas.

Daunorubicin and doxorubicin act by inhibiting DNA synthesis. Cardiotoxicity with hypotension, arrhythmias and CCF, is unique to both these drugs. They also cause vomiting, stomatitis, alopecia and bone marrow depression.

Daunorubicin is used in acute leukemias while doxorubicin is useful in solid tumors and in acute leukemias.

Epirubicin is an analog of doxorubicin which is less cardiotoxic.

Bleomycin forms free radicals and causes breakage in DNA strand. It has the advantage of the unique mechanism of action and is less toxic to the bone marrow—this is advantageous in combination regimens.

It is used in solid tumors—testicular tumors, squamous cell carcinoma of the head, neck and esophagus.

Its most serious toxicity is pulmonary fibrosis and cutaneous toxicity but does not cause significant bone marrow depression.

Microtubule Toxins

Taxanes

Paclitaxel was obtained from the bark of the western yew tree. It arrests cell division (mitosis), paclitaxel is given intravenously; it is metabolized by the liver. Adverse effects include myelosuppression, myalgia and peripheral neuropathy. **Docetaxel** is more potent and orally effective. Taxanes are useful in breast cancers and ovarian cancers. They are also found to be effective in the cancers of the head and neck, esophagus and lungs.

Vinca Alkaloids

Vincristine and vinblastine are obtained from *vinca rosea,* the periwinkle plant. They bind to microtubules in the mitotic apparatus and arrest cell division in metaphase. y are mitotic spindle poisons. The alkaloids differ in toxicity.

Vincristine: Vincristine is neurotoxic while bone marrow depression is less. It is used in leukemias, Hodgkin's lymphoma, Wilms' tumor and brain tumor.

Vinblastine causes bone marrow depression, alopecia and vomiting. It is used with bleomycin and cisplatin (VBC) in testicular tumors; it is also useful in Hodgkin's lymphoma.

Vinorelbine is a semisynthetic vinca alkaloid used in lung cancers.

Topoisomerase I Inhibitors

Topotecan and irinotecan are camptothecins. They cause breaks in DNA. They are used in ovarian and lung cancers.

Topoisomerase II Inhibitors

Etoposide is used in testicular tumors, lung cancers, lymphomas, bladder and stomach cancers.

Hormones in Cancer Chemotherapy

Glucocorticoids: Due to their lympholytic action, glucocorticoids are used in acute leukemias and lymphomas. Rapid clinical improvement is seen but duration of remission can vary from 2 weeks to 9 months. They are used for initiation of therapy due to their rapid action.

Glucocorticoids are also of value in the following:

- With radiation therapy to reduce radiation edema
- In intracranial tumors to reduce cerebral edema and
- For symptomatic relief in critically ill patients.

Prednisolone or dexamethasone are commonly used.

Estrogens are useful in (i) prostatic carcinoma as it is an androgen dependent tumor, (ii) breast cancer in males and in postmenopausal women—estrogens are used in advanced cases where surgery or radiotherapy cannot be employed.

Antiestrogens: Tamoxifen is an estrogen receptor antagonist used in estrogen receptor containing breast cancer.

Progestins are useful in the palliative management of endometrial carcinoma.

Androgens are used in the palliative treatment of breast cancer in postmenopausal women along with oophorectomy.

Antiandrogen: Flutamide is used in prostatic cancer.

Drugs which cause least/no bone marrow depression	Curable cancers
• Hormones • Vincristine • Bleomycin • L-asparaginase • Cisplatin	• Hodgkin's disease • Choriocarcinoma • Burkitt's lymphoma • Testicular tumors • Wilms' tumor • Acute leukemias in children • Ewing's sarcoma

Miscellaneous

Procarbazine is effective orally in Hodgkin's lymphoma (MOPP regimen component). It damages DNA. This may make it carcinogenic.
L-asparaginase: The amino acid asparagine is synthesized by normal cells but malignant cells are unable to synthesize asparaginase and depend on the supply from the host. Asparaginase is an enzyme that converts asparagine to aspartic acid and deprives the malignant cells of asparagine supplies resulting in inhibition of protein synthesis. It is used in acute leukemias.
Imatinib acts by inhibiting some selective enzymes (tyrosine kinases) which are involved in the pathogenesis of chronic myeloid leukemia. It can cause skin rashes and elevated liver enzymes. Imatinib is used in chronic myeloid leukemia.
Monoclonal antibodies are immunoglobulins that react specifically with antigens present on the cancer cells. Allergic reactions are common. *Trastuzumab* is useful in breast cancers. *Rituximab* attaches to antigens on the B-cells causing lysis of these cells. It is used in B-cell lymphomas.

Biological Response Modifiers

Several agents are used to beneficially influence the patients' response to treatment and to overcome some adverse effects. These have also been termed *biological response modifiers*. Some examples are:

1. **Hematopoietic growth factors**, such as erythropoietin and myeloid growth factors like GM-CSF, G-CSF, M-CSF and thrombopoietin are used to treat bone marrow suppression.
2. Interferon alpha, interleukin 2 and amifostine are also used as adjuvants to chemotherapy.

General Principles in the Treatment of Cancers (Table 12.15)

Chemotherapy in cancers is generally palliative and suppressive. Chemotherapy is just one of the modes in the treatment of cancer. Other modes like radiotherapy and surgery are also employed. Combination of drugs is preferred for synergistic effect, to

Table 12.15: Combination of drugs preferred in some malignancies.

Malignancy	*Preferred drugs*
Acute lymphatic leukemia	Vincristine + prednisolone + L-asparaginase Maintenance–mercaptopurine/ methotrexate
Acute myeloid leukemia	Cytarabine + daunorubicin
Chronic lymphatic leukemia	Chlorambucil + prednisolone
Chronic myeloid leukemia	Imatinib
Hodgkin's disease	A-Adriamycin (doxorubicin) B-Bleomycin V-Vinblastin D-Dacarbazine
Non-Hodgkin's lymphoma	(CHOP) Cyclophosphamide + doxorubicin (hydroxy daunomycin) + vincristine (oncovin) + prednisolone
Carcinoma of stomach	Fluorouracil + cisplatin
Carcinoma of colon	Fluorouracil + irinotecan
Multiple myeloma	(CYBORD) Cyclophosphamide + bortezomib + dexamethasone
Choriocarcinoma	Methotrexate
Carcinoma of testis	Etoposide + bleomycin + cisplatin
Osteogenic sarcoma	Methotrexate or doxorubicin + cisplatin
Wilms' tumor	Vincristine + actinomycin-D after surgery
Carcinoma of the head and neck	Fluorouracil + cisplatin
Carcinoma of lung	Cisplatin + paclitaxel/cemcitabine

reduce adverse effects and to prevent rapid development of resistance. Drugs which do not depress bone marrow are useful in combination regimens to avoid overlapping of adverse effects. With appropriate treatment, cure can now be achieved in a few cancers. Maintenance of good nutrition, treatment of anemia, protection against infections, adequate relief of pain and anxiety and good emotional support—all go a long way in the appropriate management of this dreaded disease.

VACCINES AND ANTISERA

Active immunization is the administration of antigen to the host in order to induce antibody production. Vaccines are used for active immunization. Vaccines are suspensions of microorganisms (dead or live attenuated) which stimulate the immunological defence of the host by developing antibodies. They impart active immunity, which takes sometime to develop and are therefore used prophylactically. The antibodies so developed destroy the specific microorganism when it enters the body (Table 12.16).

Toxoids: Bacterial exotoxins modified to remove toxicity but retain antigenicity are toxoids.

Passive immunization is providing immunity to a host passively by the transfer of antibodies, e.g., antisera and immunoglobulins (Ig). This gives immediate protection as readymade antibodies are available. Antisera like tetanus antitoxin, gas gangrene antitoxin, diphtheria and antirabies serum are obtained from serum of horses which are actively immunized against the specific organism. Sensitivity tests should be done before giving antisera.

Table 12.16: Vaccines in common use and their recommended schedules.

Vaccine	*Type of agent*	*Route of administration*	*Primary immunization*	*Booster*	*Indication*
Bacterial vaccines					
BCG	Live attenuated	ID/SC	At birth	7 and 14 years	In all children
Cholera	Inactivated	SC/IM	Adults: two doses 1 month apart	Every 6 months	People living in endemic areas
	Killed	Oral	2 doses 10–14 days apart		
Diphtheria (TRIPLE ANTIGEN)	Toxoid	IM	6, 10,14 weeks of age	18 months and at 4–6 years	For all children
Pertussis (TRIPLE ANTIGEN)	Inactivated	IM	6, 10,14 weeks of age	18 months and at 4–6 years	For all children
Tetanus (TRIPLE ANTIGEN)	Toxoid	IM	6, 10,14 weeks of age	18 months and at 4–6 years	For all children; Adults: Post-exposure prophylaxis if > 5 years has passed since last dose
Typhoid/parathyroid	Inactivated	SC	After 3 years at any age: two doses 4 weeks apart	Every 3 years	Risk of exposure to typhoid fever
Typhoid (typhoral)	Live inactivated	Oral (capsules)	Above 6 years at any age: 3 doses on alternate days 1 hour before food	Every 3 years	Risk of exposure to typhoid fever

Contd...

Contd...

Vaccine	*Type of agent*	*Route of administration*	*Primary immunization*	*Booster*	*Indication*
Meningococcal	Bacterial poly-saccharides	SC	One dose	—	1. Travellers to areas with meningococcal epidemics 2. Control of out-break in closed population
Plague	Inactivated	IM	One dose	—	In an epidemic
Viral vaccines					
Poliomyelitis (OPV)	Live virus	Oral	6, 10 and 14 weeks of age	18 months; again at 4–6 years	For all children
Measles Rubella (MR)	Live virus	SC	9 months	6–24 months	For all children
Hepatitis A	Inactivated virus	IM	1 dose (2–4 weeks before travelling to endemic areas)	After 6–12 months	1. Travellers to endemic areas 2. Homosexual men 3. Persons at occupational risk
Hepatitis B	Inactive viral antigen	IM	At birth, 1 month, 6–18 months	After 5 years but not routinely recommended	1. For all children 2. Persons at occupational risk 3. Hemophiliacs 4. Post-exposure prophylaxis
Influenza	Inactivated virus	IM	One dose	Yearly	1. High risk people like elderly, asthmatics
Rabies (Rabtpur)	Inactivated virus	IM/ID	**Pre-exposure** 3 doses at days 0,7 and 21 **Post-exposure:** 6 doses IM 0, 3, 7, 14, 30 and 90	After 1 year then at 2–5 years	1. Post-exposure treatment 2. Pre-exposure prophylaxis in persons at risk for contact with rabies virus
Varicella	Live virus	SC	2 doses 4–8 weeks apart at 18 months	—	All children from 18 months to 13 years with no history of varicella infection
Yellow fever	Live virus	SC	1 dose	Every 10 years	1. Travellers to areas where yellow fever is seen 2. Laboratory personnel at risk of exposure

(ID: intradermal; SC: subcutaneous; IM: intramuscular)

Immunoglobulins (Ig) are human gammaglobulins that carry the antibodies—like normal human gammaglobulin, tetanus Ig, rabies Ig, anti-diphtheria Ig and hepatitis-B Ig. Allergic reactions including serum sickness and anaphylaxis can occur with antiserum, while it is uncommon with **immunoglobulins**.

Primary immunization provides primary immunity and is usually given in children, e.g., DPT (triple antigen given to infants) (Table 12.17).

Secondary immunization is done to reinforce the primary immunity by giving booster doses.

Table 12.17: Passive immunization.

Preparation with source	*Dose and route*	*Indications*
Diphtheria antitoxin (horse)	IV or IM 20,000–1,20,000 units	*Diphtheria* Clinical diphtheria—to be given immediately
Tetanus immunoglobulin (human)	IM Prophylaxis: 2500 Units Treatment: 3,000–6,000 Units	*Tetanus* Treatment and postexposure prophylaxis of unclean wounds in inadequately immunized persons
Tetanus antitoxin (antitetanus serum) (ATS) (horse) (If tetanus Ig is not available)	IM/SC Prophylaxis: 1500–3000 IU Treatment: 50,000–1,00,000 IU	*Tetanus* Treatment and postexposure prophylaxis of unclean wounds in inadequately immunized persons
Rabies immunoglobulin (human)	20 IU/kg; half the dose infiltrated around the wound; remaining IM	*Rabies* Postexposure prophylaxis combined with rabies vaccine
Botulinum antitoxin	IM/IV 10,000 IU	Treatment and postexposure prophylaxis botulism
Antirabies serum (ARS) (horse)	IM 40 IU/kg	Used if rabies Ig is not available but is inferior to it
Gas gangrene antitoxin (AGS) (horse)	IM/SC/IV Prophylaxis: 10,000 IU Treatment: 30,000–75,000 IU	*Gas gangrene* Postexposure prophylaxis and treatment
Hepatitis B immunoglobulin (HBIG)	IM 0.06 mL/kg	Postexposure prophylaxis in nonimmune persons; Hepatitis B vaccine shall also be given.
Antisnake venom polyvalent (horse)	IV 20–30 mL to be given within 4 hours after the bite; additional doses may be required	Snake bite–cobra, vipers, krait
Human gammaglobulin		Gammaglobulin deficiency; prophylaxis of hepatitis A, measles, mumps, rubella
Anti-Rh (D)	Ig IM 300 μg	To the Rh negative mother after the birth of Rh positive baby or after uncompleted pregnancy with Rh positive fetus

Index

Page numbers followed by *b* refer to box, *f* refer to figure, *fc* refer to flowchart, and *t* refer to table.

D

E

J

K

L

M

Q

R

T

U

V

W

 X

 Y

Z